Pocket Guide to Diagnostic Tests

P9-AFD-506

fourth edition

Diana Nicoll, MD, PhD, MPA
Clinical Professor and Vice Chair
Department of Laboratory Medicine
University of California, San Francisco
Associate Dean
University of California, San Francisco
Chief of Staff and Chief, Laboratory Medicine Service
Veterans Affairs Medical Center, San Francisco

Stephen J. McPhee, MD
Professor of Medicine
Division of General Internal Medicine
Department of Medicine
University of California, San Francisco

Michael Pignone, MD, MPH
Assistant Professor of Medicine
Division of General Internal Medicine
Department of Medicine
University of North Carolina, Chapel Hill

With Associate Authors

Lange Medical Books/McGraw-Hill
Medical Publishing Division

New York St. Louis San Francisco Auckland Bogotá Caracas
Lisbon London Madrid Mexico City Milan Montreal New Delhi
San Juan Singapore Sydney Tokyo Toronto

Pocket Guide to Diagnostic Tests, Fourth Edition

Copyright © 2004 by **The McGraw-Hill Companies, Inc**. All rights reserved.
Printed in the United States of America. Except as permitted under the United
States Copyright Act of 1976, no part of this publication may be reproduced or distributed in any form or by any means, or stored in a data base or retrieval system,
without the prior written permission of the publisher.

Previous editions copyright © 2001 by The McGraw-Hill Companies, 1997, 1992
by Appleton & Lange

1 2 3 4 5 6 7 8 9 0   DOC/DOC   0 9 8 7 6 5 4 3

ISBN: 0-07-141184-4 (domestic)
ISSN:1061-3463

This book was set in Times Roman by Circle Graphics.
The editors were Isabel Nogueira and Barbara Holton.
The production supervisor was Catherine Saggese.
The cover designer was Mary McKeon.
R. R. Donnelley was the printer and binder.

This book was printed on acid-free paper.

INTERNATIONAL EDITION ISBN 0-07-121976-5
Copyright © 2004. Exclusive rights by *The McGraw-Hill Companies, Inc.*, for
manufacture and export.
This book cannot be re-exported from the country to which it is consigned by
McGraw-Hill.
The International Edition is not available in North America.

Contents

Associate Authors

Jane Jang, BS, MT (ASCP) SM
Laboratory Medicine Service
Veterans Affairs Medical Center, San Francisco
Microbiology: Test Selection

Fred M. Kusumoto, MD
Clinical Professor of Medicine
University of New Mexico Medical Center, Albuquerque
Director, Electrophysiology and Pacing Service
Department of Cardiology
Lovelace Medical Center, Albuquerque
Basic Electrocardiography

Susan D. Wall, MD
Professor of Radiology and Assistant Chief
Department of Radiology
Veterans Affairs Medical Center, San Francisco
Associate Dean, Graduate Medical Education
University of California, San Francisco
Diagnostic Imaging: Test Selection and Interpretation

Benjamin M. Yeh, MD
Assistant Professor of Abdominal Imaging
Department of Radiology
University of California, San Francisco
Diagnostic Imaging: Test Selection and Interpretation

Preface

Purpose

Pocket Guide to Diagnostic Tests is intended to serve as a pocket reference manual for medical and other health professional students, house officers, and practicing physicians. It is a quick reference guide to the selection and interpretation of commonly used diagnostic tests, including laboratory procedures in the clinical setting, laboratory tests (chemistry, hematology, and immunology), microbiology tests (bacteriology, virology, and serology), diagnostic imaging tests (plain radiography, CT, MRI, and ultrasonography), and electrocardiography.

This book will enable readers to understand commonly used diagnostic tests and diagnostic approaches to common disease states.

Outstanding Features

- Over 350 tests are presented in a concise, consistent, and readable format.
- Fields covered include internal medicine, pediatrics, general surgery, neurology, and gynecology.
- Costs and risks of various procedures and tests are emphasized.
- Literature references are included for most diagnostic tests.
- An index for quick reference is included on the back cover.

Organization

This pocket reference manual is not intended to include all diagnostic tests or disease states. Rather, the authors have selected those tests and diseases that are most common and relevant to the general practice of medicine.

The *Guide* is divided into 10 sections:

1. Basic Principles of Diagnostic Test Use and Interpretation
2. Laboratory Procedures in the Clinical Setting
3. Common Laboratory Tests: Selection and Interpretation
4. Therapeutic Drug Monitoring: Principles and Test Interpretation
5. Microbiology: Test Selection
6. Diagnostic Imaging: Test Selection and Interpretation
7. Basic Electrocardiography
8. Diagnostic Algorithms
9. Diagnostic Tests in Differential Diagnosis
10. Nomograms & Reference Material

Intended Audience

In this era of rapidly changing medical technology, many new diagnostic tests are being introduced every year and are replacing older tests as they are shown to be more sensitive, specific, or cost-effective. In this environment, students, house officers, and practicing physicians are looking for a pocket reference on diagnostic tests.

Medical students will find the concise summary of diagnostic laboratory, microbiologic, and imaging studies, and of electrocardiography in this pocket-sized book of great help during clinical ward rotations.

Busy house officers will find the clear organization and citations to the current literature useful in devising proper patient management.

Practitioners (internists, family physicians, pediatricians, surgeons, and other specialists who provide generalist care) may use the *Guide* as a refresher manual to update their understanding of laboratory tests and diagnostic approaches.

Nurses and other health practitioners will find the format and scope of the *Guide* valuable for understanding the use of laboratory tests in patient management.

In 2003, the contents of this book were integrated with the contents of *Current Medical Diagnosis & Treatment 2002* and *Practice Guidelines in Primary Care 2002,* in an on-line textbook called Current-med.com (available at: www.current-med.com). In 2003, the editors plan to integrate the fourth edition of *Pocket Guide to Diagnostic Tests* with *Current Medical Diagnosis & Treatment 2003* and *Practice Guidelines in Primary Care.*

Acknowledgments

The editors wish to acknowledge and express our gratitude for the invaluable editorial contributions to both information format and content of William M. Detmer, MD, and Tony M. Chou, MD, to the first three editions of this book. Dr. Detmer was the primary title page editor and a major contributor for the first edition published in 1992, and a title page editor and contributor for the second edition published in 1997, and third edition, published in 2001. Dr. Chou served as title page editor and contributor for the first and second editions, and editor for the third edition.

In addition, we wish to acknowledge G. Thomas Evans, Jr., MD (deceased) for his contribution of material on electrocardiography for the second edition, and a chapter on this topic for the third edition. In this fourth edition, this chapter has been revised by Fred M. Kusumoto, MD.

Finally, we wish to acknowledge Mary K. York, PhD (retired), for her contribution of material on microbiology for the third edition. In the present edition, this chapter has been revised by Jane Jang, BS, MT (ASCP) SM.

We wish to thank our associate authors for their contributions to this book. In addition, we are grateful to the many physicians, residents, and students who contributed useful suggestions.

We welcome comments and recommendations from our readers for future editions.

Diana Nicoll, MD, PhD, MPA
Stephen J. McPhee, MD
Michael Pignone, MD, MPH

San Francisco
September 2003

Basic Principles of Diagnostic Test Use and Interpretation*

Diana Nicoll, MD, PhD, MPA, and Michael Pignone, MD, MPH

The clinician's main task is to make reasoned decisions about patient care despite incomplete clinical information and uncertainty about clinical outcomes. Although data elicited from the history and physical examination are often sufficient for making a diagnosis or for guiding therapy, more information may be required. In these situations, clinicians often turn to diagnostic tests for help.

BENEFITS, COSTS, AND RISKS

When used appropriately, diagnostic tests can be of great assistance to the clinician. Tests can be helpful for **screening,** ie, to identify risk factors for disease and to detect occult disease in asymptomatic persons. Identification of risk factors may allow early intervention to prevent disease occurrence, and early detection of occult disease may reduce disease morbidity and mortality through early treatment. Optimal screening tests meet the criteria listed in Table 1–1.

Tests can also be helpful for **diagnosis,** ie, to help establish or exclude the presence of disease in symptomatic persons. Some tests assist in early diagnosis after onset of symptoms and signs; others assist in differential diagnosis of various possible diseases; others help determine the stage or activity of disease.

Finally, tests can be helpful in **patient management.** Tests can help to (1) evaluate the severity of disease, (2) estimate prognosis, (3) monitor the course of disease (progression, stability, or resolution), (4) detect disease recurrence, and (5) select drugs and adjust therapy.

---

*Chapter modified, with permission, from Tierney LM Jr, McPhee SJ, Papadakis MA (editors): *Current Medical Diagnosis & Treatment 2003.* McGraw-Hill, 2003.

**TABLE 1–1. CRITERIA FOR USE OF
SCREENING PROCEDURES.**

Characteristics of population
    1. Sufficiently high prevalence of disease.
    2. Likely to be compliant with subsequent tests
       and treatments.
Characteristics of disease
    1. Significant morbidity and mortality.
    2. Effective and acceptable treatment available.
    3. Presymptomatic period detectable.
    4. Improved outcome from early treatment.
Characteristics of test
    1. Good sensitivity and specificity.
    2. Low cost and risk.
    3. Confirmatory test available and practical.

When ordering diagnostic tests, clinicians should weigh the potential benefits against the potential costs and disadvantages:

(1) Some tests carry a risk of morbidity or mortality—eg, cerebral angiogram leads to stroke in 1% of cases.

(2) The potential discomfort associated with tests such as colonoscopy may deter some patients from completing a diagnostic work-up.

(3) The result of a diagnostic test may mandate further testing or frequent follow-up. For example, a patient with a positive fecal occult blood test may incur significant cost, risk, and discomfort during follow-up colonoscopy.

(4) A false-positive test may lead to incorrect diagnosis or further unnecessary testing. Classifying a healthy patient as diseased based on a falsely positive diagnostic test can cause psychologic distress and may lead to risks from unnecessary or inappropriate therapy.

(5) A diagnostic or screening test may identify cases of disease that would not otherwise have been recognized and that would not have affected the patient. For example, early-stage, low-grade prostate cancer detected by prostate-specific antigen (PSA) screening in an 84-year-old man with known severe congestive heart failure will probably not become symptomatic or require treatment during his lifetime.

(6) Total costs may be high, or cost-effectiveness may be unfavorable. An individual test such as MRI of the head can cost more than $1400, and diagnostic tests as a whole account for approximately one-fifth of health care expenditures in the USA. Even relatively inexpensive tests may have poor cost-effectiveness if they produce very small health benefits.

PERFORMANCE OF DIAGNOSTIC TESTS

Test Preparation

Factors affecting both the patient and the specimen are important. The most crucial element in a properly conducted laboratory test is an appropriate specimen.

Patient Preparation

Preparation of the patient is important for certain tests—eg, a fasting state is needed for optimal glucose and triglyceride measurements; posture and sodium intake must be strictly controlled when measuring renin and aldosterone levels; and strenuous exercise should be avoided before taking samples for creatine kinase determinations, because vigorous muscle activity can lead to falsely abnormal results.

Specimen Collection

Careful attention must be paid to patient identification and specimen labeling. Knowing when the specimen was collected may be important. For instance, aminoglycoside levels cannot be interpreted appropriately without knowing whether the specimen was drawn just before ("trough" level) or after ("peak" level) drug administration. Drug levels cannot be interpreted if they are drawn during the drug's distribution phase (eg, digoxin levels drawn during the first 6 hours after an oral dose). Substances that have a circadian variation (eg, cortisol) can be interpreted only in the context of the time of day the sample was drawn.

During specimen collection, other principles should be remembered. Specimens should not be drawn above an intravenous line, as this may contaminate the sample with intravenous fluid. Excessive tourniquet time will lead to hemoconcentration and an increased concentration of protein-bound substances such as calcium. Lysis of cells during collection of a blood specimen will result in spuriously increased serum levels of substances concentrated in cells (eg, lactate dehydrogenase and potassium). Certain test specimens may require special handling or storage (eg, blood gas specimens). Delay in delivery of specimens to the laboratory can result in ongoing cellular metabolism and therefore spurious results for some studies (eg, low blood glucose).

TEST CHARACTERISTICS

Table 1–2 lists the general characteristics of useful diagnostic tests. Most of the principles detailed below can be applied not only to laboratory and radiologic tests but also to elements of the history and physical examination.

TABLE 1–2. PROPERTIES OF USEFUL DIAGNOSTIC TESTS.

1. Test methodology has been described in detail so that it can be accurately and reliably reproduced.
2. Test accuracy and precision have been determined.
3. The reference range has been established appropriately.
4. Sensitivity and specificity have been reliably established by comparison with a gold standard. The evaluation has used a range of patients, including those who have different but commonly confused disorders and those with a spectrum of mild and severe, treated and untreated disease. The patient selection process has been adequately described so that results will not be generalized inappropriately.
5. Independent contribution to overall performance of a test panel has been confirmed if a test is advocated as part of a panel of tests.

Accuracy

The accuracy of a laboratory test is its correspondence with the true value. An inaccurate test is one that differs from the true value even though the results may be reproducible (Figures 1–1A and 1–1B). In the clinical laboratory, accuracy of tests is maximized by calibrating laboratory equipment with reference material and by participation in external quality control programs.

Precision

Test precision is a measure of a test's reproducibility when repeated on the same sample. An imprecise test is one that yields widely varying results on repeated measurements (Figure 1–1B). The precision of diagnostic tests, which is monitored in clinical laboratories by using control material, must

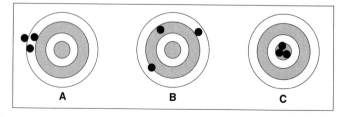

Figure 1–1. Relationship between accuracy and precision in diagnostic tests. The center of the target represents the true value of the substance being tested. **(A)** Diagnostic test that is precise but inaccurate; on repeated measurement, the test yields very similar results, but all results are far from the true value. **(B)** An imprecise and inaccurate test; repeated measurement yields widely different results and the results are far from the true value. **(C)** Ideal test—one that is both precise and accurate.

be good enough to distinguish clinically relevant changes in a patient's status from the analytic variability of the test. For instance, the manual white blood cell differential count is not precise enough to detect important changes in the distribution of cell types, because it is calculated by subjective evaluation of a small sample (100 cells). Repeated measurements by different technicians on the same sample result in widely different results. Automated differential counts are more precise because they are obtained from machines that use objective physical characteristics to classify a much larger sample (10,000 cells).

Reference Range

Reference ranges are method- and laboratory-specific. In practice, they often represent test results found in 95% of a small population presumed to be healthy; by definition, then, 5% of healthy patients will have a positive (abnormal) test (Figure 1–2). As a result, slightly abnormal results should be interpreted critically—they may be either truly abnormal or falsely abnormal. The practitioner should be aware also that the more tests ordered, the greater the chance of obtaining a falsely abnormal result. For a healthy person subjected to 20 independent tests, there is a 64% chance that one test result will lie outside the reference range (Table 1–3). Conversely, values within the reference range may not rule out the actual presence of disease because the reference range does not establish the distribution of results in patients with disease.

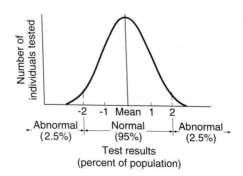

Figure 1–2. The reference range is usually defined as within 2 standard deviations of the mean test result (shown as –2 and 2) in a small population of healthy volunteers. Note that in t' example, test results are normally distributed; however, many biologic substances will ' distributions that are skewed.

TABLE 1–3. RELATIONSHIP BETWEEN THE NUMBER OF TESTS AND THE PROBABILITY THAT A HEALTHY PERSON WILL HAVE ONE OR MORE ABNORMAL RESULTS.

Number of Tests	Probability That One or More Results Will Be Abnormal
1	5%
6	26%
12	46%
20	64%

It is important to consider also whether published reference ranges are appropriate for the patient being evaluated: some ranges depend on age, sex, weight, diet, time of day, activity status, or posture. For instance, the reference ranges for hemoglobin concentration are age- and sex-dependent. Chapter 3 contains the reference ranges for commonly used chemistry and hematology tests. Test performance characteristics such as sensitivity and specificity are needed to interpret results and are discussed below.

Interfering Factors

The results of diagnostic tests can be altered by external factors, such as ingestion of drugs, and internal factors, such as abnormal physiologic states.

External interferences can affect test results in vivo or in vitro. In vivo, alcohol increases γ-glutamyl transpeptidase, and diuretics can affect sodium and potassium concentrations. Cigarette smoking can induce hepatic enzymes and thus reduce levels of substances such as theophylline that are metabolized by the liver. In vitro, cephalosporins may produce spurious serum creatinine levels due to interference with a common laboratory method of analysis.

Internal interferences result from abnormal physiologic states interfering with the test measurement. As an example, patients with gross lipemia may have spuriously low serum sodium levels if the test methodology used includes a step in which serum is diluted before sodium is measured. Because of the potential for test interference, clinicians should be wary of unexpected test results and should investigate reasons other than disease that may explain abnormal results, including laboratory error.

Sensitivity and Specificity

Clinicians should use measures of test performance such as sensitivity and specificity to judge the quality of a diagnostic test for a particular disease.

Test **sensitivity** is the likelihood that a diseased patient has a positive test. If all patients with a given disease have a positive test (ie, no diseased patients have negative tests), the test sensitivity is 100%. Generally, a test with high sensitivity is useful to exclude a diagnosis because a highly sensitive test will render few results that are falsely negative. To exclude infection with the AIDS virus, for instance, a clinician might choose a highly sensitive test such as the HIV antibody test.

A test's **specificity** is the likelihood that a healthy patient has a negative test. If all patients who do not have a given disease have negative tests (ie, no healthy patients have positive tests), the test specificity is 100%. A test with high specificity is useful to confirm a diagnosis, because a highly specific test will have few results that are falsely positive. For instance, to make the diagnosis of gouty arthritis, a clinician might choose a highly specific test, such as the presence of negatively birefringent needle-shaped crystals within leukocytes on microscopic evaluation of joint fluid.

To determine test sensitivity and specificity for a particular disease, the test must be compared against an independent "gold standard" test that defines the true disease state of the patient. For instance, the sensitivity and specificity of the ventilation/perfusion scan for pulmonary embolus are obtained by comparing the results of scans with the gold standard, pulmonary arteriography. Application of the gold standard examination to patients with positive scans establishes specificity. Failure to apply the gold standard examination following negative scans may result in an overestimation of sensitivity, because false negatives will not be identified. However, for many disease states (eg, pancreatitis), such a gold standard either does not exist or is very difficult or expensive to apply—and in such cases reliable estimates of test sensitivity and specificity are sometimes difficult to obtain.

Sensitivity and specificity can also be affected by the population from which these values are derived. For instance, many diagnostic tests are evaluated first using patients who have severe disease and control groups who are young and well. Compared with the general population, this study group will have more results that are truly positive (because patients have more advanced disease) and more results that are truly negative (because the control group is healthy). Thus, test sensitivity and specificity will be higher than would be expected in the general population, where more of a spectrum of health and disease is found. Clinicians should be aware of this **spectrum bias** when generalizing published test results to their own practice.

Test sensitivity and specificity depend on the threshold above which a test is interpreted to be abnormal (Figure 1–3). If the threshold is lowered, sensitivity is increased at the expense of lowered specificity. If the threshold is raised, sensitivity is decreased and specificity is increased.

Figure 1–4 shows how test sensitivity and specificity can be calculated using test results from patients previously classified by the gold standard as diseased or nondiseased.

The performance of two different tests can be compared by pl sensitivity and (1 minus the specificity) of each test at various

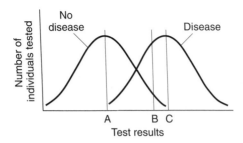

Figure 1–3. Hypothetical distribution of test results for healthy and diseased individuals. The position of the cutoff point between normal and abnormal (or negative and positive) test results determines the test's sensitivity and specificity. If point A is the cutoff point, the test would have 100% sensitivity but low specificity. If point C is the cutoff point, the test would have 100% specificity but low sensitivity. For most tests, the cutoff point is determined by the reference range, ie, the range of test results that are within 2 standard deviations of the mean (point B). In some situations, the cutoff is altered to enhance either sensitivity or specificity.

range cutoff values. The resulting **receiver operator characteristic (ROC) curve** will often show which test is better; a clearly superior test will have an ROC curve that always lies above and to the left of the inferior test curve, and, in general, the better test will have a larger area under the ROC curve. For instance, Figure 1–5 shows the ROC curves for PSA and prostatic acid phosphatase (PAP) in the diagnosis of prostate cancer. PSA is a superior test because it has higher sensitivity and specificity for all cutoff values.

USE OF TESTS IN DIAGNOSIS AND MANAGEMENT

The value of a test in a particular clinical situation depends not only on the test's sensitivity and specificity but also on the probability that the patient has the disease before the test result is known **(pretest probability).** The results of a useful test will substantially change the probability that the patient has the disease **(posttest probability).** Figure 1–4 shows how posttest probability can be calculated from the known sensitivity and specificity of the test and the estimated pretest probability of disease (or disease prevalence).

The pretest probability of disease has a profound effect on the posttest probability of disease. As demonstrated in Table 1–4, when a test with 90% sensitivity and specificity is used, the posttest probability can vary from 1% to 99% depending on the pretest probability of disease. Furthermore, as the pretest probability of disease decreases, it becomes less likely that someone with a positive test actually has the disease and more likely that the result represents a false positive.

As an example, suppose the clinician wishes to calculate the posttest probability of prostate cancer using the PSA test and a cutoff value of

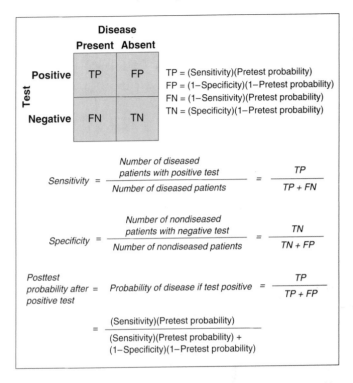

Figure 1–4. Calculation of sensitivity, specificity, and probability of disease after a positive test (posttest probability). (TP, true positive; FP, false positive; FN, false negative; TN, true negative.)

4 ng/mL. Using the data shown in Figure 1–5, sensitivity is 90% and specificity is 60%. The clinician estimates the pretest probability of disease given all the evidence and then calculates the posttest probability using the approach shown in Figure 1–4. The pretest probability that an otherwise healthy 50-year-old man has prostate cancer is equal to the prevalence of prostate cancer in that age group (probability = 10%) and the posttest probability is only 20%—ie, even though the test is positive, there is still an 80% chance that the patient does not have prostate cancer (Figure 1–6A). If the clinician finds a prostate nodule on rectal examination, the pretest probability of prostate cancer rises to 50% and the posttest probability using the same test is 69% (Figure 1–6B). Finally, if the clinician estimates the pretest

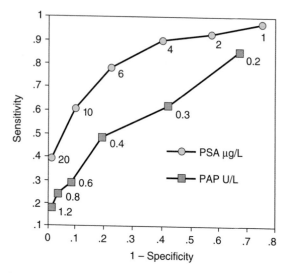

Figure 1–5. Receiver operator characteristic (ROC) curves for PSA and PAP in the diagnosis of prostate cancer. For all cutoff values, PSA has higher sensitivity and specificity; therefore, it is a better test based on these performance characteristics. *(Modified and reproduced, with permission, from Nicoll D et al: Routine acid phosphatase testing for screening and monitoring prostate cancer no longer justified. Clin Chem 1993;39:2540.)*

probability to be 98% based on a prostate nodule, bone pain, and lytic lesions on spine x-rays, the posttest probability using PSA is 99% (Figure 1–6C). This example illustrates that pretest probability has a profound effect on posttest probability and that tests provide more information when the diagnosis is truly uncertain (pretest probability about 50%) than when the diagnosis is either unlikely or nearly certain.

TABLE 1–4. INFLUENCE OF PRETEST PROBABILITY ON THE POSTTEST PROBABILITY OF DISEASE WHEN A TEST WITH 90% SENSITIVITY AND 90% SPECIFICITY IS USED.

Pretest Probability	Posttest Probability
0.01	0.08
0.50	0.90
0.99	0.999

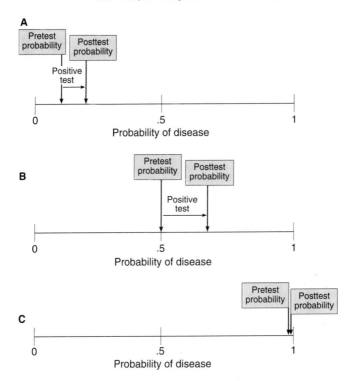

Figure 1–6. Effect of pretest probability and test sensitivity and specificity on the posttest probability of disease. (See text for explanation.)

ODDS-LIKELIHOOD RATIOS

Another way to calculate the posttest probability of disease is to use the odds-likelihood approach. Sensitivity and specificity are combined into one entity called the likelihood ratio (LR).

$$LR = \frac{\text{Probability of result in diseased persons}}{\text{Probability of result in nondiseased persons}}$$

When test results are dichotomized, every test has two likelihood ratios, one corresponding to a positive test (LR^+) and one corresponding to a negative test (LR^-):

$$LR^+ = \frac{\text{Probability that test is positive in diseased persons}}{\text{Probability that test is positive in nondiseased persons}}$$

$$= \frac{\text{Sensitivity}}{1 - \text{Specificity}}$$

$$LR^- = \frac{\text{Probability that test is negative in diseased persons}}{\text{Probability that test is negative in nondiseased persons}}$$

$$= \frac{1 - \text{Sensitivity}}{\text{Specificity}}$$

Lists of likelihood ratios can be found in some textbooks, journal articles, and computer programs (see Table 1–5 for sample values). Likelihood ratios can be used to make quick estimates of the usefulness of a contemplated diagnostic test in a particular situation. The simplest method for calculating posttest probability from pretest probability and likelihood ratios is to use a nomogram (Figure 1–7). The clinician places a straight edge through the points that represent the pretest probability and the likelihood ratio and then reads the posttest probability where the straightedge crosses the posttest probability line.

A more formal way of calculating posttest probabilities uses the likelihood ratio as follows:

$$\text{Pretest odds} \times \text{Likelihood ratio} = \text{Posttest odds}$$

To use this formulation, probabilities must be converted to odds, where the odds of having a disease are expressed as the chance of having the disease divided by the chance of not having the disease. For instance, a probability of 0.75 is the same as 3 : 1 odds (Figure 1–8).

To estimate the potential benefit of a diagnostic test, the clinician first estimates the pretest odds of disease given all available clinical information and then multiplies the pretest odds by the positive and negative likelihood ratios. The results are the **posttest odds,** or the odds that the patient has the disease if the test is positive or negative. To obtain the posttest probability, the odds are converted to a probability (Figure 1–8).

For example, if the clinician believes that the patient has a 60% chance of having a myocardial infarction (pretest odds of 3 : 2) and the creatine kinase MB test is positive ($LR^+ = 32$), then the posttest odds of having a myocardial infarction are

$$\frac{3}{2} \times 32 = \frac{96}{2} \text{ or 48:1 odds} \left(\frac{48/1}{48/1 + 1} = \frac{48}{48 + 1} = 98\% \text{ probability} \right)$$

If the CKMB test is negative ($LR^- = 0.05$), then the posttest odds of having a myocardial infarction are

TABLE 1–5. LIKELIHOOD RATIOS (LR) FOR DIAGNOSTIC TESTS.

Test	Disease	LR+	LR−
Amylase ($\uparrow$)	Pancreatitis	9.1	0.20
Anti-dsDNA ($\uparrow$)	SLE	37.0	0.28
Antinuclear antibody	SLE	4.5	0.13
Carcinoembryonic antigen	Dukes A colon cancer	1.6	0.87
Creatine kinase MB	Myocardial infarction	32.0	0.05
Esophagogastroduodenoscopy (+)	Upper GI bleeding	18.0	0.11
ESR > 30 mm/h	Temporal arteritis	3.3	0.01
Exercise echocardiography (new wall motion abnormalities)	Coronary artery disease	6.2	0.23
Exercise ECG (ST depression > 1 mm)	Coronary artery disease	5.9	0.39
Ferritin	Iron deficiency anemia	85.0	0.15
Free T$_4$ ($\uparrow$)	Hyperthyroidism	19.0	0.05
Free thyroxine index	Hyperthyroidism	6.8	0.06
Hepatitis A IgM antibody	Hepatitis A	99.0	0.01
Heterophil (+)	Infectious mononucleosis	97.0	0.03
Metanephrines ($\uparrow$)	Pheochromocytoma	11.0	0.23
Pleural fluid protein > 3 g/dL	Exudative pleural effusion	10.0	0.12
Technetium Tc 99m pyrophosphate scan (highly focal uptake)	Myocardial infarction	> 360.0	0.64
Testosterone ($\downarrow$)	Erectile dysfunction	32.0	0.03
TSH ($\uparrow$)	Hypothyroidism	99.0	0.01
24-Hour urinary free cortisol ($\uparrow$)	Hypercortisolism	10.0	0.07

$$\frac{3}{2} \times 0.05 = \frac{0.15}{2} \text{ odds} \left(\frac{0.15/2}{0.15/2 + 1} = \frac{0.15}{0.15 + 2} = 7\% \text{ probability} \right)$$

Sequential Testing

To this point, the impact of only one test on the probability of disease has been discussed, whereas during most diagnostic work-ups, clinicians obtain clinical information in a sequential fashion. To calculate the posttest odds

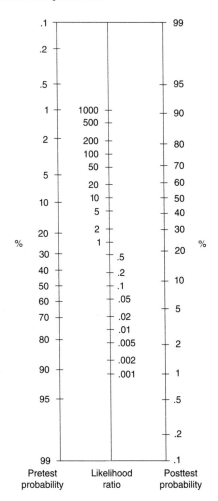

Figure 1-7. Nomogram for determining posttest probability from pretest probability and likelihood ratios. To figure the posttest probability, place a straightedge between the pretest probability and the likelihood ratio for the particular test. The posttest probability will be where the straightedge crosses the posttest probability line. *(Adapted and reproduced, with permission, from Fagan TJ: Nomogram for Bayes's theorem. N Engl J Med 1975;293:257.)*

$$\textbf{Odds} = \frac{\textbf{Probability}}{1 - \textbf{Probability}}$$

Example: If probability = 0.75,   then

$$\text{Odds} = \frac{0.75}{1 - 0.75} = \frac{0.75}{0.25} = \frac{3}{1} = 3{:}1$$

$$\textbf{Probability} = \frac{\textbf{Odds}}{\textbf{Odds} + 1}$$

Example: If odds = 3:1,   then

$$\text{Probability} = \frac{3/1}{3/1 + 1} = \frac{3}{3 + 1} = 0.75$$

Figure 1–8. Formulas for converting between probability and odds.

after three tests, for example, the clinician might estimate the pretest odds and use the appropriate likelihood ratio for each test:

$$\text{Pretest odds} \times LR_1 \times LR_2 \times LR_3 = \text{Posttest odds}$$

When using this approach, however, the clinician should be aware of a major assumption: the chosen tests or findings must be **conditionally independent.** For instance, with liver cell damage, the aspartate aminotransferase (AST) and alanine aminotransferase (ALT) enzymes may be released by the same process and are thus not conditionally independent. If conditionally dependent tests are used in this sequential approach, an inaccurate posttest probability will result.

Threshold Approach to Decision Making

A key aspect of medical decision making is the selection of a treatment threshold, ie, the probability of disease at which treatment is indicated. Figure 1–9 shows a possible way of identifying a treatment threshold by considering the value (utility) of the four possible outcomes of the treat/don't treat decision.

Use of a diagnostic test is warranted when its result could shift the probability of disease across the treatment threshold. For example, a

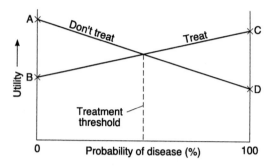

Figure 1–9. The "treat/don't treat" threshold. **(A)** Patient does not have disease and is not treated (highest utility). **(B)** Patient does not have disease and is treated (lower utility than A). **(C)** Patient has disease and is treated (lower utility than A). **(D)** Patient has disease and is not treated (lower utility than C).

clinician might decide to treat with antibiotics if the probability of strepto-coccal pharyngitis in a patient with a sore throat is greater than 25% (Figure 1–10A). If, after reviewing evidence from the history and physical examination, the clinician estimates the pretest probability of strep throat to be 15%, then a diagnostic test such as throat culture ($LR^+ = 7$) would be useful only if a positive test would shift the posttest probability above 25%. Use of the nomogram shown in Figure 1–7 indicates that the posttest probability would be 55% (Figure 1–10B); thus, ordering the test would be justified because it affects patient management. On the other hand, if the history and physical examination had suggested that the pretest probability of strep throat was 60%, the throat culture ($LR^- = 0.33$) would be indicated only if a negative test would lower the posttest probability below 25%. Using the same nomogram, the posttest probability after a negative test would be 33% (Figure 1–10C). Therefore, ordering the throat culture would not be justi-fied because it does not affect patient management.

This approach to decision making is now being applied in the clinical literature.

Decision Analysis

Up to this point, the discussion of diagnostic testing has focused on test characteristics and methods for using these characteristics to calculate the probability of disease in different clinical situations. Although useful, these methods are limited because they do not incorporate the many outcomes that may occur in clinical medicine or the values that patients and clinicians

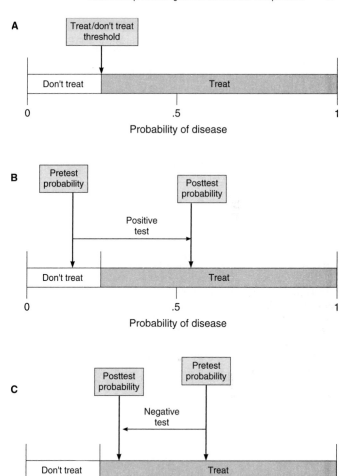

Figure 1–10. Threshold approach applied to test ordering. If the contemplated test will not change patient management, the test should not be ordered. (See text for explanation.)

place on those outcomes. To incorporate outcomes and values with characteristics of tests, decision analysis can be used.

The basic idea of decision analysis is to model the options in a medical decision, assign probabilities to the alternative actions, assign values (utilities) to the various outcomes, and then calculate which decision gives the greatest value. To complete a decision analysis, the clinician would proceed as follows:

(1) Draw a decision tree showing the elements of the medical decision.
(2) Assign probabilities to the various branches.
(3) Assign values (utilities) to the outcomes.
(4) Determine the expected utility (the product of probability and utility) of each branch.
(5) Select the decision with the highest expected utility.

Figure 1–11 shows a decision tree where the decision to be made is whether to treat without testing, perform a test and then treat based on the test result, or perform no tests and give no treatment. The clinician begins the analysis by building a decision tree showing the important elements of the decision. Once the tree is built, the clinician assigns probabilities to all the branches. In this case, all the branch probabilities can be calculated from (1) the probability of disease before the test (pretest probability), (2) the chance of a positive test if the disease is present (sensitivity), and (3) the chance of a negative test if the disease is absent (specificity). Next, the clinician assigns utility values to each of the outcomes.

After the expected utility is calculated for each branch of the decision tree by multiplying the utility of the outcome by the probability of the outcome, the clinician can identify the alternative with the highest expected utility.

Although time consuming, decision analysis can help to structure complex clinical problems and make difficult clinical decisions.

Evidence-Based Medicine

Evidence-based medicine stresses the use of evidence from clinical research—rather than intuition and pathophysiologic reasoning—as a basis for clinical decision making. Evidence-based medicine relies on the identification of methodologically sound evidence, critical appraisal of research studies, and the dissemination of accurate and useful summaries of evidence to inform clinical decision making. Systematic reviews can be used to summarize evidence for dissemination, as can evidence-based synopses of current research. Systematic reviews often use meta-analysis, a statistical technique that combines evidence from different studies to produce a more precise estimate of the effect of an intervention or accuracy of a test.

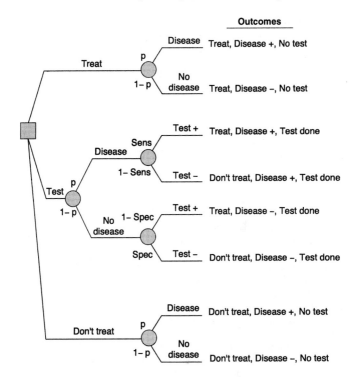

Figure 1–11. Generic tree for a clinical decision where the choices are (1) to treat the patient empirically, (2) to test and then treat if the test is positive, or (3) to withhold therapy. The square node is called a decision node, and the round nodes are called chance nodes. (p, pretest probability of disease; Sens, sensitivity; Spec, specificity.)

Clinical practice guidelines are systematically developed statements intended to assist practitioners and patients in making decisions about health care. Clinical algorithms and practice guidelines are now ubiquitous in medicine. Their utility and validity depend on the quality of the evidence that shaped the recommendations, on their being kept current, and on their acceptance and appropriate application by clinicians. Although clinicians are concerned about the effect of guidelines on professional autonomy and individual decision making, many organizations are trying to use compliance with practice guidelines as a measure of quality of care.

REFERENCES

Black ER et al (editors): *Diagnostic Strategies for Common Medical Problems,* 2nd ed. ACP-ASIM, 1999.

Detsky AS et al: Primer on decision analysis. Med Decis Making 1997; 17:123, 126, 136, 142, 152.

Elwyn G et al: Decision analysis in patient care. Lancet 2001;358:571.

Gilbert R et al: Assessing diagnostic and screening tests: Part 1. Concepts. West J Med 2001;174:405.

Gillan MG et al: Influence of imaging on clinical decision making in the treatment of lower back pain. Radiology 2001;220:393.

Guyatt G, Rennie D (editors): *Users' Guides to the Medical Literature: A Manual for Evidence-Based Clinical Practice.* Chicago, AMA Press, 2002.

Jadad AR et al: The Cochrane collaboration: Advances and challenges in improving evidence-based decision making. Med Decis Making 1998; 18:2.

Kohn MA et al: What white blood cell count should prompt antibiotic treatment in a febrile child? Tutorial on the importance of disease likelihood to the interpretation of diagnostic tests. Med Decis Making 2001;21:479.

Lijmer JG et al: Empirical evidence of design-related bias in studies of diagnostic tests. JAMA 1999;282:1061.

Mossman D, Berger JO: Intervals for posttest probabilities: A comparison of 5 methods. Med Decis Making 2001;21:498.

Omalley AJ et al: Bayesian regression methodology for estimating a receiver operating characteristic curve with two radiologic applications: Prostate biopsy and spiral CT of ureteral stones. Acad Radiol 2001;8:713.

Pauker SG et al: The threshold approach to clinical decision making. N Engl J Med 1980;301:1109.

Reid MC et al: Academic calculations versus clinical judgments: Practicing physicians' use of quantitative measures of test accuracy. Am J Med 1998;104:374.

Solomon DH et al: The rational clinical examination. Does this patient have a torn meniscus or ligament of the knee? Value of the physical examination. JAMA 2001;286:1610.

2

Laboratory Procedures in the Clinical Setting

Stephen J. McPhee, MD

This chapter presents information on how to perform common bedside laboratory procedures. Information on interpretation of results of body fluid analysis is included in some of the sections. Test results can be used for patient care only if the tests have been performed according to strict federal guidelines.

1. OBTAINING AND PROCESSING BODY FLUIDS
A. Safety Considerations
General Safety Considerations
Because all patient specimens are potentially infectious, the following precautions should be observed:

   a. Universal body fluid and needle stick precautions must be observed at all times.
   b. Disposable gloves and sometimes gown, mask, and goggles should be worn when collecting specimens.
   c. Gloves should be changed and hands washed after contact with each patient. Dispose of gloves in an appropriate biohazard waste container.
   d. Any spills should be cleaned up with 10% bleach solution.

Handling and Disposing of Needles and Gloves
   a. Do not resheathe needles.
   b. Discard needles and gloves only into designated containers.
   c. Do not remove a used needle from a syringe by hand. The needle may be removed using a specially designed waste collection system, or the entire assembly may (if disposable) be discarded as a unit into a designated container.
   d. When obtaining blood cultures, it is hazardous and unnecessary to change needles.
   e. Do not place phlebotomy or other equipment on the patient's bed.

B. Specimen Handling
Identification of Specimens
   a. Identify the patient before obtaining the specimen. (If the patient is not known to you, ask for the name and check the wristband.)
   b. Label each specimen container with the patient's name and identification number.

Specimen Tubes: Standard specimen tubes are now widely available and are easily identified by the color of the stopper (see also p 38):
   a. Red-top tubes contain no anticoagulants or preservatives and are used for chemistry tests.
   b. Marbled-top tubes contain material that allows ready separation of serum and clot by centrifugation.
   c. Lavender-top tubes contain EDTA and are used for hematology tests (eg, blood or cell counts, differentials).
   d. Green-top tubes contain heparin and are used for tests that require plasma or anticoagulation.
   e. Blue-top tubes contain citrate and are used for coagulation tests.
   f. Gray-top tubes contain fluoride and are used for some chemistry tests (eg, glucose) if the specimen cannot be analyzed immediately.

Procedure
   a. When collecting multiple specimens, fill sterile tubes used for bacteriologic tests, then tubes without additives (ie, red- or gold-top tubes) before filling those with additives to avoid the potential for bacterial contamination, transfer of anticoagulants,

etc. However, be certain to fill tubes containing anticoagulants before the blood specimen clots.
- b. The recommended order of filling tubes is (by type and color): (1) blood culture, (2) red- or gold-top, (3) blue top, (4) green top, (5) lavender top.
- c. Fill each stoppered tube completely. Tilt each tube containing anticoagulant or preservative to mix thoroughly. Place any specimens on ice as required (eg, arterial blood). Deliver specimens to the laboratory promptly.
- d. For each of the major body fluids, Table 2–1 summarizes commonly requested tests and requirements for specimen handling and provides cross-references to tables and figures elsewhere in this book for help in interpretation of the results.

2. BASIC STAINING METHODS
A. Gram Stain
Preparation of Smear
- a. Obtain a fresh specimen of the material to be stained (eg, sputum) and smear a small amount on a glass slide. Thin smears give the best results (eg, press a sputum sample between two glass slides).
- b. Let the smear air dry before heat fixing, because heating a wet smear will usually distort cells and organisms.
- c. Heat-fix the smear by passing the clean side of the slide quickly through a Bunsen burner or other flame source (no more than three or four times). The slide should be warm, not hot.
- d. Let the slide cool before staining.

Staining Technique
- a. Put on gloves.
- b. Stain with crystal violet (10 seconds).
- c. Rinse with gently running water (5 seconds).
- d. Flood with Gram iodine solution (10–30 seconds).
- e. Rinse with gently running water (5 seconds).
- f. Decolorize with acetone-alcohol solution until no more blue color leaches from the slide (5 seconds).
- g. Rinse immediately with water (5 seconds).
- h. Counterstain with safranin O (10 seconds).
- i. Rinse with water (5 seconds).
- j. Let the slide air-dry (or carefully blot with filter paper), then examine it under the microscope.

Microscopic Examination
- a. Examine the smear first using the low-power lens for leukocytes and fungi. Screen for the number and color of polymorphonuclear cells (cell nuclei should be pink, not blue).
- b. Examine using the high-power oil-immersion lens for microbial forms. Screen for intracellular organisms. Review the slide sys-

TABLE 2–1. BODY FLUID TESTS, HANDLING, AND INTERPRETATION.

Body Fluid	Commonly Requested Tests	Specimen Tube and Handling	Interpretation Guide
Arterial blood	pH, P_{O_2}, P_{CO_2}	Glass syringe. Evacuate air bubbles; remove needle; position rubber cap; place sample on ice; deliver immediately.	See acid–base nomogram p 409.
Ascitic fluid	Cell count, differential Protein, amylase Gram stain, culture Cytology (if neoplasm suspected)	Lavender top Red top Sterile Cytology	See ascitic fluid profiles, p 364.
Cerebrospinal fluid	Cell count, differential Gram stain, culture Protein, glucose VDRL or other studies (oligoclonal bands) Cytology (if neoplasm suspected)	Tube #1 Tube #2 Tube #3 Tube #4 Cytology	See cerebrospinal fluid profiles, p 368.
Pleural fluid	Cell count, differential Protein, glucose, amylase Gram stain, culture Cytology (if neoplasm suspected)	Lavender top Red top Sterile Cytology	See pleural fluid profiles, p 384.
Synovial fluid	Cell count, differential Protein, glucose Gram stain, culture Microscopic examination for crystals Cytology (if neoplasm [villonodular synovitis, metastatic disease] suspected)	Lavender top Red top Sterile Green top Cytology	See synovial fluid profiles, p 391, and Figure 2–6.

Urine	Urinalysis
	  Dipstick
	  Microscopic examination
	  Gram stain, culture
	Cytology (if neoplasm suspected)
		
		Clean tube
		Centrifuge tube
		Sterile
		Cytology
			See Table 9–25, p 400.
			See Table 2–2, p 29.
			See Figure 2–3, p 31.

tematically for (1) fungi (mycelia, then yeast), (2) small gram-negative rods (bacteroides, haemophilus, etc) (3) gram-negative cocci (neisseria, etc), (4) gram-positive rods (listeria, etc), and (5) gram-positive cocci (streptococcus, staphylococcus, etc).

  c. Label positive slides with the patient's name and identification number and save them for later review.

d. Figure 2–1 illustrates typical findings on a Gram-stained smear of sputum.

B. Wright Stain of Peripheral Blood Smear
Preparation of Smear
a. Obtain a fresh specimen of blood by pricking the patient's finger with a lancet. If alcohol is used to clean the fingertip, wipe it off first with a gauze pad.
b. Place a single drop of blood on a glass slide. Lay a second glass slide over the first one and rapidly pull it away lengthwise to leave a thin smear.
c. Let the smear air-dry. Do not heat-fix.
Staining Technique
a. Stain with fresh Wright stain (1 minute).
b. Gently add an equal amount of water and gently blow on the smear to mix the stain and water. Repeat by adding more water and blowing to mix. Look for formation of a shiny surface scum. Then allow the stain to set (3–4 minutes).
c. Rinse with gently running water (5 seconds).
d. Clean the back of the slide with an alcohol pad if necessary.

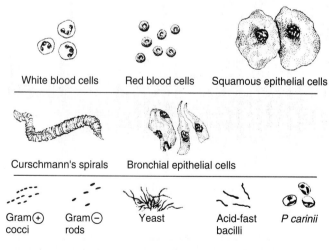

White blood cells   Red blood cells   Squamous epithelial cells

Curschmann's spirals   Bronchial epithelial cells

Gram⊕ cocci   Gram⊖ rods   Yeast   Acid-fast bacilli   *P carinii*

Figure 2–1. Common findings on microscopic examination of sputum. Most elements can be seen on Gram-stained smears except for acid-fast bacilli (auramine-rhodamine stain) and *Pneumocystis carinii* (Giemsa stain). *(Modified and reproduced, with permission from Krupp MA et al: Physician's Handbook, 21st ed. Originally published by Lange Medical Publications. Copyright © 1985 by The McGraw-Hill Companies, Inc.)*

Microscopic Examination

  a. Examine the smear first using the low-power lens to select a good area for study (red and white cells separated from one another).

  b. Then move to the high-power oil-immersion lens. Review the slide systematically for (1) platelet morphology, (2) white cells (differential types, morphology, toxic granulations and vacuoles, etc), and (3) red cells (size, shape, color, stippling, nucleation, etc).

  c. Label slides with the patient's name and identification number and save them for later review.

  d. See Figure 2–2 for examples of common peripheral blood smear abnormalities.

3. OTHER BEDSIDE LABORATORY PROCEDURES

A. Urinalysis

Collection and Preparation of Specimen

  a. Obtain a midstream urine specimen from the patient. The sample must be free of skin epithelium or bacteria, secretions, hair, lint, etc.

  b. Examine the specimen while fresh (still warm). Otherwise, bacteria may proliferate, casts and crystals may dissolve, and particulate matter may settle out. (Occasionally, amorphous crystals precipitate out, obscuring formed elements. In cold urine, they are amorphous urate crystals; these may be dissolved by gently rewarming the urine. In alkaline urine, they are amorphous phosphate crystals; these may be dissolved by adding 1 mL of acetic acid.)

  c. Place 10 mL in a tube and centrifuge at 2000–3000 rpm for 3–5 minutes.

  d. Discard the supernatant. Resuspend the sediment in the few drops that remain by gently tilting the tube.

  e. Place a drop on a glass slide, cover it with a coverslip, and examine under the microscope; no stain is needed. If bacterial infection is present, a single drop of methylene blue applied to the edge of the coverslip, or a Gram-stained smear of an air-dried, heat-fixed specimen, can assist in distinguishing gram-negative rods (eg, *E coli,* proteus, klebsiella) from gram-positive cocci (eg, enterococcus, *Staphylococcus saprophyticus*).

Procedural Technique

  a. While the urine is being centrifuged, examine the remainder of the specimen by inspection and reagent strip ("dipstick") testing.

  b. Inspect the specimen for color and clarity. Normally, urine is yellow or light orange. Dark orange urine is caused by inges-

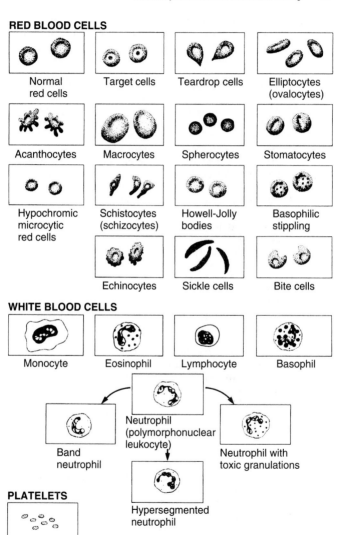

RED BLOOD CELLS

Normal red cells

Target cells

Teardrop cells

Elliptocytes (ovalocytes)

Acanthocytes

Macrocytes

Spherocytes

Stomatocytes

Hypochromic microcytic red cells

Schistocytes (schizocytes)

Howell-Jolly bodies

Basophilic stippling

Echinocytes

Sickle cells

Bite cells

WHITE BLOOD CELLS

Monocyte

Eosinophil

Lymphocyte

Basophil

Band neutrophil

Neutrophil (polymorphonuclear leukocyte)

Neutrophil with toxic granulations

Hypersegmented neutrophil

PLATELETS

Figure 2–2. Common peripheral blood smear findings.

tion of the urinary tract analgesic phenazopyridine (Pyridium, others); red urine, by hemoglobinuria, myoglobinuria, beets, senna, or rifampin therapy; green urine, by *Pseudomonas* infection or iodochlorhydroxyquin or amitriptyline therapy; brown urine, by bilirubinuria or fecal contamination; black urine, by intravascular hemolysis, alkaptonuria, melanoma, or methyldopa therapy; purplish urine, by porphyria; and milky white urine, by pus, chyluria, or amorphous crystals (urates or phosphates). Turbidity of urine is caused by pus, red blood cells, or crystals.

   c. Reagent strips provide information about specific gravity, pH, protein, glucose, ketones, bilirubin, heme, nitrite, and esterase (Table 2–2). Dip a reagent strip in the urine and compare it with the chart on the bottle. Follow the timing instructions carefully. *Note:* Reagent strips cannot be relied on to detect some proteins (eg, globulins, light chains) or sugars (other than glucose).

   d. Record the results.

Microscopic Examination

   a. Examine the area under the coverslip under the low-power and high-dry lenses for cells, casts, crystals, and bacteria. (If a Gram stain is done, examine under the oil immersion lens.)

   b. Cells may be red cells, white cells, squamous cells, transitional (bladder) epithelial cells, or atypical (tumor) cells. Red cells suggest upper or lower urinary tract infections (cystitis, prostatitis, pyelonephritis), glomerulonephritis, collagen vascular disease, trauma, renal calculi, tumors, drug reactions, and structural abnormalities (polycystic kidneys). White cells suggest inflammatory processes such as urinary tract infection (most common), collagen vascular disease, or interstitial nephritis. Red cell casts are considered pathognomonic of glomerulonephritis; white cell casts, of pyelonephritis; and fatty (lipid) casts, of nephrotic syndrome.

   c. The finding on a Gram-stained smear of unspun, clean, fresh urine of even one bacterium per field under the oil-immersion lens correlates fairly well with bacterial culture colony counts of greater than 100,000 organisms per μL.

   d. See Table 9–25, p 400, for a guide to interpretation of urinalysis; and Figure 2–3 for a guide to microscopic findings in urine.

B. Vaginal Fluid Wet Preparation
Preparation of Smear and Staining Technique

   a. Place a small amount of vaginal discharge on a glass slide.

   b. Add 2 drops of sterile saline solution.

   c. Place a coverslip over the area to be examined.

Microscopic Examination

   a. Examine under the microscope, using the high-dry lens and a low light source.

TABLE 2–2. COMPONENTS OF THE URINE DIPSTICK.[1]

Test	Values	Lowest Detectable Range	Comments
Specific gravity	1.001–1.035	1.000–1.030	Highly buffered alkaline urine may yield low specific gravity readings. Moderate protein-uria (100–750 mg/dL) may yield high readings. Loss of concentrating or diluting capacity indicates renal dysfunction.
pH	5–9 units	5.0–8.5 units	Excessive urine on strip may cause protein reagent to run over onto pH area, yielding falsely low pH reading.
Protein	0	15–30 mg/dL albumin	False-positive readings can be caused by highly buffered alkaline urine. Reagent more sensitive to albumin than other proteins. A negative result does not rule out the presence of globulins, hemoglobin, Bence Jones proteins, or mucoprotein. 1+ = 30 mg/dL 3+ = 300 mg/dL 2+ = 100 mg/dL 4+ = ≥ 2000 mg/dL
Glucose	0	75–125 mg/dL	Test is specific for glucose. False-negative results occur with urinary ascorbic acid concentrations ≥ 50 mg/dL and with ketone body levels ≥ 50 mg/dL. Test reagent reactivity also varies with specific gravity and temperature. Trace = 100 mg/dL 1 = 1000 mg/dL 1/4 = 250 mg/dL 2 = ≥ 2000 mg/dL 1/2 = 500 mg/dL
Ketone	0	5–10 mg/dL acetoacetate	Test does not react with acetone or β-hydroxy-butyric acid. (Trace) false-positive results may occur with highly pigmented urines or those containing levodopa metabolites or sulfhydryl-containing compounds (eg, mesna). Trace = 5 mg/dL Moderate = 40 mg/dL Small = 15 mg/dL Large = 80–160 mg/dL
Bilirubin	0	0.4–0.8 mg/dL	Indicates hepatitis (conjugated bilirubin). False-negative readings can be caused by ascorbic acid concentrations ≥ 25 mg/dL. False-positive readings can be caused by etodolac metabolites. Test is less sensitive than Ictotest Reagent tablets.

(continued)

TABLE 2–2 (CONTINUED).

Test	Values	Lowest Detectable Range	Comments
Blood	0[2]	0.015–0.062 mg/dL hemoglobin	Test equally sensitive to myoglobin and hemoglobin (including both intact erythrocytes and free hemoglobin). False-positive results can be caused by oxidizing contaminants (hypochlorite) and microbial peroxidase (urinary tract infection). Test sensitivity is reduced in urines with high specific gravity, captopril, or heavy proteinuria.
Nitrite	0	0.06–0.10 mg/dL nitrite ion	Test depends on the conversion of nitrate (derived from the diet) to nitrite by gram-negative bacteria in urine. Test specific for nitrite. False-negative readings can be caused by ascorbic acid. Test sensitivity is reduced in urines with high specific gravity.
Leukocytes (esterase)	0[3]	6–15 WBCs/hpf	Indicator of urinary tract infection. Test detects esterases contained in granulocytic leukocytes. Test sensitivity is reduced in urines with high specific gravity, elevated glucose concentrations (≥ 4 g/dL), or presence of cephalexin, cephalothin, tetracycline, or high concentrations of oxalate.

[1] Package insert, revised 9/95. Bayer Diagnostics Reagent Strips for Urinalysis, Bayer Corporation.
[2] Except in menstruating females.
[3] Except in females with vaginitis.

      b. Look for motile trichomonads (undulating protozoa propelled by four flagella). Look for clue cells (vaginal epithelial cells with large numbers of organisms attached to them, obscuring cell borders), pathognomonic of *Gardnerella vaginalis*-associated vaginosis.

      c. See Figure 2–4 for an example of a positive wet prep (trichomonads, clue cells) and Table 9–26, p 402 for the differential diagnosis of vaginal discharge.

C. Skin or Vaginal Fluid KOH Preparation
Preparation of Smear and Staining Technique

      a. Obtain a skin specimen by using a No. 15 scalpel blade to scrape scales from the skin lesion onto a glass slide or to remove the top of a vesicle onto the slide. Or place a single drop of vaginal discharge on the slide.

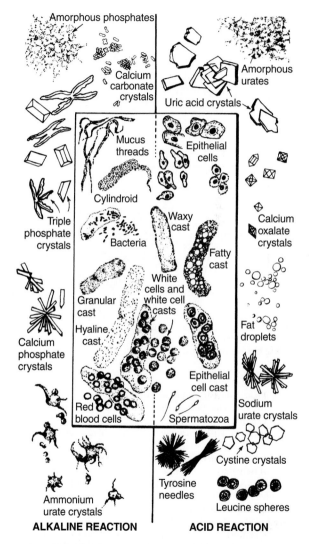

Figure 2–3. Microscopic findings on examination of the urine. *(Modified and reproduced, with permission from Krupp MA et al: Physician's Handbook, 21st ed. Originally published by Lange Medical Publications. Copyright © 1985 by The McGraw-Hill Companies, Inc.)*

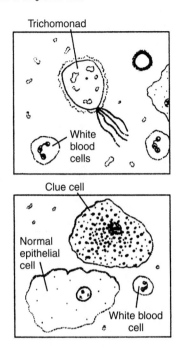

Figure 2–4. Wet preparation showing trichomonads, white blood cells, and clue cells.

   b. Place 1 or 2 drops of potassium hydroxide (10–20%) on top of
      the specimen on the slide. Lay a coverslip over the area to be
      examined.
   c. Heat the slide from beneath with a match or Bunsen burner
      flame until the slide contents begin to bubble.
   d. Clean carbon off the back side of the slide with an alcohol pad
      if necessary.
      Note: A fishy amine odor upon addition of KOH to a vaginal dis-
      charge is typical of bacterial vaginosis caused by *Gardnerella
      vaginalis.*

Microscopic Examination
   a. Examine the smear under the high-dry lens for mycelial
      forms. Branched, septate hyphae are typical of dermatophyto-
      sis (eg, trichophyton, epidermophyton, microsporum species);
      branched, septate pseudohyphae with or without budding yeast

forms are seen with candidiasis (candida species); and short, curved hyphae plus clumps of spores ("spaghetti and meatballs") are seen with tinea versicolor *(Malassezia furfur)*.
   b. See Figure 2–5 for an example of a positive KOH prep.

D. Synovial Fluid Examination for Crystals
Preparation of Smear
   a. No stain is necessary.
   b. Place a small amount of synovial fluid on a glass slide.
   c. Place a coverslip over the area to be examined.
Microscopic Examination
   a. Examine under a polarized light microscope with a red compensator, using the high-dry lens and a moderately bright light source.

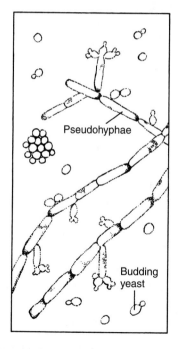

Figure 2–5. KOH preparation showing mycelial forms (pseudohyphae) and budding yeast typical of *Candida albicans*.

b. Look for needle-shaped, negatively birefringent urate crystals (crystals parallel to the axis of the compensator appear yellow) in gout or rhomboidal, positively birefringent calcium pyrophosphate crystals (crystals parallel to the axis of the compensator appear blue) in pseudogout.

c. See Figure 2–6 for examples of positive synovial fluid examinations for these two types of crystals.

E. Pulse Oximetry

Indications

To measure oxygen saturation in a noninvasive and often continuous fashion.

Contraindications

a. Hypotension, hypothermia, low perfusion states, severe or rapid desaturation, and severe anemia (hemoglobin < 5 g/dL) cause inaccurate readings.

b. Hyperbilirubinemia, methemoglobinemia, fetal hemoglobinemia, and carboxyhemoglobinemia can falsely elevate oxygen saturation measurements.

c. Excessive ambient light, simultaneous use of a blood pressure cuff, the presence of intravascular dyes (eg, methylene blue),

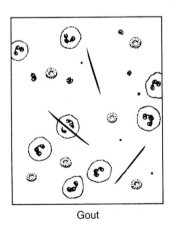
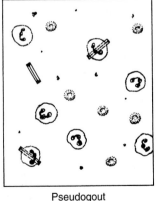

Gout   Pseudogout

Figure 2–6. Examination of synovial fluid for crystals using a compensated, polarized microscope. In gout, crystals are needle shaped, negatively birefringent, and composed of monosodium urate. In pseudogout, crystals are rhomboidal, positively birefringent, and composed of calcium pyrophosphate dihydrate. In both diseases, crystals can be found free-floating or within polymorphonuclear cells.

and electrical interference (eg, MRI scanners, electrosurgery) can also cause erroneous readings.

Approach to the Patient

The patient should be positioned close to the pulse oximeter and should hold the probe site still. The sampling area should have good circulation and be free of skin irritation.

Procedural Technique

a. Plug the pulse oximeter into a grounded AC power outlet or make sure that sufficient battery power is available. Turn the oximeter on and wait until self-calibration is complete.

b. Select the probe to be used and connect it to the pulse oximeter. The probe consists of a light source (a red light-emitting device in most cases) and a photodetector. Probes are available for the ear, finger, and, in neonates, the foot, ankle, palm, calf, and forearm.

c. Attach the probe to the patient after cleansing the surrounding skin with an alcohol swab. Some probes come with double-sided adhesive disks that improve probe signal.

d. Watch the waveform and pulse indicators to assess the quality of the signal. Readjust if a poor signal is present.

e. Set alarm warnings on the device.

f. Check the probe site at least every 4 hours. Care should be taken not to apply tension to the probe cables.

Possible Complications

Allergic reaction to adhesives.

Comments

Because of the curvilinear nature of the oxygen-hemoglobin dissociation curve, oxygen saturation (SaO_2) is not directly proportionate to oxygen partial pressure (PaO_2). Therefore, a relatively small change in oxygen saturation (eg, from 94% to 83%) can represent a large change in PaO_2 (eg, from 80 mm Hg to 50 mm Hg). In addition, the dissociation curve varies markedly from patient to patient and with pH, temperature, and altitude. To ensure accurate assessment of oxygenation, one should correlate pulse oximetry with arterial blood gas analysis.

REFERENCES

Gram Stain

Fournier AM: The Gram stain. Ann Intern Med 1998;128:776.

Hirschmann JV: The sputum Gram stain. J Gen Intern Med 1991;6:261.

Popescu A, Doyle RJ: The Gram stain after more than a century. Biotech Histochem 1996;71:145.

Reed WW et al: Sputum gram's stain in community-acquired pneumococcal pneumonia. A meta-analysis. West J Med 1996;165:197.

Urinalysis

Jou WW, Powers RD: Utility of dipstick urinalysis as a guide to management of adults with suspected infection or hematuria. South Med J 1998;91:266.

Lorincz AE et al: Urinalysis: Current status and prospects for the future. Ann Clin Lab Sci 1999;29:169.

Misdraji J, Nguyen PL: Urinalysis. When—and when not—to order. Postgrad Med 1996;100:173.

Semeniuk H et al: Evaluation of the leukocyte esterase and nitrite urine dipstick screening tests for detection of bacteriuria in women with suspected uncomplicated urinary tract infections. J Clin Microbiol 1999;37:3051.

Vaginal Wet Prep

Ferris DG et al: Office laboratory diagnosis of vaginitis. Clinician-performed tests compared with a rapid nucleic acid hybridization test. J Fam Pract 1995;41:575.

Thihnkhamrop J: Vaginal fluid pH as a screening test for vaginitis. Int J Gynaecol Obstet 1999;66:143.

Wiesenfeld HC et al: The infrequent use of office-based diagnostic tests for vaginitis. Am J Obstet Gynecol 1999;181:39.

Synovial Fluid Examination

Schumacher HR: Crystal-induced arthritis: An overview. Am J Med 1996;100:46S.

Pulse Oximetry

Franklin ML: Transcutaneous measurement of partial pressure of oxygen and carbon dioxide. Respir Care Clin North Am 1995;1:11.

Grap MJ: Pulse oximetry. Crit Care Nurs 1998;18:94.

Jensen LA, Onyskiw JE, Prasad NG: Meta-analysis of arterial oxygen saturation monitoring by pulse oximetry in adults. Heart Lung 1998;27:387.

Ortiz FO et al: Accuracy of pulse oximetry in sickle cell disease. Am J Respir Crit Care Med 1999;159:447.

Sinex JE: Pulse oximetry: Principles and limitations. Am J Emerg Med 1999;17:59.

Smatlak P et al: Clinical evaluation of noninvasive monitoring of oxygen saturation in critically ill patients. Am J Crit Care 1998;7:370.

3

Common Laboratory Tests: Selection and Interpretation

Diana Nicoll, MD, PhD, MPA, Stephen J. McPhee, MD, and Michael Pignone, MD, MPH

HOW TO USE THIS SECTION

This section contains information about commonly used laboratory tests. It includes most of the blood, urine, and cerebrospinal fluid tests found in this book, with the exception of drug levels. Entries are in outline format and are arranged alphabetically.

Test/Reference Range/Collection

This first outline listing begins with the common test name, the specimen analyzed, and any test name abbreviation (in parentheses).

Below this in the first outline listing is the reference range for each test. The first entry is in conventional units, and the second entry (in [brackets]) is in SI units (Système International d'Unités). Any panic values for a particular test are placed here after the word *Panic*. The reference ranges provided are from several large medical centers; consult your own clinical laboratory for those used in your institution.

This outline listing also shows which tube to use for collecting blood and other body fluids, how much the test costs (in relative symbolism; see below), and how to collect the specimen. Listed below are the common collection tubes and their contents:

Tube Top Color	Tube Contents	Typically Used In
Lavender	EDTA	Complete blood count
Gold or Marbled	Serum separator	Serum chemistry tests

(continued)

Tube Top Color	Tube Contents	Typically Used In
Red	None	Blood banking (serum)
Blue	Citrate	Coagulation studies
Green	Heparin	Plasma studies
Yellow	Acid citrate	HLA typing
Navy	Trace metal free	Trace metals (eg, lead)
Gray	Inhibitor of glycolysis (sodium fluoride)	Lactic acid

The scale used for the cost of each test is:

Approximate Cost	Symbol Used in Tables
$1–20	$
$21–50	$$
$51–100	$$$
> $100	$$$$

Physiologic Basis

This outline listing contains physiologic information about the substance being tested. Information on classification and biologic importance, as well as interactions with other biologic substances and processes, is included.

Interpretation

This outline lists clinical conditions that affect the substance being tested. Generally, conditions with higher prevalence will be listed first. When the sensitivity of the test for a particular disease is known, that information will follow the disease name in parentheses, eg, "rheumatoid arthritis (83%)." Some of the common drugs that can affect the test substance in vivo will also be included in this outline listing.

Comments

This outline listing sets forth general information pertinent to the use and interpretation of the test and important in vitro interferences with the test procedure. Appropriate general references are also listed.

Test Name

The test name is placed as a header to the rest of the outline list to allow for quick referencing.

Test/Range/Collection	Physiologic Basis	Interpretation	Comments
		ABO Grouping	
ABO grouping, serum and red cells (ABO) Red $ Properly identified and labeled blood specimens are critical.	The four blood groups A, B, O, and AB are determined by the presence of antigens A and B or their absence (O) on a patient's red blood cells. Antibodies are present in serum for which red cells lack antigen.	In the US white population, 45% are type O, 40% A, 11% B, 4% AB. In the African-American population, 49% are type O, 27% A, 20% B, 4% AB. In the US Asian population, 40% are type O, 28% A, 27% B, 5% AB. In the Native American population, 79% are type O, 16% A, 4% B, <1% AB.	For both blood donors and recipients, routine ABO grouping includes both red cell and serum testing, as checks on each other. Tube testing is as follows: patient's red cells are tested with anti-A and anti-B for the presence or absence of agglutination (forward or cell grouping), and patient's serum is tested against known A and B cells (reverse or serum grouping). *Technical Manual of the American Association of Blood Banks,* 14th ed. American Association of Blood Banks, 2002. Curr Opin Hematol 2001;8:397.
		Acetaminophen	
Acetaminophen, serum (Tylenol; others) 10–20 mg/L [66–132 µmol/L] *Panic:* >50 mg/L Marbled $$ For suspected overdose, draw two samples at least 4 hours apart, at least 4 hours after ingestion. Note time of ingestion, if known. Order test stat.	In overdose, liver and renal toxicity are produced by the hydroxylated metabolite if it is not conjugated with glutathione in the liver.	**Increased in:** Acetaminophen overdose. Interpretation of serum acetaminophen level depends on time since ingestion. Levels drawn <4 hours after ingestion cannot be interpreted since the drug is still in the absorption and distribution phase. Use nomogram (Figure 10–1, p 408 to evaluate possible toxicity. Levels >150 mg/dL at 4 hours or >50 mg/dL at 12 hours after ingestion suggest toxicity. Nomogram inaccurate for chronic ingestions.	Do not delay acetylcysteine (Mucomyst) treatment (140 mg/kg orally) if stat levels are unavailable. Drug Saf 2001;24(7):503. Crit Care 2002;6(2):108.

		Acetoacetate	Acetylcholine receptor antibody
Acetoacetate, serum or urine 0 mg/dL, [μmol/L] Marbled or urine container $ Urine sample should be fresh.	Acetoacetate, acetone, and β-hydroxybutyrate contribute to ketoacidosis when oxidative hepatic metabolism of fatty acids is impaired. Proportions in serum vary but are generally 20% acetoacetate, 78% β-hydroxybutyrate, and 2% acetone.	**Present in:** Diabetic ketoacidosis, alcoholic ketoacidosis, prolonged fasting, severe carbohydrate restriction with normal fat intake.	Nitroprusside test is semiquantitative; it detects acetoacetate and is sensitive down to 5–10 mg/dL. Trace = 5 mg/dL, small = 15 mg/dL, moderate = 40 mg/dL, large = 80 mg/dL [1 mg/dL = 100 μmol/L]. β-Hydroxybutyrate is not a ketone and is not detected by the nitroprusside test. Acetone is also not reliably detected by this method. Failure of test to detect β-hydroxybutyrate in ketoacidosis may produce a seemingly paradoxical increase in ketones with clinical improvement as nondetectable β-hydroxybutyrate is replaced by detectable acetoacetate. Br Med J 1972;2:565.
Acetylcholine receptor antibody, serum Negative Marbled $$	Acetylcholine receptor antibodies are involved in the pathogenesis of myasthenia gravis. Sensitive radioassay or ELISA is available based on inhibition of binding of ^{125}I alpha-bungarotoxin to the acetylcholine receptor.	**Positive in:** Myasthenia gravis (73%). Single fiber EMG may have best sensitivity.	Titer has been found to correlate with clinical severity. Clin Chem 1993;39:2053. Lancet 2001;357:2122. Curr Opin Neurol 2001;14:583.

Test/Range/Collection	Physiologic Basis	Interpretation	Comments
Adrenocorticotropic hormone	**Adrenocorticotropic hormone**		**Alanine aminotransferase**
Adrenocorticotropic hormone, plasma (ACTH) 20–100 pg/mL [4–22 pmol/L] Heparinized plastic container $$$$ Send promptly to laboratory on ice. ACTH is unstable in plasma, is inactivated at room temperature, and adheres strongly to glass. Avoid all contact with glass.	Pituitary ACTH (release stimulated by hypothalamic corticotropin-releasing factor) stimulates cortisol release from the adrenal gland. There is feedback regulation of the system by cortisol. ACTH is secreted episodically and shows circadian variation, with highest levels at 6:00–8:00 AM; lowest levels at 9:00–10:00 PM.	**Increased in:** Pituitary (40–200 pg/mL) and ectopic (200–71,000 pg/mL) Cushing syndrome, primary adrenal insufficiency (>250 pg/mL), adrenogenital syndrome with impaired cortisol production. **Decreased in:** Adrenal Cushing syndrome (<20 pg/mL), pituitary ACTH (secondary adrenal) insufficiency (<50 pg/mL).	ACTH levels (RIA) can only be interpreted when measured with cortisol after standardized stimulation or suppression tests (see Adrenocortical insufficiency algorithm, p 340, and Cushing syndrome algorithm, p 343). Postgrad Med 1998;104:61. Endocrinol Metab Clin North Am 2001;30:729. Ann Endocrinol (Paris) 2001;62:173. Am J Med Sci 2001;321:137.
Alanine aminotransferase, serum (ALT, SGPT, GPT) 0–35 U/L [0–0.58 µkat/L] (laboratory specific) Marbled $	Intracellular enzyme involved in amino acid metabolism. Present in large concentrations in liver, kidney; in smaller amounts, in skeletal muscle and heart. Released with tissue damage, particularly liver injury.	**Increased in:** Acute viral hepatitis (ALT > AST), biliary tract obstruction (cholangitis, choledocholithiasis), alcoholic hepatitis and cirrhosis (AST > ALT), liver abscess, metastatic or primary liver cancer; right heart failure, ischemia or hypoxia, injury to liver ("shock liver"), extensive trauma. Drugs that cause cholestasis or hepatotoxicity. **Decreased in:** Pyridoxine (vitamin B_6) deficiency.	ALT is the preferred enzyme for evaluation of liver injury. Screening ALT in low-risk populations has a low (12%) positive predictive value. Dig Dis Sci 1993;38:2145. Clin Chem 2001;46:2050.

Albumin		
Albumin, serum 3.4–4.7 g/dL [34–47 g/L] Marbled $	Major component of plasma proteins; influenced by nutritional state, hepatic function, renal function, and various diseases. Major binding protein. While there are more than 50 different genetic variants (alloalbumins), only occasionally does a mutation cause abnormal binding (eg, in familial dysalbuminemic hyperthyroxinemia).	**Increased in:** Dehydration, shock, hemoconcentration. **Decreased in:** Decreased hepatic synthesis (chronic liver disease, malnutrition, malabsorption, malignancy, congenital analbuminemia [rare]). Increased losses (nephrotic syndrome, burns, trauma, hemorrhage with fluid replacement, fistulas, enteropathy, acute or chronic glomerulonephritis). Hemodilution (pregnancy, CHF). Drugs: estrogens.	Serum albumin gives an indication of severity in chronic liver disease. Useful in nutritional assessment if there is no impairment in production or increased loss of albumin and is an independent risk factor for all-cause mortality in the elderly (age >70). There is a 10% reduction in serum albumin level in late pregnancy (related to hemodilution). Clin Nutr 2001;20:477. Am Fam Physician 2000;62:308. J Nutr Health and Aging 2000;41:42.

	Aldosterone, plasma		
Test/Range/Collection	Physiologic Basis	Interpretation	Comments
Aldosterone, plasma *Salt-loaded* (120 meq Na⁺/d): Supine: 3–10 Upright: 5–30 ng/dL *Salt-depleted* (10 meq Na⁺/d): Supine: 12–36 Upright: 17–137 ng/dL [1 ng/dL = 27.7 pmol/L] Lavender or green $$$ Early AM fasting speci- men. Separate imme- diately and freeze.	Aldosterone is the major mineralocor- ticoid hormone and is a major regu- lator of extracellular volume and serum potassium concentration. For evaluation of hyperaldosteronism (associated with hypertension and hypokalemia), patients should be salt-loaded and recumbent when specimen is drawn. For evaluation of hypoaldosteronism (associated with hyperkalemia), patients should be salt-depleted and upright when specimen is drawn.	**Increased in:** Primary hyper- aldosteronism (72%). **Decreased in:** Primary or secondary hypoaldosteronism.	Testing for hyperaldosteronism and hypoaldosteronism must be done using specific protocols, and results must be interpreted based on refer- ence values from the laboratory performing the test. 24-hour urinary excretion of aldos- terone is the most sensitive test for hyperaldosteronism. (See Aldosterone, urine, below.) The significance of an elevated plasma aldosterone level is difficult to inter- pret without simultaneous determina- tion of plasma renin activity (PRA). In primary aldosteronism, plasma aldosterone is usually elevated while PRA is low; in secondary hyperaldo- steronism, both plasma aldosterone and PRA are usually elevated. Semin Nephrol 2002;22:44.

Aldosterone, urine		
Aldosterone, urine* *Salt-loaded* (120 meq Na⁺/d for 3–4 days): 1.5–12.5 µg/24 h *Salt-depleted* (20 meq Na⁺/d for 3–4 days): 18–85 µg/24 h [1 µg/24 h = 2.77 nmol/d] Bottle containing boric acid $$$$	Secretion of aldosterone is controlled by the renin-angiotensin system. Renin (synthesized and stored in juxtaglomerular cells of kidney) is released in response to both decreased perfusion pressure at the juxtaglomerular apparatus and negative sodium balance. Renin then hydrolyses angiotensinogen to angiotensin I, which is converted to angiotensin II, which then stimulates the adrenal gland to produce aldosterone.	**Increased in:** Primary and secondary hyperaldosteronism, some patients with essential hypertension. **Decreased in:** Primary hypoaldosteronism (eg, 18-hydroxylase deficiency), secondary hypoaldosteronism (hyporeninemic hypoaldosteronism).	Urinary aldosterone is the most sensitive test for primary hyperaldosteronism. Levels >14 µg/24 h after 3 days of salt-loading have a 96% sensitivity and 93% specificity for primary hyperaldosteronism. Only 7% of patients with essential hypertension have urinary aldosterone levels >14 µg/24 h after salt-loading. Neither serum potassium nor PRA is a satisfactory screening test for hyperaldosteronism. Hypokalemia is present in only 73% of patients with hyperaldosteronism on a normal sodium diet, and in 86% after salt loading. Suppressed PRA has only a 64% sensitivity and 83% specificity for hyperaldosteronism. Endocrinol Metab Clin North Am 1994;23:271. J Clin Hypertens (Greenwich) 2001;3:189.

* To evaluate hyperaldosteronism, patient is salt-loaded and recumbent. Obtain 24-hour urine for aldosterone (and for sodium to check that sodium excretion is >250 meq/day). To evaluate hypoaldosteronism, patient is salt-depleted and upright; check patient for hypotension before 24-hour urine collected.

Test/Range/Collection	Physiologic Basis	Interpretation	Comments
		Alkaline phosphatase	
Alkaline phosphatase, serum 41–133 IU/L [0.7–2.2 μkat/L] (method- and age-dependent) Marbled $	Alkaline phosphatases are found in liver, bone, intestine, and placenta.	**Increased in:** Obstructive hepatobiliary disease, bone disease (physiologic bone growth, Paget disease, osteomalacia, osteogenic sarcoma, bone metastases), hyperparathyroidism, rickets, benign familial hyperphosphatasemia, pregnancy (third trimester), GI disease (perforated ulcer or bowel infarct), hepatotoxic drugs. **Decreased in:** Hypophosphatasia.	Alkaline phosphatase performs well in measuring the extent of bone metastases in prostate cancer. Normal in osteoporosis. Alkaline phosphatase isoenzyme separation by electrophoresis or differential heat inactivation is unreliable. Use γ-glutamyl transpeptidase, which increases in hepatobiliary disease but not in bone disease, to infer origin of increased alkaline phosphatase (ie, liver or bone). Endocrinol Metab Clin North Am 1990;19:1. Int J Urol 1997;4:572. Clin Cornerstone 2001;3:1.
		Amebic serology	
Amebic serology, serum <1:64 titer Marbled $$	Test for presence of *Entamoeba histolytica* by detection of antibodies which develop 2–4 weeks after infection. Tissue invasion by the organism may be necessary for antibody production.	**Increased in:** Current or past infection with *E histolytica*. Amebic abscess (91%), amebic dysentery (84%), asymptomatic cyst carriers (9%), patients with other diseases, and healthy people (2%).	In some endemic areas, as many as 44% of those tested have positive serologies. Precipitin or indirect hemagglutination and recombinant antigen-based ELISA tests are available. Am J Trop Parasitol 1993;87:31. Gastroenterol Clin North Am 2001;30:797.

Ammonia		
Ammonia, plasma (NH_3) 18–60 µg/dL [11–35 µmol/L] Green $$ Separate plasma from cells immediately. Avoid hemolysis. Analyze immediately. Place on ice.	Ammonia is liberated by bacteria in the large intestine or by protein metabolism and is rapidly converted to urea in the liver. In liver disease or portal-systemic shunting, the blood ammonia concentration increases. In acute liver failure, elevation of blood ammonia may cause brain edema; in chronic liver failure, it may be responsible for hepatic encephalopathy.	**Increased in:** Liver failure, hepatic encephalopathy (especially if protein consumption is high or if there is GI bleeding), fulminant hepatic failure, Reye syndrome, portacaval shunting, cirrhosis, urea cycle metabolic defects, urea-splitting urinary tract infection with urinary diversion, and organic acidemias. Drugs: diuretics, acetazolamide, asparaginase, fluorouracil (transient), others. Spuriously increased by any ammonia-containing detergent on laboratory glassware. **Decreased in:** Decreased production by gut bacteria (kanamycin, neomycin). Decreased gut absorption (lactulose).	Correlates poorly with degree of hepatic encephalopathy. Test not useful in adults with known liver disease. Test is not as useful as CSF glutamine (see p 96). Proc Soc Exp Biol Med 1994;206:329. Am J Kidney Dis 2001;37:1069.

Test/Range/Collection	Physiologic Basis	Interpretation	Comments
Amylase, serum 20–110 U/L [0.33–1.83 µkat/L] (laboratory specific) Marbled $	Amylase hydrolyzes complex carbohydrates. Serum amylase is derived primarily from pancreas and salivary glands and is increased with inflammation or obstruction of these glands. Other tissues have some amylase activity, including ovaries, small and large intestine, and skeletal muscle.	**Increased in:** Acute pancreatitis (70–95%), pancreatic pseudocyst, pancreatic duct obstruction (cholecystitis, choledocholithiasis, pancreatic carcinoma, stone, stricture, duct sphincter spasm), bowel obstruction and infarction, mumps, parotitis, diabetic ketoacidosis, penetrating peptic ulcer, peritonitis, ruptured ectopic pregnancy, macroamylasemia. Drugs: azathioprine, hydrochlorothiazide. **Decreased in:** Pancreatic insufficiency, cystic fibrosis. Usually normal or low in chronic pancreatitis.	Macroamylasemia is indicated by high serum but low urine amylase. Serum lipase is an alternative test for acute pancreatitis. Amylase isoenzymes are not of practical use because of technical problems. Pancreas 1998;16:45. J Clin Gastroenterol 2002;34:459.
Angiotensin-converting enzyme, serum (ACE) 12–35 U/L [<590 nkat/L] (method dependent) Marbled $$	ACE is a dipeptidyl carboxypeptidase that converts angiotensin I to the vasopressor, angiotensin II. ACE is normally present in the kidneys and other peripheral tissues. In granulomatous disease, ACE levels increase, derived from epithelioid cells within granulomas.	**Increased in:** Sarcoidosis (sensitivity = 63%, specificity = 93%, LR+ = 9.0) (when upper limit of normal is 50), hyperthyroidism, acute hepatitis, primary biliary cirrhosis, diabetes mellitus, multiple myeloma, osteoarthritis, amyloidosis, Gaucher's disease, pneumoconiosis, histoplasmosis, miliary tuberculosis. Drugs: dexamethasone. **Decreased in:** Renal disease, obstructive pulmonary disease, hypothyroidism.	Test is not useful as a screening test for sarcoidosis (low sensitivity). Specificity is compromised by positive tests in diseases more common than sarcoidosis. Some advocate measurement of ACE to follow disease activity in sarcoidosis. Curr Rheumatol Rep 2000;2:343.

	Antibody screen	Antidiuretic hormone
Antibody screen, serum Red $ Properly identified and labeled blood specimens are critical.	Detects antibodies to non-ABO red blood cell antigens in recipient's serum, using reagent red cells selected to possess antigens against which common antibodies can be produced. Further identification of the specificity of any antibody detected (using panels of red cells of known antigenicity) makes it possible to test donor blood for the absence of the corresponding antigen.	**Positive in:** Presence of alloantibody, autoantibody.	In practice, a type and screen (ABO and Rh grouping and antibody screen) is adequate work-up for patients undergoing operative procedures unlikely to require transfusion. A negative antibody screen implies that a recipient can receive type-specific (ABO-Rh identical) blood with minimal risk. *Technical Manual of the American Association of Blood Banks*, 14th ed. American Association of Blood Banks, 2002.
Antidiuretic hormone, plasma (ADH) If serum osmolality >290 mosm/kg H_2O: 2–12 pg/mL If serum osmolality <290 mosm/kg H_2O: <2 pg/mL Lavender $$$$ Draw in two chilled tubes and deliver to lab on ice. Specimen for serum osmolality must be drawn at same time.	Antidiuretic hormone (vasopressin) is a hormone secreted from the posterior pituitary that acts on the distal nephron to conserve water and regulate the tonicity of body fluids. Water deprivation provides both an osmotic and a volume stimulus for ADH release by increasing plasma osmolality and decreasing plasma volume. Water administration lowers plasma osmolality and expands blood volume, inhibiting the release of ADH by the osmoreceptor and the atrial volume receptor mechanisms.	**Increased in:** Nephrogenic diabetes insipidus, syndrome of inappropriate antidiuretic hormone (SIADH). Drugs: nicotine, morphine, chlorpropamide, clofibrate, cyclophosphamide. **Normal relative to plasma osmolality in:** Primary polydipsia. **Decreased in:** Central (neurogenic) diabetes insipidus. Drugs: ethanol, phenytoin.	Test very rarely indicated. Measurement of serum and urine osmolality usually suffices. Test not indicated in diagnosis of SIADH. Patients with SIADH show decreased plasma sodium and decreased plasma osmolality relative to plasma. These findings in a normovolemic patient with normal thyroid and adrenal function are sufficient to make the diagnosis of SIADH without measuring ADH itself. Semin Nephrol 1994;14:368. Crit Care Clin 2001;17:11. Am J Ther 2000;7:23.

Test/Range/Collection	Physiologic Basis	Interpretation	Comments
Antiglobulin test, direct, red cells (Direct Coombs, DAT) Negative Lavender or red $ Blood anticoagulated with EDTA is used to prevent in vitro uptake of complement components. A red top tube may be used, if necessary.	Direct antiglobulin test demonstrates in vivo coating of washed red cells with globulins, in particular IgG and C3d. Washed red cells are tested directly with antihuman globulin reagent. DAT is positive (shows agglutination) immediately when IgG coats red cells. Complement or IgA coating may only be demonstrated after incubation at room temperature.	**Positive in:** Autoimmune hemolytic anemia, hemolytic disease of the newborn, alloimmune reactions to recently transfused cells, and drug-induced hemolysis. Drugs: cephalosporins, levodopa, methadone, methyldopa, penicillin, phenacetin, quinidine.	A positive DAT implies in vivo red cell coating by immunoglobulins or complement. Such red cell coating may or may not be associated with immune hemolytic anemia. Poly-specific and anti-IgG reagents detect approximately 500 molecules of IgG per red cell, but autoimmune hemolytic anemia has been reported with IgG coating below this level. 10% of hospital patients have a positive DAT without clinical manifestations of immune-mediated hemolysis. A false-positive DAT is often seen in patients with hypergammaglobulinemia, eg, in some HIV-positive patients. *Technical Manual of the American Association of Blood Banks*, 14th ed. American Association of Blood Banks, 2002.
Antiglobulin test, indirect, serum (Indirect Coombs) Negative Red $	Demonstrates presence in patient's serum of unexpected antibody to ABO and Rh-compatible red blood cells. First, the patient's serum is incubated in vitro with reagent red cells and washed to remove unbound globulins. Then antihuman globulin (AHG, Coombs) reagent is added. Agglutination of red cells indicates that serum contains antibodies to antigens present on the reagent red cells.	**Positive in:** Presence of alloantibody or autoantibody. Drugs: methyldopa.	The technique is used in antibody detection and identification and in the major cross-match prior to transfusion (see Type and Cross-Match, p 178). *Technical Manual of the American Association of Blood Banks*, 14th ed. American Association of Blood Banks, 2002.

	α_1-Antiprotease	Antistreptolysin O titer
α_1-Antiprotease (α_1-antitrypsin), serum 110–270 mg/dL [1.1–2.7 g/L] Marbled $$	α_1-Antiprotease is an α_1 globulin glycoprotein serine protease inhibitor (Pi) whose deficiency leads to excessive protease activity and panacinar emphysema in adults or liver disease in children (seen as ZZ and SZ phenotypes). Cirrhosis of the liver and liver cancer in adults are also associated with the Pi Z phenotype.	**Increased in:** Inflammation, infection, rheumatic disease, malignancy, and pregnancy because it is an acute phase reactant. **Decreased in:** Congenital α_1-antiprotease deficiency, nephrotic syndrome.	Smoking is a much more common cause of chronic obstructive pulmonary disease in adults than is α_1-antiprotease deficiency. Curr Opin Pulm Med 1996;2:155. Am J Med Sci 2001;321:33.
Antistreptolysin O titer, serum (ASO) Children <5 years: <85; 5–19 years: <170 Adults: <85 Todd units (laboratory-specific) Marbled $$	Detects the presence of antibody to the antigen streptolysin O produced by group A streptococci. Streptococcal antibodies appear about 2 weeks after infection. Titer rises to a peak at 4–6 weeks and may remain elevated for 6 months to 1 year. Test is based on the neutralization of hemolytic activity of streptolysin O toxin by antistreptolysin O antibodies in serum.	**Increased in:** Recent infection with group A β-hemolytic streptococci: scarlet fever, erysipelas, streptococcal pharyngitis/tonsillitis (40–50%), rheumatic fever (80–85%), poststreptococcal glomerulonephritis. Some collagen-vascular diseases. Certain serum lipoproteins, bacterial growth products, or oxidized streptolysin O may result in inhibition of hemolysis and thus cause false-positive results.	Standardization of (Todd) units may vary significantly from laboratory to laboratory. ASO titers are not useful in management of acute streptococcal pharyngitis. In patients with rheumatic fever, test may be a more reliable indicator of recent streptococcal infection than throat culture. An increasing titer is more suggestive of acute streptococcal infection than a single elevated level. Even with severe infection, ASO titers will rise in only 70–80% of patients. N Engl J Med 1970;282:23.78. J Clin Epidemiol 1993;46:1181.

Test/Range/Collection	Physiologic Basis	Interpretation	Comments		
				Antithrombin III	**Aspartate aminotransferase**
Antithrombin III (AT III), plasma 84–123% (qualitative) 22–39 mg/dL (quantitative) Blue $$ $$ Transport to lab on ice. Plasma must be separated and frozen in a polypropylene tube within 2 hours.	Antithrombin III is a serine protease inhibitor that protects against thrombus formation by inhibiting thrombin and factors IXa, Xa, XIa, XIIa, plasmin, and kallikrein. It accounts for 70–90% of the anticoagulant activity of human plasma. Its activity is enhanced 100-fold by heparin. There are two types of assay: functional (qualitative) and immunologic (quantitative). Since the immunologic assay cannot rule out functional AT III deficiency, a functional assay should be ordered first. Functional assays test AT III activity in inhibiting thrombin or factor Xa. Given an abnormal functional assay, the quantitative immunologic test indicates whether there is decreased synthesis of AT III or intact synthesis of a dysfunctional protein.	**Increased by:** Oral anticoagulants. **Decreased in:** Congenital and acquired AT III deficiency (renal disease, chronic liver disease), oral contraceptive use, chronic disseminated intravascular coagulation, acute venous thrombosis (consumption), and heparin therapy.	Congenital and acquired AT III deficiency results in a hypercoagulable state, venous thromboembolism, and heparin resistance. Congenital AT III deficiency is present in 1:2000–1:5000 people and is autosomal codominant. Heterozygotes have AT III levels 20–60% of normal. Thromb Haemost 1993;69:231. Emerg Med Clin North Am 2001;19:839.		
Aspartate aminotransferase, serum (AST, SGOT, GOT) 0–35 IU/L [0–0.58 μkat/L] (laboratory-specific) Marbled $	Intracellular enzyme involved in amino acid metabolism. Present in large concentrations in liver, skeletal muscle, brain, red cells, and heart. Released into the bloodstream when tissue is damaged, especially in liver injury.	**Increased in:** Acute viral hepatitis (ALT > AST), biliary tract obstruction (cholangitis, choledocholithiasis), alcoholic hepatitis and cirrhosis (AST > ALT), liver abscess, metastatic or primary liver cancer; right heart failure, ischemia or hypoxia, injury to liver ("shock liver"), extensive trauma. Drugs that cause cholestasis or hepatotoxicity. **Decreased in:** Pyridoxine (vitamin B_6) deficiency.	Test is not indicated for diagnosis of myocardial infarction. AST/ALT ratio > 1 suggests cirrhosis in patients with hepatitis C. Am J Gastroenterol 1998;93:44. Ann Clin Biochem 2001;38:652.		

	B cell immunoglobulin heavy chain gene rearrangement	*bcr/abl* translocation
B cell immunoglobulin heavy chain gene rearrangement Whole blood, bone marrow, or frozen tissue Lavender $$$$	In general, the percentage of B lymphocytes with identical immunoglobulin heavy chain gene rearrangements is very low; in malignancies, however, the clonal expansion of one population leads to a large number of cells with identical B cell immunoglobulin heavy chain gene rearrangements. Southern blot is used to identify a monoclonal population.	**Positive in:** B cell neoplasms such as lymphoma.
	Samples with >10% of cells showing a given B cell rearrangement are considered positive. However, a large monoclonal population is consistent with—but not diagnostic of—malignancy. Arch Pathol Lab Med 1988;112:117.	
bcr/abl translocation Blood Lavender $$$$	Approximately 95% of chronic myelogenous leukemia (CML) is associated with the "Philadelphia chromosome," a translocation that moves the *c-abl* proto-oncogene from chromosome 9 to the breakpoint cluster (*bcr*) region of chromosome 22. Southern blot is used to identify the translocation.	**Positive in:** Chronic myelogenous leukemia (sensitivity 95%) and acute lymphocytic leukemia (sensitivity 10–15%).
	This assay will detect the 9;22 translocation if it has taken place in >10% of the cells. CML patients with bone marrow transplants can be monitored for recurrence of disease with this test. N Engl J Med 1988;319:990. Best Pract Res Clin Hematol 2001;14:553. Leuk Res 2002;26:713. Acta Hematol 2002;107:57.	

Test/Range/Collection	Physiologic Basis	Interpretation	Comments
Bilirubin, serum 0.1–1.2 mg/dL [2–21 μmol/L] Direct (conjugated to glucuronide) bilirubin: 0.1–0.4 mg/dL [<7 μmol/L]; Indirect (unconjugated) bilirubin: 0.2–0.7 mg/dL [<12 μmol/L] Marbled $$	Bilirubin, a product of hemoglobin metabolism, is conjugated in the liver to mono- and diglucuronides and excreted in bile. Some conjugated bilirubin is bound to serum albumin, so-called D (delta) bilirubin. Elevated serum bilirubin occurs in liver disease, biliary obstruction, or hemolysis.	**Increased in:** Acute or chronic hepatitis, cirrhosis, biliary tract obstruction, toxic hepatitis, neonatal jaundice, congenital liver enzyme abnormalities (Dubin-Johnson, Rotor, Gilbert, Crigler-Najjar syndromes), fasting, hemolytic disorders. Hepatotoxic drugs.	Assay of total bilirubin includes conjugated (direct) and unconjugated (indirect) bilirubin plus delta bilirubin (conjugated bilirubin bound to albumin). It is usually clinically unnecessary to fractionate total bilirubin. The fractionation is unreliable by the diazo reaction and may underestimate unconjugated bilirubin. Only conjugated bilirubin appears in the urine, and it is indicative of liver disease; hemolysis is associated with increased unconjugated bilirubin. Persistence of delta bilirubin in serum in resolving liver disease means that total bilirubin does not effectively indicate the time course of resolution. Pediatrics 1992;89:80. Br J Hosp Med 1994;51:181. Pediatr Rev 1994;15:233. Clin Cornerstone 2001;3:1.

Bleeding time		
Bleeding time 2–10 minutes $$ Test done by laboratory personnel. Simplate (presterilized device with spring-loaded blade) is used to make single cut 1 mm deep and 6 mm long on dorsal aspect of forearm after inflation of sphygmomanometer to 40 mm Hg. Filter paper is used to absorb blood from wound margins every 30 seconds, and time to cessation of bleeding is noted.	This is a test of platelet function, not a test of coagulation factors.	**Increased in:** Platelet disorders, thrombocytopenia, Bernard-Soulier syndrome, thrombasthenia. Also elevated in some forms of von Willebrand disease, which is a disorder of factor VIII coagulant activity and not primarily a platelet disorder. Drugs: aspirin and other preparations containing aspirin.	Test is useful as a screening test (with aspirin challenge) for diagnosis of von Willebrand's disease and platelet disorders. Test adds no clinically useful information to the prediction of clinically significant bleeding beyond that obtained from the history, physical examination, and other laboratory tests—platelet count, blood urea nitrogen (BUN), prothrombin time (PT), and partial thromboplastin time (PTT). In patients with no history of bleeding and no intake of nonsteroidal anti-inflammatory drugs, an increased bleeding time does not correlate with actual surgical bleeding. Semin Thromb Hemost 1990;16:1. Blood 1994;84:3363. Med Clin North Am 1994;78:577. Mayo Clinic Proc 2002;77:181.

Test/Range/Collection	Physiologic Basis	Interpretation	Comments
Blood urea nitrogen, serum (BUN) 8–20 mg/dL [2.9–7.1 mmol/L] Marbled $	Urea, an end product of protein metabolism, is excreted by the kidney. BUN is directly related to protein intake and nitrogen metabolism and inversely related to the rate of excretion of urea. Urea concentration in glomerular filtrate is the same as in plasma, but its tubular reabsorption is inversely related to the rate of urine formation. Thus, the BUN is a less useful measure of glomerular filtration rate than the serum creatinine (Cr).	**Increased in:** Renal failure (acute or chronic), urinary tract obstruction, dehydration, shock, burns, CHF, GI bleeding. Nephrotoxic drugs (eg, gentamicin). **Decreased in:** Hepatic failure, nephrotic syndrome, cachexia (low-protein and high-carbohydrate diets).	Urease assay method commonly used. BUN/Cr ratio (normally 12:1–20:1) is decreased in acute tubular necrosis, advanced liver disease, low protein intake, and following hemodialysis. BUN/Cr ratio is increased in dehydration, GI bleeding, and increased catabolism. Ann Emerg Med 1992;21:713. Nursing 1994;24:88. Cleve Clin J Med 2002;69:569.
β-Natriuretic peptide (BNP), blood <50 pg/mL Lavender $$	BNP is released from the heart in response to increased wall tension and has natriuretic/diuretic effects.	**Increased in:** CHF (BNP levels >100 pg/ml sensitivity of 90%, specificity of 73%, BNP 1 <50 pg/ml has negative predictive value of 96%).	BNP testing is not a substitute for careful cardiopulmonary evaluation and should not be the sole criterion for admission/discharge of a patient. Although normal levels indicate a low probability of CHF, they do not exclude it or other serious cardiopulmonary disorders. Increased levels are not specific for CHF and can occur with pulmonary embolism, pulmonary hypertension and acute myocardial infarction. BNP is not recommended for screening for left ventricular dysfunction or hypertrophy in the general population. Treatment of CHF has been reported to decrease BNP levels in parallel with improving clinical symptoms.

ß-Natriuretic peptide	*Brucella* antibody	C-reactive protein
In patients with acute coronary syndromes, increased BNP levels are associated with increased risk of death during the subsequent 10 months and with increased risk of myocardial infarction. NEJM 2001; 345:1014. NEJM 2002; 347:161. Circulation 2002; 106:416. JAMA 2002; 288:1252.	This test will detect antibodies against all of the *Brucella* species except *B canis*. A fourfold or greater rise in titer in separate specimens drawn 1–4 weeks apart is indicative of recent exposure. Final diagnosis depends on isolation of organism by culture. J Infect Dis 1989;159:219. Rev Infect Dis 1991;13:359.	Elevated C-reactive protein level appears to be an independent risk factor for coronary heart disease events. High levels appear to be predictive of progression of rheumatoid arthritis. Ann Intern Med 1999;130:933. Clin Chem Lab Med 2001;39:907. Rheumatology (Oxford) 2003;39(Suppl 1):24.
	Increased in: *Brucella* infection (except *B canis*) (97% within 3 weeks of illness); recent brucellergin skin test; infections with *Francisella tularensis*, *Yersinia enterocolitica*, salmonella. Rocky Mountain spotted fever; vaccinations for cholera and tularemia. **Normal in:** *B canis* infection.	**Increased in:** Inflammatory states.
	Patients with acute brucellosis generally develop an agglutinating antibody titer of ≥ 1 : 160 within 3 weeks. The titer may rise during the acute infection, with relapses, brucellergin skin testing, or use of certain vaccines (see Interpretation). The agglutinin titer usually declines after 3 months or after successful therapy. Low titers may persist for years.	Marker of inflammation.
	Brucella antibody, serum <1 : 80 titer Marbled $	**C-reactive protein,** serum 0–2 mg/dL Marbled $

	C1 esterase inhibitor		
Test/Range/Collection	Physiologic Basis	Interpretation	Comments
C1 esterase inhibitor (C1 INH), serum Method-dependent Marbled $$	C1 esterase inhibitor (C1 INH) is an alpha-globulin, which controls the first stage of the classic complement pathway and inhibits thrombin, plasmin, and kallikrein. Deficiency results in spontaneous activation of C1, leading to consumption of C2 and C4. The functional assay involves the measurement of C1 INH as it inhibits the hydrolysis of a substrate ester by C1 esterase. Immunoassay of C1 INH is also available.	**Decreased in:** Hereditary angioedema (HAE) (85%) (15% of patients with HAE will have normal levels by immunoassay, but the protein is nonfunctional and levels determined by the functional assay will be low).	C1 esterase inhibitor deficiency is an uncommon cause of angioedema. There are two subtypes of hereditary angioedema. In one, the protein is absent; in the other, it is nonfunctional. Acquired angioedema has been attributed to massive consumption of C1 INH (presumably by tumor or lymphoma-related immune complexes) or to anti-C1 INH autoantibody. When clinical suspicion exists, a serum C4 level screens for HAE. Low levels of C4 are present in all cases during an attack. C1 esterase inhibitor levels are not indicated unless either the C4 level is low or there is a very high clinical suspicion of HAE in a patient with normal C4 during an asymptomatic phase between attacks. In acquired C1 INH deficiency, the C1 level is also significantly decreased (often 10% of normal), whereas in HAE the C1 level is normal or only slightly decreased. Med Clin North Am 2000;76:805. Am Intern Med 2000;132:144. J Clin Pathol 2002;55:266.

	C-peptide		**Calcitonin**
C-peptide, serum 0.8–4.0 ng/mL [μg/L] Marbled $$$ Fasting sample preferred.	C-peptide is an inactive by-product of the cleavage of proinsulin to active insulin. Its presence indicates endogenous release of insulin. C-peptide is largely excreted by the kidney.	**Increased in:** Renal failure, ingestion of oral hypoglycemic drugs, insulinomas, B cell transplants. **Decreased in:** Factitious hypoglycemia due to insulin administration, pancreatectomy, type I diabetes mellitus (decreased or undetectable).	Test is most useful to detect factitious insulin injection (increased insulin, decreased C-peptide) or to detect endogenous insulin production in diabetic patients receiving insulin (C-peptide present). A molar ratio of insulin to C-peptide in peripheral venous blood >1.0 in a hypoglycemic patient is consistent with surreptitious or inadvertent insulin administration but not insulinoma. Am J Med 1989;86:335. Arch Intern Med 1993;153:650. Am J Physiol Endocrinol Metab 2002;278:E759.
Calcitonin, plasma Male: <90 pg/mL [ng/L] Female: <70 pg/mL [ng/L] Green $$$ Fasting sample required. Place on ice.	Calcitonin is a 32-amino-acid polypeptide hormone secreted by the parafollicular C cells of the thyroid. It decreases osteoclastic bone resorption and lowers serum calcium levels.	**Increased in:** Medullary thyroid carcinoma (>500 pg/mL on two occasions), Zollinger-Ellison syndrome, pernicious anemia, pregnancy (at term), newborns, carcinoma (breast, lung, pancreas), chronic renal failure.	Test is useful to diagnose and monitor medullary thyroid carcinoma, although stimulation tests may be necessary (eg, pentagastrin test). Genetic testing is now available for the diagnosis of multiple endocrine neoplasia type II. (MEN II is the most common familial form of medullary thyroid carcinoma.) Ann Intern Med 1995;122:118. Curr Treat Options Oncol 2000;1:359.

Test/Range/Collection	Physiologic Basis	Interpretation	Comments
Calcium, serum (Ca^{2+}) 8.5–10.5 mg/dL [2.1–2.6 mmol/L] **Panic:** <6.5 or >13.5 mg/dL Marbled $ Prolonged venous sta- sis during collection causes false increase in serum calcium.	Serum calcium is the sum of ionized calcium plus complexed calcium and calcium bound to proteins (mostly albumin). Level of ionized calcium is regulated by parathyroid hormone and vitamin D.	**Increased in:** Hyperparathyroidism, malignancies secreting parathyroid hormone–related protein (PTHrP) (especially squamous cell carcinoma of lung and renal cell carcinoma), vitamin D excess, milk-alkali syndrome, multiple myeloma, Paget disease of bone with immobilization, sarcoidosis, other granulomatous disorders, familial hypocalciuria, vitamin A intoxication, thyrotoxicosis, Addison disease. Drugs: antacids (some), calcium salts, chronic diuretic use (eg, thiazides), lithium, others. **Decreased in:** Hypoparathyroidism, vitamin D deficiency, renal insufficiency, pseudohypoparathyroidism, magnesium deficiency, hyperphosphatemia, massive transfusion, hypoalbuminemia.	Need to know serum albumin to interpret calcium level. For every decrease in albumin by 1 mg/dL, calcium should be corrected upward by 0.8 mg/dL. In 10% of patients with malignancies, hypercalcemia is attributable to coexistent hyperparathyroidism, suggesting that serum PTH levels should be measured at initial presentation of all hypercalcemic patients (see pp 139 and 416). J Am Soc Nephrol 2001; 12(Suppl 17):53. Rev Endocr Metab Disord 200;1:247. Curr Treat Options Oncol 2001;2:365.

| | | | **Calcium, serum** |

Calcium, ionized		
Calcium, ionized, serum 4.4–5.4 mg/dL (at pH 7.4) [1.1–1.3 mmol/L] Whole blood specimen must be collected anaerobically and anticoagulated with standardized amounts of heparin. Tourniquet application must be brief. Specimen should be analyzed promptly. Marbled $$	Calcium circulates in three forms: as free Ca^{2+} (47%), protein-bound to albumin and globulins (43%), and as calcium–ligand complexes (10%) (with citrate, bicarbonate, lactate, phosphate, and sulfate). Protein binding is highly pH-dependent, and acidosis results in an increased free calcium fraction. Ionized Ca^{2+} is the form that is physiologically active. Ionized calcium is a more accurate reflection of physiologic status than total calcium in patients with altered serum proteins (renal failure, nephrotic syndrome, multiple myeloma, etc), altered concentrations of calcium-binding ligands, and acid–base disturbances. Measurement of ionized calcium is by ion-selective electrodes.	**Increased in:** ↓ blood pH. **Decreased in:** ↑ blood pH, citrate, heparin, EDTA.	Ionized calcium measurements are not needed except in special circumstances, eg, massive blood transfusion, liver transplantation, neonatal hypocalcemia, and cardiac surgery. Validity of test depends on sample integrity. Ann Clin Lab Sci 1991;21:297.

Test/Range/Collection	Physiologic Basis	Interpretation	Comments
Calcium, urine (U_{Ca}) 100–300 mg/24 h [2.5–7.5 mmol/24 h or 2.3–3.3 mmol/12 h] Urine bottle containing hydrochloric acid $$$ Collect 24-hour urine or 12-hour overnight urine.	Ordinarily there is moderate urinary calcium excretion, the amount depending on dietary calcium, parathyroid hormone (PTH) level, and protein intake. Renal calculi occur much more often in hyperparathyroidism than in other hypercalcemic states.	**Increased in:** Hyperparathyroidism, osteolytic bone metastases, myeloma, osteoporosis, vitamin D intoxication, distal RTA, idiopathic hypercalciuria, thyrotoxicosis, Paget disease, Fanconi syndrome, hepatolenticular degeneration, schistosomiasis, sarcoidosis, malignancy (breast, bladder), osteitis deformans, immobilization. Drugs: acetazolamide, calcium salts, cholestyramine, corticosteroids, dihydrotachysterol, initial diuretic use (eg, furosemide), others. **Decreased in:** Hypoparathyroidism, pseudohypoparathyroidism, rickets, osteomalacia, nephrotic syndrome, acute glomerulonephritis, osteoblastic bone metastases, hypothyroidism, celiac disease, steatorrhea, hypocalciuric hypercalcemia, other causes of hypocalcemia. Drugs: aspirin, bicarbonate, chronic diuretic use (eg, thiazides, chlorthalidone), estrogens, indomethacin, lithium, neomycin, oral contraceptives.	Approximately one-third of patients with hyperparathyroidism have normal urine calcium excretion. The extent of calcium excretion can be expressed as a urine calcium (U_{Ca})/urine creatinine (U_{Cr}) ratio. Normally, $$\frac{U_{Ca}(mg/dL)}{U_{Cr}(mg/dL)} < 0.14$$ and $$\frac{U_{Ca}(mmol/L)}{U_{Cr}(mmol/L)} < 0.40$$ respectively. Hypercalciuria is defined as a ratio >0.20 or >0.57, respectively. Test is useful in the evaluation of renal stones but is not usually needed for the diagnosis of hyperparathyroidism, which can be made using serum calcium (see above) and PTH measurements (see pp 139 and 416). It may be useful in hypercalcemic patients to rule out familial hypocalciuric hypercalcemia. In the diagnosis of hypercalciuria, U_{Ca}/U_{Cr} ratios in random single-voided urine specimens correlate well with 24-hour calcium excretions. Endocrinol Metab Clin North Am 2000;29:503. Lancet 2001;358:651.

	Carbon dioxide		Carboxyhemoglobin
Carbon dioxide (CO_2), total (bicarbonate) serum 22–28 meq/L [mmol/L] **Panic:** <15 or >40 meq/L [mmo/L] Marbled $ Do not leave exposed to air because this will cause falsely low CO_2 levels.	Bicarbonate–carbonic acid buffer is one of the most important buffer systems in maintaining normal body fluid pH. Total CO_2 is measured as the sum of bicarbonate concentration plus carbonic acid concentration plus dissolved CO_2. Because bicarbonate makes up 90–95% of the total CO_2 content, total CO_2 is a useful surrogate for bicarbonate concentration.	**Increased in:** Primary metabolic alkalosis, compensated respiratory acidosis, volume contraction, mineralocorticoid excess, congenital chloridorrhea. Drugs: diuretics (eg, thiazide, furosemide). **Decreased in:** Metabolic acidosis, compensated respiratory alkalosis. Fanconi's syndrome, volume overload. Drugs: acetazolamide, outdated tetracycline.	Total CO_2 determination is indicated for all seriously ill patients on admission. If arterial blood gas studies are done, total CO_2 test is redundant. Simultaneous measurement of pH and Pco_2 is required to fully characterize a patient's acid–base status. Postgrad Med 2000;107(3):249, 253, 257. Respir Care 2001;46:366. Respir Care 2001;46:342.
Carboxyhemoglobin, whole blood (HbCO) <9% [<0.09] Lavender $$ Do not remove stopper.	Carbon monoxide (CO) combines irreversibly with hemoglobin at the sites that normally bind oxygen. This produces a decrease in oxygen saturation and a shift in the oxyhemoglobin dissociation curve, resulting in decreased release of oxygen to the tissues.	**Increased in:** Carbon monoxide poisoning. Exposure to automobile exhaust or smoke from fires. Cigarette smokers can have up to 9% carboxyhemoglobin, nonsmokers have <2%.	Test (if available within minutes, together with O_2 saturation by oximeter) is useful in evaluation of CO poisoning. Po_2 is usually normal in CO poisoning. Test measures carboxyhemoglobin spectrophotometrically. Toxicology 2001;145:1

	Carcinoembryonic antigen		
Test/Range/Collection	**Physiologic Basis**	**Interpretation**	**Comments**
Carcinoembryonic antigen, serum (CEA) 0–2.5 ng/mL [μg/L] Marbled $$	CEA is an oncofetal antigen, a glyco-protein associated with certain malignancies, particularly epithelial tumors.	**Increased in:** Colon cancer (72%), lung cancer (76%), pancreatic cancer (91%) stomach cancer (61%), cigarette smokers, benign liver disease (acute 50% and chronic 90%), benign GI disease (peptic ulcer, pancreatitis, colitis). Elevations >20 ng/mL are generally associated with malignancy. For breast cancer recurrence (using 5 ng/mL cutoff), sensitivity = 44.4% and specificity = 95.5%.	**Screening:** Test is not sensitive or specific enough to be useful in cancer screening. **Monitoring after surgery:** Test is used to follow progression of colon cancer after surgery (elevated CEA levels suggest recurrence 3–6 months before other clinical indicators), although such monitoring has not yet been shown to improve survival rates. If monitoring is done, the same assay method must be used consistently in order to eliminate any method-dependent variability. Br Cancer Treat 1995;37:209. Dig Surg 2000;17:209. Clin Chem 2001;47:624.

	CD4

| CD4 cell count, absolute, whole blood | Lymphocyte identification depends on specific cell surface antigens (clusters of differentiation, CD), which can be detected with monoclonal antibodies using flow cytometry. CD4 cells are predominantly helper-inducer cells of the immunologic system. They react with peptide class II major histocompatibility complex antigens and augment B cell responses and T cell lymphokine secretion. CD4 cells are the major target of HIV-1. | **Increased in:** Rheumatoid arthritis, type I diabetes mellitus, SLE without renal disease, primary biliary cirrhosis, atopic dermatitis, Sézary syndrome, psoriasis, chronic autoimmune hepatitis.
Decreased in: AIDS/HIV infection, SLE with renal disease, acute CMV infection, burns, graft-versus-host disease, sunburn, myelodysplasia syndromes, acute lymphocytic leukemia in remission, recovery from bone marrow transplantation, herpes infection, infectious mononucleosis, measles, ataxia-telangiectasia, vigorous exercise. | Progressive decline in the number and function of CD4 lymphocytes seems to be the most characteristic immunologic defect in AIDS. Absolute CD4 measurement is particularly useful (more useful than the CD4/CD8 ratio) in determining eligibility for antiretroviral therapy (usually when CD4 < 500 cells/µL) and in monitoring the progress of the disease.
Most AIDS-defining infections occur when the CD4 count drops below 200 cells/µL.
Absolute CD4 count depends, analytically, on the reliability of the white blood cell differential count, as well as on the percentage of CD4 cells identified using the appropriate monoclonal antibody.
HIV Med 2001;2:146.
Ann Intern Med 2001;134:761.
Clin Lab Med 2001;21:841. |
| CD4: 359–1725 cells/µL (29–61%)

Lavender
$$$
For an absolute CD4 count, order a CBC and differential also. | | | |

Test/Range/Collection	Physiologic Basis	Interpretation	Comments
Centromere antibody, serum (ACA) Negative Marbled $$	Anticentromere antibodies are antibodies to nuclear proteins of the kinetochore plate.	**Positive in:** CREST (70–90%), scleroderma (10–15%), Raynaud disease (10–30%).	In patients with connective tissue disease, the predictive value of a positive test is >95% for scleroderma or related disease (CREST, Raynaud disease). Diagnosis of CREST is made clinically (calcinosis, Raynaud disease, esophageal dysmotility, sclerodactyly, and telangiectasia). In the absence of clinical findings, the test has low predictive value. (See also Autoantibodies table, p 366) Clin Rheumatol 1994;13:427. Ann Rheum Dis 1995;54:148. Ann Rheum Dis 2002;61:121.
Ceruloplasmin, serum 20–35 mg/dL [200–350 mg/L] Marbled $$	Ceruloplasmin, a 120,000–160,000 MW α_2-glycoprotein synthesized by the liver, is the main (95%) copper-carrying protein in human serum.	**Increased in:** Acute and chronic inflammation, pregnancy. Drugs: oral contraceptives, phenytoin. **Decreased in:** Wilson disease (hepatolenticular degeneration) (95%), liver disease other than Wilson (15%), liver disease other than Wilson (23%), malabsorption, malnutrition, primary biliary cirrhosis, nephrotic syndrome, severe copper deficiency, Menkes disease (X-linked inherited copper deficiency).	Slitlamp examination for Kayser-Fleischer rings and serum ceruloplasmin level recommended for diagnosis of Wilson disease. Serum copper level is very rarely indicated. Screening all patients with liver disease is ineffective. 5% of patients with Wilson disease have low-normal levels of ceruloplasmin. J Hepatol 1997;27:358. Semin Liver Dis 2000;20:353.

	Chloride	
Chloride, serum (Cl⁻) 98–107 meq/L [mmol/L] Marbled $	Chloride, the principal inorganic anion of extracellular fluid, is important in maintaining normal acid–base balance and normal osmolality. If chloride is lost (as HCl or NH₄Cl), alkalosis ensues; if chloride is ingested or retained, acidosis ensues.	**Increased in:** Renal failure, nephrotic syndrome, renal tubular acidosis, dehydration, overtreatment with saline, hyperparathyroidism, diabetes insipidus, metabolic acidosis from diarrhea (loss of HCO₃), respiratory alkalosis, hyperadrenocorticism. Drugs: acetazolamide (hyperchloremic acidosis), androgens, hydrochlorothiazide, salicylates (intoxication). **Decreased in:** Vomiting, diarrhea, gastrointestinal suction, renal failure combined with salt deprivation, overtreatment with diuretics, chronic respiratory acidosis, diabetic ketoacidosis, excessive sweating, SIADH, salt-losing nephropathy, acute intermittent porphyria, water intoxication, expansion of extracellular fluid volume, adrenal insufficiency, hyperaldosteronism, metabolic alkalosis. Drugs: chronic laxative or bicarbonate ingestion, corticosteroids, diuretics.	Test is helpful in assessing normal and increased anion gap metabolic acidosis and in distinguishing hypercalcemia due to primary hyperparathyroidism (high serum chloride) from that due to malignancy (normal serum chloride). Crit Care Med 1992;20:227. Am J Med Sci 2000;319:10.

	Cholesterol		
Test/Range/Collection	**Physiologic Basis**	**Interpretation**	**Comments**
Cholesterol, serum

Desirable: <200 mg/dL [<5.2 mmol/L]
Borderline: 200–239 mg/dL [5.2–6.1 mmol/L]
High risk: >240 mg/dL [>6.2 mmol/L]

Marbled
$

Fasting preferred for LDL cholesterol.
HDL and total cholesterol can be measured nonfasting. | Cholesterol level is determined by lipid metabolism, which is in turn influenced by heredity, diet, and other liver, kidney, thyroid, and endocrine organ functions.
Total cholesterol (TC) = low density lipoprotein (LDL) cholesterol + high density lipoprotein (HDL) cholesterol + (triglycerides [TG] / 5) (valid only if TG < 400).
Because LDL cholesterol is the clinically important entity, it is calculated as

$$LDL = TC - HDL - \frac{TG}{5}$$

This calculation is valid only if specimen is obtained fasting (to obtain relevant triglyceride level). | **Increased in:** Primary disorders: polygenic hypercholesterolemia, familial hypercholesterolemia (deficiency of LDL receptors), familial combined hyperlipidemia, familial dysbetalipoproteinemia. Secondary disorders: hypothyroidism, uncontrolled diabetes mellitus, nephrotic syndrome, biliary obstruction, anorexia nervosa, hepatoma, Cushing's syndrome, acute intermittent porphyria. Drugs: corticosteroids.
Decreased in: Severe liver disease (acute hepatitis, cirrhosis, malignancy), hyperthyroidism, severe acute or chronic illness, malnutrition, malabsorption (eg, HIV), extensive burns, familial (Gaucher disease, Tangier disease), abetalipoproteinemia, intestinal lymphangiectasia. | It is important to treat the cause of secondary hypercholesterolemia (eg, hypothyroidism). Need to check total cholesterol and HDL cholesterol because cardiovascular risk may be increased with relatively modest total cholesterol elevation if HDL cholesterol is low.
National Cholesterol Education Program Expert Panel has published clinical recommendations for cholesterol management (see JAMA 1993 reference).
JAMA 1993;260:3015.
Geriatrics 2000;55:48.
Prev Cardiol 2002;5:131.
Circulation 2002;105:886.
Clin Chim Acta 2002;315:49. |

Chorionic gonadotropin, β-subunit, quantitative		
Chorionic gonadotropin, β-subunit, quantitative, serum (β-hCG) Males and nonpregnant females: undetectable or <2 mIU/mL [IU/L] Marbled $$	Human chorionic gonadotropin is a glycoprotein made up of two sub-units (α and β). Human glycoproteins such as LH, FSH, and TSH share the α subunit of hCG, but the β subunit is specific for hCG. hCG is produced by trophoblastic tissue, and its detection in serum or urine is the basis for pregnancy testing. Serum hCG can be detected as early as 24 hours after implantation at a concentration of 5 mIU/mL. During normal pregnancy, serum levels double every 2–3 days and are 50–100 mIU/mL at the time of the first missed menstrual period. Peak levels are reached 60–80 days after the last menstrual period (LMP) (30,000–100,000 mIU/mL), and levels then decrease to a plateau of 5,000–10,000 mIU/mL at about 120 days after LMP and persist until delivery.	**Increased in:** Pregnancy (including ectopic pregnancy), hyperemesis gravi-darum, trophoblastic tumors (hydatidi-form mole, choriocarcinoma of uterus), some germ cell tumors (teratomas of ovary or testicle, seminoma), ectopic hCG production by other malignancies (stomach, pancreas, lung, colon, liver). Failure of elevated serum levels to decrease after surgical resection of trophoblastic tumor indicates metasta-tic tumor; levels rising from normal indicate tumor recurrence. **Decreasing over time:** Threatened abortion.	Routine pregnancy testing is done by *qualitative* serum or urine hCG test. Test will be positive (>50 mIU/mL) in most pregnant women at the time of or shortly after the first missed menstrual period. *Quantitative* hCG testing is indicated for (1) the evaluation of suspected ectopic pregnancy (where levels are lower than in normal pregnancy at the same gestational age) if the routine pregnancy test is negative; and (2) the evaluation of threatened abortion. In both situations, hCG levels fail to demonstrate the normal early preg-nancy increase. Test is also indicated for following the course of trophoblastic and germ cell tumors. Urology 1994;44:392. Am Fam Physician 2000;61:1080. J Reprod Med 2000;45:692.

Test/Range/Collection	Physiologic Basis	Interpretation	Comments
		Clostridium difficile enterotoxin	**Clotting time, activated**
***Clostridium difficile* enterotoxin**, stool Negative (≤1 : 10 titer) Urine or stool container $$$ Must be tested within 12 hours of collection as toxin (B) is labile.	*Clostridium difficile*, a motile, gram-positive rod, is the major recognized agent of antibiotic-associated diarrhea, which is toxigenic in origin (see Antibiotic-associated colitis, p 226). There are two toxins (A and B) produced by *C difficile*. Cell culture is used to detect the cytopathic effect of the toxins, whose identity is confirmed by neutralization with specific antitoxins. Toxin A (more weakly cytopathic in cell culture) is enterotoxic and produces enteric disease. Toxin B (more easily detected in standard cell culture assays) fails to produce intestinal disease.	**Positive in:** Antibiotic-associated diarrhea (15–25%), antibiotic-associated colitis (50–75%), and pseudomembranous colitis (90–100%). About 3% of healthy adults and 10–20% of hospitalized patients have *C difficile* in their colonic flora. There is also a high carrier rate of *C difficile* and its toxin in healthy neonates.	Definitive diagnosis of disease caused by *C difficile* toxin is by endoscopic detection of pseudomembranous colitis. Direct examination of stool for leukocytes, gram-positive rods, or blood is not helpful. Culture of *C difficile* is not routinely performed, because it would isolate numerous nontoxigenic *C difficile* strains. Clin Microbiol Infect 2001;7:411. Gastroenterol Clin North Am 2001;30:753. Dig Dis 2000;18:147. Arch Intern Med 2001;161:525.
Clotting time, activated, whole blood (ACT) 114–186 seconds Special black tube $$ Performed at patient bedside. Avoid traumatic venipuncture, which may cause contamination with tissue juices and decrease clotting time.	A bedside or operating room test that assesses heparinization by measuring time taken for whole blood to clot.	**Prolonged in:** Heparin therapy, severe deficiency of clotting factors (except factors VII and XIII), functional platelet disorders, afibrinogenemia, circulating anticoagulants. **Normal in:** Thrombocytopenia, factor VII deficiency, von Willebrand disease.	Many consider this test unreliable. Reproducibility of prolonged ACTs is poor. Increasingly, the ACT has been used in the operating room, dialysis units, critical care centers, and during interventional cardiology/radiology procedures to monitor anticoagulation and titrate heparin dosages. At centers without experience, should not be used to regulate therapeutic heparin dosage adjustments; use PTT instead. Am J Crit Care 1993;2:81. Clin Cardiol 1994;17:357.

		Coccidioides antibodies	**Cold agglutinins**
Coccidioides antibodies, serum or CSF Negative Marbled $$	Screens for presence of antibodies to *Coccidioides immitis*. Some centers use the mycelial-phase antigen, coccidioidin, to detect antibody. IgM antibodies appear early in disease in 75% of patients, begin to decrease after week 3, and are rarely seen after 5 months. They may persist in disseminated cases, usually in the immunocompromised. IgG antibodies appear later in the course of the disease. Meningeal disease may have negative serum IgG and require CSF IgG antibody titers.	**Positive in:** Infection by coccidioides (90%). **Negative in:** Coccidioidin skin testing, many patients with chronic cavitary coccidioides; 5% of meningeal coccidioides is negative by CSF complement fixation (CF) test.	Diagnosis is based on culture and serologic testing. Precipitin and CF tests detect 90% of primary symptomatic cases. Precipitin test is most effective in detecting early primary infection or an exacerbation of existing disease. Test is diagnostic but not prognostic. CF test becomes positive later than precipitin test, and titers can be used to assess severity of infection. Titers rise as the disease progresses and decline as the patient improves. Enzyme immunoassay now available; data suggest good performance. N Engl J Med 1995;332:1077. Am J Clin Pathol 1997;107:148. Semin Respir Infect 2001;16:242.
Cold agglutinins, plasma < 1:20 titer Lavender or blue $$ Specimen should be kept at 37°C.	Detects antibodies that agglutinate red blood cells in the cold (strongly at 4°C, weakly at 24°C, and weakly or not at all at 37°C). These antibodies are present in primary atypical pneumonias due to *Mycoplasma pneumoniae*, in certain autoimmune hemolytic anemias, and in normal persons (not clinically significant).	**Increased in:** Chronic cold agglutinin disease, lymphoproliferative disorders (eg, Waldenström macroglobulinemia), autoimmune hemolytic anemia, collagen-vascular diseases, *M pneumoniae* pneumonia, infectious mononucleosis, mumps orchitis, cytomegalovirus, tropical diseases (eg, trypanosomiasis).	In *Mycoplasma* pneumonia, titers rise early, are maximal at 3–4 weeks after onset, and then disappear rapidly. These antibodies are usually IgM anti-I antibodies distinct from antibodies to *M pneumoniae*. A rise in cold agglutinin antibody titer is suggestive of recent mycoplasma infection but is found in other diseases. N Engl J Med 1977;297:583. Transfus Sci 2000;22:125. Curr Opin Hematol 2001;8:411.

Test/Range/Collection	Physiologic Basis	Interpretation	Comments
Complement C3		
Complement C3, serum 64–166 mg/dL [640–1660 mg/L] Marbled $$	The classic and alternative complement pathways converge at the C3 step in the complement cascade. Low levels indicate activation by one or both pathways. Most diseases with immune complexes will show decreased C3 levels. Test is usually performed as an immunoassay (by radial immunodiffusion or nephelometry).	**Increased in:** Many inflammatory conditions as an acute phase reactant, active phase of rheumatic diseases (eg, rheumatoid arthritis, SLE), acute viral hepatitis, myocardial infarction, cancer, diabetes mellitus, pregnancy, sarcoidosis, amyloidosis, thyroiditis. **Decreased by:** Decreased synthesis (protein malnutrition, congenital deficiency, severe liver disease), increased catabolism (immune complex disease, membranoproliferative glomerulonephritis [75%], SLE, Sjögren syndrome, rheumatoid arthritis, disseminated intravascular coagulation, paroxysmal nocturnal hemoglobinuria, autoimmune hemolytic anemia, gram-negative bacteremia), increased loss (burns, gastroenteropathies).	Complement C3 levels may be useful in following the activity of immune complex diseases. The best test to detect inherited deficiencies is CH50. N Engl J Med 1987;316:1525. Intern Med 2001;40:1254.
Complement C4		
Complement C4, serum 15–45 mg/dL [150–450 mg/L] Marbled $$	C4 is a component of the classic complement pathway. Depressed levels usually indicate classic pathway activation. Test is usually performed as an immunoassay and not a functional assay.	**Increased in:** Various malignancies (not clinically useful). **Decreased by:** Decreased synthesis (congenital deficiency), increased catabolism (SLE, rheumatoid arthritis, proliferative glomerulonephritis, hereditary angioedema), and increased loss (burns, protein-losing enteropathies).	Low C4 accompanies acute attacks of hereditary angioedema, and C4 is used as a first-line test for the disease. C1 esterase inhibitor levels are not indicated for the evaluation of hereditary angioedema unless C4 is low. Congenital C4 deficiency occurs with an SLE-like syndrome. N Engl J Med 1987;316:1525. Am J Med 1990;88:656.

	Complement CH50	**Cortisol**
Complement CH50, plasma or serum (CH50) 22–40 U/mL (laboratory-specific) Marbled $$$	The quantitative assay of hemolytic complement activity depends on the ability of the classic complement pathway to induce hemolysis of red cells sensitized with optimal amounts of anti-red cell antibodies. For precise titrations of hemolytic complement, the dilution of serum that will lyse 50% of the indicator red cells is determined as the CH50. This arbitrary unit depends on the conditions of the assay and is therefore laboratory-specific.	Release of corticotropin-releasing factor (CRF) from the hypothalamus stimulates release of ACTH from the pituitary, which in turn stimulates release of cortisol from the adrenal. Cortisol provides negative feedback to this system. Test measures both free cortisol and cortisol bound to cortisol-binding globulin (CBG). Morning levels are higher than evening levels.
	Decreased with: >50–80% deficiency of classic pathway complement components (congenital or acquired deficiencies). **Normal in:** Deficiencies of the alternative pathway complement components.	**Increased in:** Cushing syndrome, acute illness, surgery, trauma, septic shock, depression, anxiety, alcoholism, starvation, chronic renal failure, increased CBG (congenital, pregnancy, estrogen therapy). **Decreased in:** Addison disease; decreased CBG (congenital, liver disease, nephrotic syndrome).
	This is a functional assay of biologic activity. Sensitivity to decreased levels of complement components depends on exactly how the test is performed. It is used to detect congenital and acquired severe deficiency disorders of the classic complement pathway. N Engl J Med 1987;316:1525. Pediatr Clin North Am 2000;47:1339.	Cortisol levels are useful only in the context of standardized suppression or stimulation tests. (See Cosyntropin stimulation test, p 74, and Dexamethasone suppression tests, pp 80–81.) Circadian fluctuations in cortisol levels limit usefulness of single measurements. Analysis of diurnal variation of cortisol is not useful diagnostically. Endocrinol Metab Clin North Am 1994;23:511. J Clin Endocrinol Metab 2001;86:2909.

Corresponding left-column descriptor for Cortisol row: **Cortisol,** plasma or serum
8:00 AM: 5–20 µg/dL [140–550 nmol/L]
Marbled, lavender, or green
$$

Test/Range/Collection	Physiologic Basis	Interpretation	Comments
Cortisol (urinary free), urine 10–110 μg/24 h [30–300 nmol/d] Urine bottle containing boric acid. $$$ Collect 24-hour urine.	Urinary free cortisol measurement is useful in the initial evaluation of suspected Cushing syndrome (see Cushing syndrome algorithm, p 343).	**Increased in:** Cushing syndrome, acute illness, stress. **Not Increased in:** Obesity.	This test replaces both the assessment of 17-hydroxycorticosteroids and the 17-ketogenic steroids in the initial diagnosis of Cushing syndrome. Not useful for the diagnosis of adrenal insufficiency. A shorter (12-hour) overnight collection and measurement of the ratio of urine free cortisol to urine creatinine appears to perform nearly as well as a 24-hour collection for urine free cortisol. Clin Endocrinol 1998;48:503. Ann Endocrinol (Paris) 2001;62:173. Ann Endocrinol (Paris) 2001;62:168. Endocrinol Metab Clin North Am 2001;30:729.
Cosyntropin stimulation test, serum or plasma Marbled, green, or lavender $$$ First draw a cortisol level. Then administer cosyntropin (1 μg or 0.25 mg IV). Draw another cortisol level in 30 minutes.	Cosyntropin (synthetic ACTH preparation) stimulates the adrenal to release cortisol. A normal response is a doubling of basal levels or an increment of 7 μg/dL (200 nmol/L) to a level above 18 μg/dL (>504 nmol/L). A poor cortisol response to cosyntropin indicates adrenal insufficiency (see Adrenocortical insufficiency algorithm, Figure 8–2, p 340).	**Decreased in:** Adrenal insufficiency, pituitary insufficiency, AIDS.	Test does not distinguish primary from secondary (pituitary) adrenal insufficiency, because in secondary adrenal insufficiency the atrophic adrenal may be unresponsive to cosyntropin. Test may not reliably detect pituitary insufficiency. Metyrapone test (p 130) may be useful to assess the pituitary-adrenal axis. AIDS patients with adrenal insufficiency may have normal ACTH stimulation tests. J Clin Endocrinol Metab 1998;83:2726. Neth J Med 2000;56:91. Am J Med Sci 2001;321:137.

Creatine kinase		
Creatine kinase, serum (CK) 32–267 IU/L [0.53–4.45 µkat/L] (method-dependent) Marbled $	Creatine kinase splits creatine phosphate in the presence of ADP to yield creatine and ATP. Skeletal muscle, myocardium, and brain are rich in the enzyme. CK is released by tissue damage.	**Increased in:** Myocardial infarction (MI), myocarditis, muscle trauma, rhabdomyolysis, muscular dystrophy, polymyositis, severe muscular exertion, malignant hyperthermia, hypothyroidism, cerebral infarction, surgery, Reye syndrome, tetanus, generalized convulsions, alcoholism, IM injections, DC countershock. Drugs: clofibrate, HMG-CoA reductase inhibitors.	CK is as sensitive a test as aldolase for muscle damage, so aldolase is not needed. During an MI, serum CK level rises rapidly (within 3–5 hours); elevation persists for 2–3 days post-MI. Total CK is not specific enough for use in diagnosis of MI, but a normal total CK has a high negative predictive value. A more specific test is needed for diagnosis of MI (eg, CK-MB or cardiac troponin I). Cardiac troponin I and CK-MB or CK-MB mass concentration are better markers for myocardial infarction. Br Heart J 1994;72:112. Med J Aust 2001;175:486.

	Creatine kinase MB		
Test/Range/Collection	**Physiologic Basis**	**Interpretation**	**Comments**
Creatine kinase MB, serum enzyme activity (CK-MB) <16 IU/L [<0.27 μkat/L] or <4% of total CK or <7 μg/L mass units (laboratory-specific) Marbled $$	CK consists of 3 isoenzymes, made up of 2 subunits, M and B. The fraction with the greatest electrophoretic mobility is CK1 (BB); CK2 (MB) is intermediate, and CK3 (MM) moves slowest toward the anode. Skeletal muscle is characterized by isoenzyme MM and brain by isoenzyme BB. Myocardium has approximately 40% MB isoenzyme. Assay techniques include isoenzyme separation by electrophoresis (isoenzyme activity units) or immunoassay using antibody specific for MB fraction (mass units).	**Increased in:** Myocardial infarction, cardiac trauma, certain muscular dystrophies, and polymyositis. Slight persistent elevation reported in a few patients on hemodialysis.	CK-MB is a relatively specific test for MI. It appears in serum approximately 4 hours after infarction, peaks at 12–24 hours, and declines over 48–72 hours. CK-MB mass concentration is a more sensitive marker of MI than CK-MB isoenzymes or total CK within 4–12 hours after infarction. Cardiac troponin I levels are useful in the late (after 48 hours) diagnosis of MI because, unlike CK-MB levels, they remain elevated for 5–7 days. Within 48 hours, sensitivity and specificity of troponin I are similar to CK-MB. Specificity of troponin I is higher than CK-MB in patients with skeletal muscle injury or renal failure, or postoperatively. Cardiac troponin I is therefore the preferred test. Estimation of CK-MM and CK-BB is not clinically useful. Use total CK. N Engl J Med 1994;330:670. N Engl J Med 1994;331:561. Ann Emerg Med 2001;37:478.

Creatinine		
Creatinine, serum (Cr) 0.6–1.2 mg/dL [50–100 µmol/L] Marbled $	Endogenous creatinine is excreted by filtration through the glomerulus and by tubular secretion. Creatinine clearance is an acceptable clinical measure of glomerular filtration rate (GFR), although it sometimes overestimates GFR (eg, in cirrhosis). For each 50% reduction in GFR, serum creatinine approximately doubles.	**Increased in:** Acute or chronic renal failure, urinary tract obstruction, nephrotoxic drugs, hypothyroidism. **Decreased in:** Reduced muscle mass.	In alkaline picrate method, substances other than Cr (eg, acetoacetate, acetone, β-hydroxybutyrate, α-ketoglutarate, pyruvate, glucose) may give falsely high results. Therefore, patients with diabetic ketoacidosis may have spuriously elevated Cr. Cephalosporins may spuriously increase or decrease Cr measurement. Increased bilirubin may spuriously decrease Cr. Chronic renal insufficiency may be underrecognized. Age, male gender, and black race are predictors of kidney disease. Serum creatinine levels frequently do not reflect decreased renal function because creatinine production rate is decreased with reduced lean body mass. Increased intravascular volume and increased volume of distribution associated with anasarca may also mask decreased renal function by reducing serum creatinine levels. Am J. Kidney Dis 2000; 36(6 Suppl 3):S4. Med Clin North Am 2001;85:1241.

Test/Range/Collection	Physiologic Basis	Interpretation	Comments
Creatinine clearance			
Creatinine clearance, (Cl$_{Cr}$) Adults: 90–130 mL/min/1.73 m^2 BSA \$\$ Collect carefully timed 24-hour urine and simultaneous serum/plasma creatinine sample. Record patient's weight and height.	Widely used test of GFR. Theoretically reliable, but often compromised by incomplete urine collection. Creatinine clearance is calculated from measurement of urine creatinine (U$_{Cr}$ [mg/dL]), plasma/serum creatinine (P$_{Cr}$ [mg/dL]), and urine flow rate (V [mL/min]) according to the formula: $$Cl_{Cr}(mL/min) = \frac{U_{Cr} \times V}{P_{Cr}}$$ where $$V(mL/min) = \frac{24\text{-hour urine volume(mL)}}{1440}$$ Creatinine clearance is often "corrected" for body surface area (BSA [m^2]) according to the formula: $$Cl_{Cr} = Cl_{Cr} \times \frac{1.73}{BSA}$$ (corrected) (uncorrected)	**Increased in:** High cardiac output, exercise, acromegaly, diabetes mellitus (early stage), infections, hypothyroidism. **Decreased in:** Acute or chronic renal failure, decreased renal blood flow (shock, hemorrhage, dehydration, CHF). Drugs: nephrotoxic drugs.	Serum Cr may, in practice, be a more reliable indicator of renal function than 24-hour Cl$_{Cr}$ unless urine collection is carefully monitored. An 8-hour collection provides results similar to those obtained by a 24-hour collection. Cl$_{Cr}$ will overestimate GFR to the extent that Cr is secreted by the renal tubules (eg, in cirrhosis). Cl$_{Cr}$ can be estimated from the serum creatinine using the following formula: $$\frac{Cl_{Cr}}{(mL/min)} = \frac{(140 - Age) \times Wt(kg)}{72 \times P_{Cr}}$$ Serial decline in Cl$_{Cr}$ is the most reliable indicator of progressive renal dysfunction. Arch Intern Med 1994;154:201. Anesthesiol Clin North America 2000;18:739. Postgrad Med 2001;10:55.

	Cryoglobulins		Cryptococcal antigen
Cryoglobulins, serum <0.12 mg/dL Marbled $ Must be immediately transported to lab at 37°C	Cryoglobulins are immunoglobulins (IgG, IgM, IgA, or light chains) which precipitate on exposure to the cold. Type I cryoglobulins (25%) are monoclonal proteins, most commonly IgM, occasionally IgG, and rarely IgA or Bence Jones protein, seen in multiple myeloma and Waldenström macroglobulinemia. Type II (25%) are mixed cryoglobulins with a monoclonal component (usually IgM but occasionally IgG or IgA) that complexes with autologous normal IgG in the cryoprecipitate. Type III (50%) are mixed polyclonal cryoglobulins (IgM and IgG).	**Increased in:** Immunoproliferative disorders (multiple myeloma, Waldenström macroglobulinemia, chronic lymphocytic leukemia, lymphoma), collagen-vascular disease (SLE, polyarteritis nodosa, rheumatoid arthritis), hemolytic anemia, essential mixed cryoglobulinemia, hepatitis B and C infection.	All types of cryoglobulins may cause cold-induced symptoms, including Raynaud phenomenon, vascular purpura, and urticaria. Patients with type II and III cryoglobulinemia often have immune complex disease, with vascular purpura, arthritis, and nephritis. Typing of cryoglobulins by electrophoresis is not necessary for diagnosis or clinical management. About 50% of essential mixed cryoglobulinemia patients have evidence of hepatitis C infection. Am J Med 1994;96:124. J Clin Pathol 2002;55:4.
Cryptococcal antigen, serum or CSF Negative Marbled (serum) or glass or plastic tube (CSF) $$	The capsular polysaccharide of *Cryptococcus neoformans* potentiates opportunistic infections by the yeast. The cryptococcal antigen test used is often a latex agglutination test.	**Increased in:** Cryptococcal infection.	False-positive and false-negative results have been reported. False-positives due to rheumatoid factor can be reduced by pretreatment of serum using pronase before testing. Sensitivity and specificity of serum cryptococcal antigen titer for cryptococcal meningitis are 91% and 83%, respectively. Ninety-six percent of cryptococcal infections occur in AIDS patients. Infect Immun 1994;62:1507. J Clin Microbiol 1994;32:2158. Infect Dis Clin North Am 2001;15:567.

	Cytomegalovirus antibody	Dexamethasone suppression test (low dose)
Test/Range/Collection	**Physiologic Basis**	**Interpretation**	**Comments**

Test/Range/Collection	Physiologic Basis	Interpretation	Comments
Cytomegalovirus antibody, serum (CMV) Negative Marbled $$$	Detects the presence of antibody to CMV, either IgG or IgM. CMV infection is usually acquired during childhood or early adulthood. By age 20–40 years, 40–90% of the population has CMV antibodies.	**Increased in:** Previous or active CMV infection. False-positive CMV IgM tests occur when rheumatoid factor or infectious mononucleosis is present.	Serial specimens exhibiting a greater than fourfold titer rise suggest a recent infection. Active CMV infection must be documented by viral isolation. Useful for screening of potential organ donors and recipients. Detection of CMV IgM antibody in the serum of a newborn usually indicates congenital infection. Detection of CMV IgG antibody is not diagnostic, because maternal CMV IgG antibody passed via the placenta can persist in newborn's serum for 6 months. Rev Infect Dis 1988;10:S468. Obstet Gynecol Surv 2002;57:245. J Am Soc Nephrol 2001;12:848. Expert Rev Mol Diagn 2001;1:19. Herpes 2001;8:37.
Dexamethasone suppression test (single low-dose, overnight), serum 8:00 AM serum cortisol level: <5 µg/dL [<140 nmol/L] $$ Give 1 mg dexamethasone at 11:00 PM. At 8:00 AM, draw serum cortisol level.	In normal patients, dexamethasone suppresses the 8:00 AM serum cortisol level to below 5 µg/dL. Patients with Cushing syndrome have 8:00 AM levels >10 µg/dL (>276 nmol/L).	**Positive in:** Cushing syndrome (98% sensitivity, 98% specificity in lean outpatients), obese patients (13%), hospitalized or chronically ill patients (23%).	Good screening test for Cushing syndrome. If this test is abnormal, use high-dose test (see below) to determine etiology. (See also Cushing syndrome algorithm, p 343.) Patients taking phenytoin may fail to suppress because of enhanced dexamethasone metabolism. Depressed patients may also fail to suppress morning cortisol level. Ann Clin Biochem 1997;34(Part 3):222. Ann Endocrinol (Paris) 2001;62:173.

	Dexamethasone suppression test (high dose)	Double-stranded DNA antibody
Dexamethasone suppression test (high-dose, overnight), serum 8:00 AM serum cortisol level: <5 µg/dL [<140 nmol/L] $$ Give 8 mg dexamethasone dose at 11:00 PM. At 8:00 AM, draw cortisol level.	Suppression of plasma cortisol levels to < 50% of baseline with dexamethasone indicates Cushing disease (pituitary-dependent ACTH hypersecretion) and differentiates this from adrenal and ectopic Cushing syndrome (see Cushing syndrome algorithm, p 343).	**Positive in:** Cushing disease (88–92% sensitivity; specificity 57–100%).	Test indicated only after a positive low-dose dexamethasone suppression test. Sensitivity and specificity depend on sampling time and diagnostic criteria. The ovine corticotropin-releasing hormone (CRH) stimulation test and bilateral sampling of the inferior petrosal sinuses combined with CRH administration are being evaluated for the definitive diagnosis of Cushing disease. Measurement of urinary 17-hydroxycorticosteroids has been replaced in this test by measurement of serum cortisol. J Clin Endocrinol Metab 1994;78:418. N Engl J Med 1994;331:629. Ann Intern Med 1994;121:318. Medicine 1995;74:74. J Neurooncol 2001;54:151.
Double-stranded-DNA antibody (ds-DNA Ab), serum <1 : 10 titer Marbled $$	IgG or IgM antibodies directed against host double-stranded DNA.	**Increased in:** Systemic lupus erythematosus (60–70% sensitivity, 95% specificity) based on >1 : 10 titer. **Not increased in:** Drug-induced lupus.	High titers are seen only in SLE. Titers of ds-DNA antibody correlate well with disease activity and with occurrence of glomerulonephritis. (See also Autoantibodies table, p 366.) Clin Immunol Immunopathol 1988;47:121. Curr Opin Rheumatol 2000;12:364.

Test/Range/Collection	Physiologic Basis	Interpretation	Comments	
			Epstein-Barr virus antibodies	**Erythrocyte count**
Epstein-Barr virus antibodies, serum (EBV Ab) Negative Marbled $$	Antiviral capsid antibodies (anti-VCA) (IgM) often reach their peak at clinical presentation and last up to 3 months; anti-VCA IgG antibodies last for life. Early antigen antibodies (anti-EA) are next to develop, are most often positive at 1 month after presentation, typically last for 2–3 months, and may last up to 6 months in low titers. Anti-EA may also be found in some patients with Hodgkin disease, chronic lymphocytic leukemia, and some other malignancies. Anti-EB nuclear antigen (anti-EBNA) antibody begins to appear in a minority of patients in the third or fourth week but is uniformly present by 6 months.	**Increased in:** EB virus infection, infectious mononucleosis. Antibodies to the diffuse (D) form of antigen (detected in the cytoplasm and nucleus of infected cells) are greatly elevated in nasopharyngeal carcinoma. Antibodies to the restricted (R) form of antigen (detected only in the cytoplasm of infected cells) are greatly elevated in Burkitt lymphoma.	Most useful in diagnosing infectious mononucleosis in patients who have the clinical and hematologic criteria for the disease but who fail to develop the heterophile agglutinins (10%) (see Heterophile agglutination, p 108). EBV antibodies cannot be used to diagnose "chronic" mononucleosis. Chronic fatigue syndrome is not caused by EBV. The best indicator of primary infection is a positive anti-VCA IgM (check for false-positives caused by rheumatoid factor). *J Clin Microbiol* 1996;34:3240. *Postgrad Med* 2000;107:175, 183, 186. *Clin Otolaryngol* 2001;26:3. Rose NR et al (eds.): *Manual of Clinical Laboratory Immunology,* 6th ed. American Society for Microbiology, 2002.	
Erythrocyte count, whole blood (RBC count) 4.2–5.6 × 10⁶/μL [× 10¹²/L] Lavender $	Erythrocytes are counted by automated instruments using electrical impedance or light scattering.	**Increased in:** Secondary polycythemia (hemoconcentration), polycythemia vera. Spurious increase with increased white blood cells. **Decreased in:** Anemia. Spurious decrease with autoagglutination.	*Lab Med* 1983;14:509. *Nephrol Dial Transplant* 2000;15(Suppl 3):36. *Semin Hematol* 2001;38(1 Suppl 2):25. *Semin Hematol* 2001;38(1 Suppl 2):21.	

Test / Specimen / Cost	Physiologic Basis	Interpretation	Comments
Erythrocyte sedimentation rate, whole blood (ESR) Male: <10 Female: <15 mm/h (laboratory-specific) Lavender $ Test must be run within 2 hours after sample collection.	In plasma, erythrocytes (red blood cells [RBCs]) usually settle slowly. However, if they aggregate for any reason (usually because of plasma proteins called acute phase reactants, eg, fibrinogen), they settle rapidly. Sedimentation of RBCs occurs because their density is greater than plasma. ESR measures the distance in millimeters that erythrocytes fall during 1 hour.	**Increased in:** Infections (osteomyelitis, pelvic inflammatory disease [75%]), inflammatory disease (temporal arteritis, polymyalgia rheumatica, rheumatic fever), malignant neoplasms, paraproteinemias, anemia, pregnancy, chronic renal failure, GI disease (ulcerative colitis, regional ileitis). For endocarditis, sensitivity = 93%. **Decreased in:** Polycythemia, sickle cell anemia, spherocytosis, anisocytosis, hypofibrinogenemia, hypogammaglobulinemia, congestive heart failure, microcytosis. Drugs: high-dose corticosteroids.	There is a good correlation between ESR and C-reactive protein, but ESR is less expensive. Test is useful and indicated only for diagnosis and monitoring of temporal arteritis and polymyalgia rheumatica. The test is not sensitive or specific for other conditions. ESR is higher in women, blacks, and older persons. Low value is of no diagnostic significance. Ann Intern Med 1986;104:515. Clin Exp Rheumatol 2000; 18(4 Suppl 20):S29. JAMA 2002;287:92.
Erythropoietin, serum (EPO) 5–20 mIU/mL [5–20 IU/L] Marbled $$$	Erythropoietin is a glycoprotein hormone produced in the kidney that induces red blood cell production by stimulating proliferation, differentiation, and maturation of erythroid precursors. Hypoxia is the usual stimulus for production of EPO. In conditions of bone marrow hyporesponsiveness, EPO levels are elevated. In chronic renal failure, EPO production is decreased.	**Increased in:** Anemias associated with bone marrow hyporesponsiveness (aplastic anemia, iron deficiency anemia), secondary polycythemia (high-altitude hypoxia, COPD, pulmonary fibrosis), erythropoietin-producing tumors (cerebellar hemangioblastomas, pheochromocytomas, renal tumors), pregnancy, polycystic kidney disease. **Decreased in:** Anemia of chronic disease, renal failure, inflammatory states, primary polycythemia (polycythemia vera) (39%).	Test is not very useful in differentiating polycythemia vera from secondary polycythemia. Because virtually all patients with severe anemia due to chronic renal failure respond to EPO therapy, pretherapy EPO levels are not indicated. Patient receiving EPO as chronic therapy should have iron deficiency screening routinely. Haematologica 1997;82:406. Semin Hematol 2000;37(4 Suppl 6):1. Blood 2000;96:823. Semin Hematol 2001;38(1 Suppl 2):21.

Test/Range/Collection	Physiologic Basis	Interpretation	Comments
Ethanol, serum (EtOH) 0 mg/dL [mmol/L] Marbled $$ Do not use alcohol swab. Do not remove stopper.	Measures serum level of ethyl alcohol (ethanol).	**Present in:** Ethanol ingestion.	Whole blood alcohol concentrations are about 15% lower than serum concentrations. Each 0.1 mg/dL of ethanol contributes about 22 mosm/kg to serum osmolality. Legal intoxication in many states is defined as >80 mg/dL (>17 mmol/L). N Engl J Med 1976;294:757.
Factor V (Leiden) mutation Blood Lavender or blue $$$$	The Leiden mutation is a single nucleotide base substitution leading to an amino acid substitution (glutamine replaces arginine) at one of the sites where coagulation factor V is cleaved by activated protein C. The mutation causes factor V to be partially resistant to protein C, which is involved in inhibiting coagulation. Factor V mutations may be present in up to half of the cases of unexplained venous thrombosis and are seen in 95% of patients with activated protein C resistance.	**Positive in:** Hypercoagulability secondary to factor V mutation (specificity approaches 100%).	The presence of mutation is only a risk factor for thrombosis, not an absolute marker for disease. Homozygotes have a 50- to 100-fold increase in risk of thrombosis (relative to the general population), and heterozygotes have a 7-fold increase in risk. The current PCR and reverse dot blot assay only detects the Leiden mutation of factor V; other mutations may yet be discovered. Ann Intern Med 1999;130:643. Am J Med Sci 2001;322:88. Emerg Med Clin North Am 2001;19:839. Arch Pathol Lab Med 2002;126:577.

Test / Specimen	Physiologic Basis	Interpretation	Comments
Factor VIII assay, plasma 40–150% of normal, (varies with age) Blue $$$ Deliver immediately to laboratory on ice. Stable for 2 hours.	Measures activity of factor VIII (antihemophilic factor), a key factor of the intrinsic clotting cascade.	**Increased in:** Inflammatory states (acute phase reactant, last trimester of pregnancy, oral contraceptives). **Decreased in:** Hemophilia A, von Willebrand disease, disseminated intravascular coagulation, acquired factor VIII antibodies.	Normal hemostasis requires at least 25% of factor VIII activity. Symptomatic hemophiliacs usually have levels ≤5%. Disease levels are defined as severe (<1%), moderate (1–5%), and mild (>5%). Factor VIII assays are used to guide replacement therapy in patients with hemophilia. Factor deficiency can be distinguished from factor inhibitors by a PTT mixing study. Semin Hematol 1967;4:93. Semin Thromb Hemost 2000;26:195.
Fecal fat, stool Random: <60 droplets of fat/high power field 72 hour: <7 g/d $$$ Qualitative: random stool sample is adequate. Quantitative: dietary fat should be at least 50–150 g/d for 2 days before collection. Then all stools should be collected for 72 hours and refrigerated.	In healthy people, most dietary fat is completely absorbed in the small intestine. Normal small intestinal lining, bile acids, and pancreatic enzymes are required for normal fat absorption.	**Increased in:** Malabsorption from small bowel disease (regional enteritis, celiac disease, tropical sprue), pancreatic insufficiency, diarrhea with or without fat malabsorption.	A random, qualitative fecal fat (so-called Sudan stain) is only useful if positive. Furthermore, it does not correlate well with quantitative measurements. Sudan stain appears to detect triglycerides and lipolytic by-products, whereas 72-hour fecal fat measures fatty acids from a variety of sources, including phospholipids, cholesteryl esters, and triglycerides. The quantitative method can be used to measure the degree of fat malabsorption initially and then after a therapeutic intervention. A normal quantitative stool fat reliably rules out pancreatic insufficiency and most forms of generalized small intestine disease. Gastroenterol Clin North Am 1989;18:467. Gastroenterology 1992;102:1936. Am J Gastroenterol 2001;96:3237.

Test/Range/Collection	Physiologic Basis	Interpretation	Comments
Fecal occult blood, stool Negative $ Patient should be on a special diet free of exogenous peroxidase activity (meat, fish, turnips, horseradish), GI irritants (aspirin, nonsteroidal anti-inflammatory drugs), and iron. To avoid false-negatives, patients should avoid taking vitamin C. Patient collects two specimens from three consecutive bowel movements.	Measures blood in the stool using gum guaiac as an indicator reagent. In the Hemoccult test, gum guaiac is impregnated in a test paper that is smeared with stool using an applicator. Hydrogen peroxide is used as a developer solution. The resultant phenolic oxidation of guaiac in the presence of blood in the stool yields a blue color.	**Positive in:** Upper GI disease (peptic ulcer, gastritis, variceal bleeding, esophageal and gastric cancer), lower GI disease (diverticulosis, colonic polyps, colon carcinoma, inflammatory bowel disease, vascular ectasias, hemorrhoids).	Although fecal occult blood testing is an accepted screening test for colon carcinoma, the sensitivity and specificity of an individual test are low. The utility of fecal occult blood testing after digital rectal examination has not been well studied. Three randomized controlled trials have shown reductions in colon cancer mortality with yearly (33% reduction) or biennial (15–21% reduction) testing. About 1000 fifty-year-olds must be screened for 10 years to save one life. In patients older than 50 years, annual fecal occult blood testing with flexible sigmoidoscopy at 5-year intervals is recommended by the American Cancer society. Ann Intern Med 1997;126:811. BMJ 1998;317:559. Am Fam Physician 2001;63:1101. Gastrointest Endosc Clin North Am 2002;12:11.

Ferritin		
Ferritin, serum Males 16–300 ng/mL [μg/L] Females 4–161 ng/mL [μg/L] Marbled $$	Ferritin is the body's major iron storage protein. The serum ferritin level correlates with total body iron stores. The test is used to detect iron deficiency, to monitor response to iron therapy, and, in iron overload states, to monitor iron removal therapy. It is also used to predict homozygosity for hemochromatosis in relatives of affected patients. In the absence of liver disease, it is a more sensitive test for iron deficiency than serum iron and iron-binding capacity (transferrin saturation).	**Increased in:** Iron overload (hemochromatosis [sensitivity 85%, specificity 95%], hemosiderosis), acute or chronic liver disease, alcoholism, various malignancies (eg, leukemia, Hodgkin disease), chronic inflammatory disorders (eg, rheumatoid arthritis, adult Still disease), thalassemia minor, adult Still disease), thalassemia minor, hyperthyroidism, HIV infection, non-insulin-dependent diabetes mellitus, and postpartum state. **Decreased in:** Iron deficiency (60–75%).	Serum ferritin is clinically useful in distinguishing between iron deficiency anemia (serum ferritin levels diminished) and anemia of chronic disease or thalassemia (levels usually normal or elevated). Test of choice for diagnosis of iron deficiency anemia. Ferritin (ng/mL) / LR for Iron Deficiency: >100 — 0.08 45–100 — 0.54 35–45 — 1.83 25–35 — 2.54 15–25 — 8.83 ≤15 — 52.00 Liver disease will increase serum ferritin levels and mask the diagnosis of iron deficiency. J Gen Intern Med 1992;7:145 Am J Hematol 1993;42:177. Br J Haematol 1993;85:787. J Intern Med 1994;236:315. Am Fam Physician 2000;62:1565. Eur J Gastroenterol Hepatol 2002;14:217.

Test/Range/Collection	Physiologic Basis	Interpretation	Comments
α-Fetoprotein, serum (AFP) 0–15 ng/mL [μg/L] Marbled $$ Avoid hemolysis.	α-Fetoprotein is a glycoprotein produced both early in fetal life and by some tumors.	**Increased in:** Hepatocellular carcinoma (72%), massive hepatic necrosis (74%), viral hepatitis (34%), chronic active hepatitis (29%), cirrhosis (11%), regional enteritis (5%), benign gynecologic diseases (22%), testicular carcinoma (embryonal) (70%), teratocarcinoma (64%), teratoma (37%), ovarian carcinoma (57%), endometrial cancer (50%), cervical cancer (53%), pancreatic cancer (23%), gastric cancer (18%), colon cancer (5%). **Negative in:** Seminoma.	The test is not sensitive or specific enough to be used as a general screening test for hepatocellular carcinoma. However, screening may be justified in populations at very high risk for hepatocellular cancer. In hepatocellular cancer or germ cell tumors associated with elevated AFP, the test may be helpful in detecting recurrence after therapy. AFP is also used to screen pregnant women at 15–20 weeks gestation for possible fetal neural tube defects. AFP level in maternal serum or amniotic fluid is compared with levels expected at a given gestational age. Can J Urol 2001;8:1184. Clin Liver Dis 2001;5:145. Clin Perinatol 2001;28:279. Pediatr Hematol Oncol 2001;18:11.

α-Fetoprotein

Fibrin D-dimers		
Fibrin D-dimers, plasma Negative Blue $$	Plasmin acts on fibrin to form various fibrin degradation products. The D-dimer level can be used as a measure of activation of the fibrinolytic system.	**Increased in:** Disseminated intravascular coagulation (DIC), other thrombotic disorders, pulmonary embolism, venous or arterial thrombosis.	Fibrin D-dimer assay has replaced the Fibrin(ogen) Split Products test as a screen for DIC, because the D-dimer assay can distinguish fibrin degradation products (in DIC) from fibrinogen degradation products (in primary fibrinogenolysis). Because the presence of fibrin D-dimer is not specific for DIC, the definitive diagnosis of DIC must depend on other tests, including the platelet count and serum fibrinogen level. Absence of fibrin D-dimers cannot reliably exclude venous thromboembolism unless the sensitivity of the test has been established in the local laboratory. Am Intern Med 1998;129:1006. Thromb Res 2001;103:V225. Semin Thromb Hemost 2001;27:657. Arch Intern Med 2002;162:747.

Test/Range/Collection	Physiologic Basis	Interpretation	Comments
Fibrinogen (functional), plasma 175–433 mg/dL [1.75–4.3 g/L] *Panic:* <75 mg/dL Blue $$	Fibrinogen is synthesized in the liver and has a half-life of about 4 days. Thrombin cleaves fibrinogen to form insoluble fibrin monomers, which polymerize to form a clot.	**Increased in:** Inflammatory states (acute phase reactant), use of oral contraceptives, pregnancy. **Decreased in:** Decreased hepatic synthesis, increased consumption (DIC, thrombolysis). Hereditary: Afibrinogenemia (rare), hypofibrinogenemia, dysfibrinogenemia.	Hypofibrinogenemia is an important diagnostic laboratory feature of DIC. Diagnosis of dysfibrinogenemia depends upon the discrepancy between measurable antigenic and low functional (clottable) fibrinogen levels. Preliminary data suggest that plasma levels of fibrinogen and fibrin D-dimers are independent predictors of ischemic heart disease. Blood 1982;60:284. Ann Intern Med 1993;118:956. Ann NY Acad Sci 2001;936:560.
Fluorescent treponemal antibody-absorbed, serum (FTA-ABS) Nonreactive Marbled $$	Detects specific antibodies against *Treponema pallidum.* Patient's serum is first diluted with nonpathogenic treponemal antigens (to bind nonspecific antibodies). The absorbed serum is placed on a slide that contains fixed *T pallidum.* Fluorescein-labeled antihuman gamma globulin is then added to bind to and visualize (under a fluorescence microscope) the patient's antibody on treponemes.	**Reactive in:** Syphilis: primary (95%), secondary (100%), late (96%), latent (100%); also rarely positive in collagen-vascular diseases in the presence of antinuclear antibody.	Used to confirm a reactive nontreponemal screening serologic test for syphilis such as RPR or VDRL (see pp 157 and 182, respectively). Once positive, the FTA-ABS may remain positive for life. However, one study found that at 36 months after treatment, 24% of patients had nonreactive FTA-ABS tests. In a study of HIV-infected men with a prior history of syphilis, 38% of patients with AIDS or ARC had loss of reactivity to treponemal tests, compared with 7% of HIV-seropositive asymptomatic men and 0% of HIV-seronegative men. J Infect Dis 1990;162:862. Ann Intern Med 1991;114:1005. Sex Transm Infect 2000;76:73.

Folic acid (RBC)		
Folic acid (RBC), whole blood 165–760 ng/mL [370–1720 nmol/L] Lavender $$$	Folate is a vitamin necessary for methyl group transfer in thymidine formation, and hence DNA synthesis. Deficiency can result in megaloblastic anemia.	**Decreased in:** Tissue folate deficiency (from dietary folate deficiency), B_{12} deficiency (50–60%, since cellular uptake of folate depends on B_{12}).	Red cell folate level correlates better than serum folate level with tissue folate deficiency. A low red cell folate level may indicate either folate or B_{12} deficiency. A therapeutic trial of folate (and not red cell or serum folate testing) is indicated when the clinical and dietary history is strongly suggestive of folate deficiency and the peripheral smear shows hypersegmented polymorphonuclear leukocytes. However, the possibility of vitamin B_{12} deficiency must always be considered in the setting of megaloblastic anemia, since folate therapy will treat the hematologic, but not the neurologic, sequelae of vitamin B_{12} deficiency. Blood 1983;61:624. Clin Chem 2000;46:1277.

Test/Range/Collection	Physiologic Basis	Interpretation	Comments
	Follicle-stimulating hormone		**Free erythrocyte protoporphyrin**
Follicle-stimulating hormone, serum (FSH) Male: 1–10 mIU/mL Female: (mIU/mL) Follicular 4–13 Luteal 2–13 Midcycle 5–22 Postmenopausal 20–138 (laboratory-specific) Marbled $$	FSH is stimulated by the hypothalamic hormone GnRH and is then secreted from the anterior pituitary in a pulsatile fashion. Levels rise during the preovulatory phase of the menstrual cycle and then decline. FSH is necessary for normal pubertal development and fertility in males and females.	**Increased in:** Primary (ovarian) gonadal failure, ovarian or testicular agenesis, castration, postmenopause, Klinefelter syndrome, drugs. **Decreased in:** Hypothalamic disorders, pituitary disorders, pregnancy, anorexia nervosa. Drugs: corticosteroids, oral contraceptives.	Test indicated in the work-up of amenorrhea in women (see Amenorrhea algorithm, p 341), delayed puberty, impotence, and infertility in men. Impotence work-ups should begin with serum testosterone measurement. Basal FSH levels in premenopausal women depend on age, smoking history, and menstrual cycle length and regularity. Because of its variability, FSH is an unreliable guide to menopausal status during the transition into menopause. Endocrinol Metab Clin North Am 1992;21:921. JAMA 1993;270:83. J Clin Endocrinol Metab 1994; 79:1105. Semin Reprod Med 2000;18:5. Recent Prog Horm Res 2002;57:257.
Free erythrocyte protoporphyrin, whole blood (FEP) <35 μg/dL (method-dependent) Lavender $$$	Protoporphyrin is produced in the next to last step of heme synthesis. In the last step, iron is incorporated into protoporphyrin to produce heme. Enzyme deficiencies, lack of iron, or presence of interfering substances (lead) can disrupt this process and cause elevated FEP.	**Increased in:** Decreased iron incorporation into heme (iron deficiency, infection, and lead poisoning), erythropoietic protoporphyria.	FEP can be used to screen for lead poisoning in children provided that iron deficiency has been ruled out. Test does not discriminate between uroporphyrin, coproporphyrin, and protoporphyrin, but protoporphyrin is the predominant porphyrin measured. Clin Pediatr 1991;30:74. Am J Dis Child 1993;147:66.

	Fructosamine	Gamma-glutamyl transpeptidase	Gastrin
	Fructosamine correlates well with fasting plasma glucose ($r = .74$) but cannot be used to predict precisely the HbA$_{1c}$. Acta Diabetologica 1998;35:48. Nurs Clin North Am 2001;36:361.	GGT is useful in follow-up of alcoholics undergoing treatment because the test is sensitive to modest alcohol intake. GGT is elevated in 90% of patients with liver disease. GGT is used to confirm hepatic origin of elevated serum alkaline phosphatase. Ann Clin Biochem 2001;38:652. Crit Rev Clin Lab Sci 2001;38:263. Semin Gastrointest Dis 2001;12:89. Ann Clin Biochem 2002;39:22.	Gastrin is the first-line test for determining whether a patient with active ulcer disease has a gastrinoma. Gastric analysis is not indicated. Before interpreting an elevated level, be sure that the patient is not taking antacids, H$_2$ blockers, or proton pump inhibitors. Both fasting and post-secretin infusion levels may be required for diagnosis. Endocrinol Metab Clin North Am 1993;22:823. Lancet 1996;347:270. Curr Treat Options Oncol 2001;2:337.
	Increased in: Diabetes mellitus.	**Increased in:** Liver disease: acute viral or toxic hepatitis, chronic or subacute hepatitis, alcoholic hepatitis, cirrhosis, biliary tract obstruction (intrahepatic or extrahepatic), primary or metastatic liver neoplasm, mononucleosis. Drugs (by enzyme induction): phenytoin, carbamazepine, barbiturates, alcohol.	**Increased in:** Gastrinoma (Zollinger-Ellison syndrome) (80–93% sensitivity), antral G cell hyperplasia, hypochlorhydria, achlorhydria, chronic atrophic gastritis, pernicious anemia. Drugs: antacids, cimetidine, and other H$_2$ blockers; omeprazole and other proton pump inhibitors. **Decreased in:** Antrectomy with vagotomy.
	Glycation of albumin produces fructosamine, a less expensive marker of glycemic control than HbA$_{1c}$.	GGT is an enzyme present in liver, kidney, and pancreas. It is induced by alcohol intake and is an extremely sensitive indicator of liver disease, particularly alcoholic liver disease.	Gastrin is secreted from G cells in the stomach antrum and stimulates acid secretion from the gastric parietal cells. Values fluctuate throughout the day but are lowest in the early morning.
	Fructosamine, serum 1.6–2.6 mmol/L Marbled $	**Gamma-glutamyl transpeptidase,** serum (GGT) 9–85 U/L [0.15–1.42 µkat/L] (laboratory specific) Marbled $	**Gastrin,** serum <100 pg/mL [ng/L] Marbled $$ Overnight fasting required.

	Glucose		
Test/Range/Collection	Physiologic Basis	Interpretation	Comments
Glucose, serum 60–110 mg/dL [3.3–6.1 mmol/L] *Panic:* <40 or >500 mg/dL Marbled $ Overnight fasting usually required.	Normally, the glucose concentration in extracellular fluid is closely regulated so that a source of energy is readily available to tissues and so that no glucose is excreted in the urine.	**Increased in:** Diabetes mellitus, Cushing syndrome (10–15%), chronic pancreatitis (30%). Drugs: corticosteroids, phenytoin, estrogen, thiazides. **Decreased in:** Pancreatic islet cell disease with increased insulin, insulinoma, adrenocortical insufficiency, hypopituitarism, diffuse liver disease, malignancy (adrenocortical, stomach, fibrosarcoma), infant of a diabetic mother, enzyme deficiency diseases (eg, galactosemia). Drugs: insulin, ethanol, propranolol; sulfonylureas, tolbutamide, and other oral hypoglycemic agents.	Diagnosis of diabetes mellitus requires a fasting plasma glucose of >126 mg/dL on more than one occasion. Hypoglycemia is defined as a glucose of <50 mg/dL in men and <40 mg/dL in women. While random serum glucose levels correlate with home glucose monitoring results (weekly mean capillary glucose values), there is wide fluctuation within individuals. Thus, glycosylated hemoglobin levels are favored to monitor glycemic control. The American Diabetes Association recommends that adults age 45 years or older should be evaluated for diabetes by measuring fasting glucose levels. Long-term outcomes studies are needed to provide evidence for this recommendation.. JAMA 1999;281:1203. Diabetes Care 2000;23:1563. Diabetes Metab Res Rev 2000;16:230. Geriatrics 2001;56:20,32. Clin Chim Acta 2002;315:61.

Glucose tolerance test		

Glucose tolerance test, serum
 	
Fasting: <110
1-hour: <200
2-hour: <140 mg/dL
[Fasting: <6.4
1-hour: <11.0
2-hour: <7.7 mmol/L]
 	
Marbled
$$
 	
Subjects should receive a 150- to 200-g/d carbohydrate diet for at least 3 days prior to test. A 75-g glucose dose is dissolved in 300 mL of water for adults (1.75 g/kg for children) and given after an overnight fast. Serial determinations of plasma or serum venous blood glucoses are obtained at baseline, 1 hour, and 2 hours.
	The test determines the ability of a patient to respond appropriately to a glucose load.	**Increased glucose rise (decreased glucose tolerance) in:** Diabetes mellitus, impaired glucose tolerance, gestational diabetes, severe liver disease, hyperthyroidism, stress (infection), increased absorption of glucose from GI tract (hyperthyroidism, gastrectomy, gastroenterostomy, vagotomy, excess glucose intake), Cushing syndrome, pheochromocytoma. Drugs: diuretics, oral contraceptives, glucocorticoids, nicotinic acid, phenytoin.
		
		Decreased glucose rise (flat glucose curve) in: Intestinal disease (celiac sprue, Whipple disease), adrenal insufficiency (Addison disease, hypopituitarism), pancreatic islet cell tumors or hyperplasia.
			Test is not generally required for diagnosis of diabetes mellitus.
			In screening for gestational diabetes, the glucose tolerance test is performed between 24 and 28 weeks of gestation. After a 50-g oral glucose load, a 2-hour postprandial blood glucose is measured as a screen. If the result is >140 mg/dL, then the full test with 100-g glucose load is done using the following reference ranges:
			
			    Fasting: <105
			    1-hour: <190
			    2-hour: <165
			    3-hour: <145 mg/dL
			
			Routine screening for gestational diabetes has not been found to be cost-effective, and is not recommended by the Canadian Task Force on the Periodic Health Examination.
			Diabetes Care 1999;22(Suppl 1):55.
			Obstet Gynecol Clin North Am 2001;28:513.

Test/Range/Collection	Physiologic Basis	Interpretation	Comments
G6PD screen			
Glucose-6-phosphate dehydrogenase screen, whole blood (G6PD) 5–14 units/g Hb [0.1–0.28 µkat/L] Green or blue $$	G6PD is an enzyme in the hexose monophosphate shunt that is essential in generating reduced glutathione and NADPH, which protect hemoglobin from oxidative denaturation. Numerous G6PD isoenzymes have been identified. Most African-Americans have G6PD-A(+) isoenzyme. 10–15% have G6PD-A(−), which has only 15% of normal enzyme activity. It is transmitted in an X-linked recessive manner. Some Mediterranean people have the B− variant that has extremely low enzyme activity (1% of normal).	**Increased in:** Young erythrocytes (reticulocytosis). **Decreased in:** G6PD deficiency.	In deficient patients, hemolytic anemia can be triggered by oxidant agents: antimalarial drugs (eg, chloroquine), nalidixic acid, nitrofurantoin, dapsone, phenacetin, vitamin C, and some sulfonamides. Any African-American about to be given an oxidant drug should be screened for G6PD deficiency. (Also screen people from certain Mediterranean areas: Greece, Italy, etc.) Hemolytic episodes can also occur in deficient patients who eat fava beans, in patients with diabetic acidosis, and in infections. G6PD deficiency may be the cause of hemolytic disease of newborns in Asians and Mediterraneans. Baillieres Best Pract Res Clin Hematol 2000;13:21. Mayo Clin Proc 2001;76:285.
Glutamine			
Glutamine, CSF Glass or plastic tube 6–15 mg/dL ***Panic:*** >40 mg/dL $$$	Glutamine is synthesized in the brain from ammonia and glutamic acid. Elevated CSF glutamine is associated with hepatic encephalopathy.	**Increased in:** Hepatic encephalopathy.	Test is not indicated if albumin, ALT, bilirubin, and alkaline phosphatase are normal or if there is no clinical evidence of liver disease. Hepatic encephalopathy is essentially ruled out if the CSF glutamine is normal. Arch Intern Med 1971;127:1033. Science 1974;183:81.

Glycohemoglobin		
Glycohemoglobin; glycated (glycosylated) hemoglobin, serum (HbA$_{1c}$) 3.9–6.9% (method-dependent) Lavender $$	During the life span of each red blood cell, glucose combines with hemoglobin to produce a stable glycated hemoglobin. The level of glycated hemoglobin is related to the mean plasma glucose level during the prior 1–3 months. There are three glycated A hemoglobins: HbA$_{1a}$, HbA$_{1b}$, and HbA$_{1c}$. Some assays quantitate HbA$_{1c}$, some quantitate total HbA$_1$, and some quantitate all glycated hemoglobins, not just A.	**Increased in:** Diabetes mellitus, splenectomy. Falsely high results can occur depending on the method used and may be due to presence of hemoglobin F or uremia. **Decreased in:** Any condition that shortens red cell life span (hemolytic anemias, congenital spherocytosis, acute or chronic blood loss, sickle cell disease, hemoglobinopathies).	Test is not currently recommended for diagnosis of diabetes mellitus, although it performs well. It is used to monitor long-term control of blood glucose level. Reference ranges are method-specific. Hemoglobin variants may interfere with HbA$_{1c}$ determinations. Development and progression of chronic complications of diabetes are related to the degree of altered glycemia. Measurement of HbA$_{1c}$ can improve metabolic control by leading to changes in diabetes treatment. Diabetes Care 1994;17:938. JAMA 1996;246:1246. Clin Chem 2001;47:1157. Diabetes Metab Res Rev 2001;17:94. Mayo Clin Proc 2001;76:1137.

Test/Range/Collection	Physiologic Basis	Interpretation	Comments
		Growth hormone	**Haptoglobin**
Growth hormone, serum (GH) 0–5 ng/mL [μg/L] Marbled $$$	Growth hormone is a single-chain polypeptide of 191 amino acids that induces the generation of somatomedins, which directly stimulate collagen and protein synthesis. GH levels are subject to wide fluctuations during the day.	**Increased in:** Acromegaly (90% have GH levels >10 ng/mL), Laron dwarfism (defective GH receptor), starvation. Drugs: dopamine, levodopa. **Decreased in:** Pituitary dwarfism, hypopituitarism.	Nonsuppressibility of GH levels to <2 ng/mL after 100 g oral glucose and elevation of IGF-1 levels are the two most sensitive tests for acromegaly. Random determinations of GH are rarely useful in the diagnosis of acromegaly. For the diagnosis of hypopituitarism or GH deficiency in children, an insulin hypoglycemia test has been used. Failure to increase GH levels to >5 ng/mL after insulin (0.1 unit/kg) is consistent with GH deficiency. Clin Endocrinol 1997;46:531. Lancet 1998;352:1455. Endocr Rev 2001;22:425. Horm Res 2001;55(Suppl 2):73. Horm Res 2001;55(Suppl 2):100.
Haptoglobin, serum 46–316 mg/dL [0.5–3.2 g/L] Marbled $$	Haptoglobin is a glycoprotein synthesized in the liver that binds free hemoglobin.	**Increased in:** Acute and chronic infection (acute phase reactant), malignancy, biliary obstruction, ulcerative colitis, myocardial infarction, and diabetes mellitus. **Decreased in:** Newborns and children, posttransfusion intravascular hemolysis, autoimmune hemolytic anemia, liver disease (10%). May be decreased following uneventful transfusion (10%) for unknown reasons.	Low haptoglobin is considered an indicator of hemolysis, but it is of uncertain clinical predictive value because of the greater prevalence of other conditions associated with low levels and because of occasional normal individuals who have very low levels. It thus has low specificity. High normal levels probably rule out significant intravascular hemolysis. Low haptoglobin levels aid in early recognition of hemolysis in the HELLP syndrome. Clin Chem 1987;33:1265. J Perinat Med 2000;28:249.

Helicobacter pylori antibody		
Helicobacter pylori antibody, serum Negative Marbled $$	*Helicobacter pylori* is a gram-negative spiral bacterium that is found on gastric mucosa. It induces acute and chronic inflammation in the gastric mucosa and a positive serologic antibody response. Serologic testing for *H pylori* antibody (IgG) is by ELISA.	**Increased (positive) in:** Histologic (chronic or chronic active) gastritis due to *H pylori* infection (with or without peptic ulcer disease). Sensitivity 98%, specificity 48%. Asymptomatic adults: 15–50%.	95% of patients with duodenal ulcers and >70% of patients with gastric ulcers have chronic infection with *H pylori* along with associated histologic gastritis. All patients with peptic ulcer disease and positive *H pylori* serology should be treated to eradicate *H pylori* infection. The prevalence of *H pylori*-positive serologic tests in asymptomatic adults is approximately 35% overall but is >50% in patients over age 60. Fewer than one in six adults with *H pylori* antibody develop peptic ulcer disease. Treatment of asymptomatic adults is not currently recommended. The role of *H pylori* in patients with chronic dyspepsia is controversial. There is currently no role for treatment of such patients except in clinical trials. After successful eradication, serologic titers fall over a 3- to 6-month period but remain positive in up to 50% of patients at 1 year. Gastroenterol Clin North Am 1993;22:105. Gut 1994;35:19. Ann Intern Med 1994;120:977. JAMA 1994;272:65. Can J Infect Dis 1998;9:277. J Clin Lab Anal 2001;15:301.

Test/Range/Collection	Physiologic Basis	Interpretation	Comments
Hematocrit, whole blood (Hct) Male: 39–49% Female: 35–45% (age dependent) Lavender $	The Hct represents the percentage of whole blood volume composed of erythrocytes. Laboratory instruments calculate the Hct from the erythrocyte count (RBC) and the mean corpuscular volume (MCV) by the formula: $$Hct = RBC \times MCV$$	**Increased in:** Hemoconcentration (as in dehydration, burns, vomiting), polycythemia, extreme physical exercise. **Decreased in:** Macrocytic anemia (liver disease, hypothyroidism, vitamin B_{12} deficiency, folate deficiency), normocytic anemia (early iron deficiency, anemia of chronic disease, hemolytic anemia, acute hemorrhage) and microcytic anemia (iron deficiency, thalassemia).	Conversion from hemoglobin (Hb) to hematocrit is roughly Hb × 3 = Hct. Hematocrit reported by clinical laboratories is not a spun hematocrit. The spun hematocrit may be spuriously high if the centrifuge is not calibrated, if the specimen is not spun to constant volume, or if there is "trapped plasma." In determining transfusion need, the clinical picture must be considered in addition to the hematocrit. Point-of-care instruments may not measure hematocrit accurately in all patients. In hemodialysis patients, maintaining a hematocrit in the range of 33–36% provides best outcomes in studies of hospitalizations and mortality. JAMA 1988;259:2433. Arch Pathol Lab Med 1994;118:429. Clin Chem 1995;41:306. Semin Nephrol 2000;20:345.

Hemoglobin A_2, whole blood (HbA_2) 1.5–3.5% of total hemoglobin (Hb) Lavender $$	HbA_2 is a minor component of normal adult hemoglobin (<3.5% of total Hb).	**Increased in:** β-Thalassemia major (HbA_2 levels 4–10% of total Hb), β-thalassemia minor (HbA_2 levels 4–8% of total Hb). **Decreased in:** Untreated iron deficiency, hemoglobin H disease.	Test is useful in the diagnosis of β-thalassemia minor (in absence of iron deficiency, which decreases HbA_2 and can mask the diagnosis). Quantitated by column chromatographic or automated HPLC techniques. Normal HbA_2 levels are seen in delta β-thalassemia or very mild β-thalassemias. Blood 1988;72:1107. J Clin Pathol 1993;46:852. Hematol Pathol 1994;8:25. Clin Chem 2000;46:1284. Semin Hematol 2001;38:343.	**Hemoglobin A_2**
Hemoglobin electrophoresis, whole blood HbA: > 95 HbA_2: 1.5–3.5% Lavender, blue, or green $$	Hemoglobin electrophoresis is used as a screening test. It is used to detect and differentiate hemoglobin variants. Separation of hemoglobins by electrophoresis is based on different rates of migration of charged hemoglobin molecules in an electric field.	↑HbS: HbA > HbS = sickle cell trait (HbAS) or sickle α-thalassemia; HbS and F, no HbA = sickle cell anemia (HbSS) or sickle β-thalassemia; HbS > HbA and F: sickle β+-thalassemia. ↑HbC: HbA > HbC = HbC trait (HbAC); HbC and F, no HbA = HbC disease; HbC > HbA = HbC β+-thalassemia. ↑HbH: HbH disease. ↑HbA_2, F: See HbA_2, above, and HbF, below.	Evaluation of a suspected hemoglobinopathy should include electrophoresis of a hemolysate to detect an abnormal hemoglobin and quantitation of hemoglobins A_2 and F. Automated HPLC instruments are proving to be useful alternative methods for hemoglobinopathy screening. Molecular diagnosis aids in genetic counseling of patients with thalassemia and combined hemoglobinopathies. Semin Perinatol 1990;14:483. Clin Chem 2000;46:1284.	**Hemoglobin electrophoresis**

	Hemoglobin, fetal		
Test/Range/Collection	Physiologic Basis	Interpretation	Comments
Hemoglobin, fetal, whole blood (HbF) Adult: <2% (varies with age) Lavender, blue, or green $$	Fetal hemoglobin constitutes about 75% of total hemoglobin at birth and declines to 50% at 6 weeks, 5% at 6 months, and <1.5% by 1 year. During the first year, adult hemoglobin (HbA) becomes the predominant hemoglobin.	**Increased in:** Hereditary disorders: eg, β-thalassemia major (60–100% of total Hb is HbF), β-thalassemia minor (2–5% HbF), HbE β-thalassemia (10–80%), sickle cell anemia (1–3% HbF), hereditary persistence of fetal hemoglobin (10–40% HbF). Acquired disorders <10% HbF): aplastic anemia, megaloblastic anemia, leukemia. **Decreased in:** Hemolytic anemia of the newborn.	Semiquantitative acid elution test provides an estimate of fetal hemoglobin only and varies widely between laboratories. It is useful in distinguishing hereditary persistence of fetal hemoglobin (all RBCs show an increase in fetal hemoglobin) from β-thalassemia minor (only a portion of RBCs are affected). Enzyme-linked antiglobulin test and flow cytometry are used to detect fetal red cells in the Rh(−) maternal circulation in suspected cases of Rh sensitization and to determine the amount of RhoGAM to administer (1 vial/15 mL fetal RBC). Prenatal diagnosis of hemoglobinopathies may be accomplished by quantitative hemoglobin levels by HPLC or molecular diagnostic techniques. Clin Chem 1992;38:1906. J Pediatr Hematol Oncol 2000;22:567. Clin Lab Med 2001;21:829.

	Hemoglobin, total	Hemosiderin
Hemoglobin, total, whole blood (Hb) Male: 13.6–17.5 Female: 12.0–15.5 g/dL (age-dependent) [Male: 136–175 Female: 120–155 g/L] ***Panic:*** ≤7 g/dL Lavender $	Hemoglobin is the major protein of erythrocytes and transports oxygen from the lungs to peripheral tissues. It is measured by spectrophotometry on automated instruments after hemolysis of red cells and conversion of all hemoglobin to cyanmethemoglobin.	Hemosiderin is a protein produced by the digestion of hemoglobin. Its presence in the urine indicates acute or chronic release of free hemoglobin into the circulation with accompanying depletion of the scavenging proteins, hemopexin and haptoglobin. Presence of hemosiderin usually indicates intravascular hemolysis or recent transfusion.
	Increased in: Hemoconcentration (as in dehydration, burns, vomiting), polycythemia, extreme physical exercise. **Decreased in:** Macrocytic anemia (liver disease, hypothyroidism, vitamin B$_{12}$ deficiency, folate deficiency), normocytic anemia (early iron deficiency, anemia of chronic disease, hemolytic anemia, acute hemorrhage), and microcytic anemia (iron deficiency, thalassemia).	**Increased in:** Intravascular hemolysis: hemolytic transfusion reactions, paroxysmal nocturnal hemoglobinuria, microangiopathic hemolytic anemia, mechanical destruction of erythrocytes (heart valve hemolysis), sickle cell anemia, thalassemia major, oxidant drugs with G6PD deficiency (eg, dapsone). Hemochromatosis.
Hemosiderin, urine Negative Urine container $$ Fresh, random sample.	Hypertriglyceridemia and very high white blood cell counts can cause false elevations of Hb. There is still controversy over the optimal target hemoglobin in patients with anemia due to chronic renal failure who are treated with erythropoietin. Recent studies suggest that patients developing anemia from cancer chemotherapy have better outcomes if treated with erythropoietin. JAMA 1988;259:2433. Lancet 2000;355:1169. Semin Nephrol 2000;20:382. Semin Oncol 2001;28(2 Suppl 8):49.	Hemosiderin can be qualitatively detected in urinary sediment using Prussian blue stain. Med Clin North Am 1992;76:649.

		Hepatitis A antibody	Hepatitis B surface antigen
Test/Range/Collection	**Physiologic Basis**	**Interpretation**	**Comments**
Hepatitis A antibody, serum (Anti-HAV) Negative Marbled $$	Hepatitis A is caused by a non-enveloped 27-nm RNA virus of the enterovirus-picornavirus group and is usually acquired by the fecal–oral route. IgM antibody is detectable within a week after symptoms develop and persists for 6 months. IgG appears 4 weeks later than IgM and persists for years (see Figure 10–4, p 412, for time course of serologic changes).	**Positive in:** Acute hepatitis A (IgM), convalescence from hepatitis A (IgG).	The most commonly used test for hepatitis A antibody is an immunoassay that detects total IgG and IgM antibodies. This test can be used to establish immune status. Specific IgM testing is necessary to diagnose acute hepatitis A. IgG antibody positivity is found in 40–50% of adults in the United States and Europe (higher rates in developing nations). Testing for anti-HAV (IgG) may reduce cost of HAV vaccination programs. Arch Intern Med 1994;154:663.
Hepatitis B surface antigen, serum (HBsAg) Negative Marbled $$	In hepatitis B virus infection, surface antigen is detectable 2–5 weeks before onset of symptoms, rises in titer, and peaks at about the time of onset of clinical illness. Generally it persists for 1–5 months, declining in titer and disappearing with resolution of clinical symptoms (see Figure 10–5, p 413, for time course of serologic changes).	**Increased in:** Acute hepatitis B, chronic hepatitis B (persistence of HBsAg for >6 months, positive HBcAb [total]). HBsAg-positive carriers. May be undetectable in acute hepatitis B infection. If clinical suspicion is high, HBcAb (IgM) test is then indicated.	First-line test for the diagnosis of acute or chronic hepatitis B. If positive, no other test is needed. HBeAg is a marker of extensive viral replication found only in HBsAg-positive sera. Persistently HBeAg-positive patients are more infectious than HBeAg-negative patients and more likely to develop chronic liver disease. Clin Microbiol Rev 1999;12:351. Semin Liver Dis 2000;20(Suppl 1):3. Postgrad Med J 2001;77:498. Hosp Med 2002;63:16.

Test/Range/Collection	Physiologic Basis	Interpretation	Comments
Hepatitis B surface antibody, serum (HBsAb, anti-HBs) Negative Marbled $$	Test detects antibodies to hepatitis B virus (HBV), which are thought to confer immunity to hepatitis B. Because several subtypes of hepatitis B exist, there is a possibility of subsequent infection with a second subtype.	**Increased in:** Hepatitis B immunity due to HBV infection or hepatitis B vaccination. **Absent in:** Hepatitis B carrier state, non-exposure.	**Hepatitis B surface antibody** Test indicates immune status. It is not useful for the evaluation of acute or chronic hepatitis. (See Figure 10–5, p 413, for time course of serologic changes.) Clin Microbiol Rev 1999;12:351. J Infect 2000;41:130.
Hepatitis B core antibody, total, serum (HBcAb, anti-HBc) Negative Marbled $$	HBcAb (IgG and IgM) will be positive (as IgM) about 2 months after exposure to hepatitis B. Its persistent positivity may reflect chronic hepatitis (IgM) or recovery (IgG). (See Figure 10–5, p 413, for time course of serologic changes.)	**Positive in:** Hepatitis B (acute and chronic), hepatitis B carriers (high levels), prior hepatitis B (immune) when IgG present in low titer with or without HBsAb. **Negative:** After hepatitis B vaccination.	**Hepatitis B core antibody** HBcAb (total) is useful in evaluation of acute or chronic hepatitis only if HBsAg is negative. An HBcAb (IgM) test is then indicated only if the HBcAb (total) is positive. HBcAb (IgM) may be the only serologic indication of acute HBV infection. Clin Microbiol Rev 1999;12:351. J Infect 2000;41:130.

	Hepatitis B e antigen		
Test/Range/Collection	Physiologic Basis	Interpretation	Comments
Hepatitis B e antigen/antibody (HBeAg/Ab), serum Negative Marbled $$	HBeAg is a soluble protein secreted by hepatitis B virus, related to HBcAg, indicating viral replication and infectivity. Two distinct serologic types of hepatitis B have been described, one with a positive HBeAg and the other with a negative HBeAg and a positive anti-HBe antibody.	**Increased (positive) in:** HBV (acute, chronic) hepatitis.	The assumption has been that loss of HBeAg and accumulation of HBeAb are associated with decreased infectivity. Testing has proved unreliable, and tests are not routinely needed as indicators of infectivity. All patients positive for HBsAg must be considered infectious. Anti-HBeAb is used to select patients for clinical trials of interferon therapy or liver transplantation. Proc Natl Acad Sci U S A 1991;88:4186. J Med Microbiol 1994;41:374. J Med Virol 2000;61:374. Cochrane Database Syst Rev 2002;2:CD000345.

Hepatitis C antibody		
Hepatitis C antibody, serum (HCAb) Negative Marbled $$	Detects antibody to hepatitis C virus. Current screening test (ELISA) detects antibodies to proteins expressed by putative structural (HC34) and nonstructural (HC31, C100-3) regions of the HCV genome. The presence of these antibodies indicates that the patient has been infected with HCV, and may be capable of transmitting HCV. A recombinant immunoblot assay (RIBA) is available as a confirmatory test.	**Increased in:** Acute hepatitis C (only 20–50%; seroconversion may take 6 months or more), posttransfusion chronic non-A, non-B hepatitis (70–90%), sporadic chronic non-A, non-B hepatitis (30–80%), blood donors (0.5–1%), non-blood-donating general public (2–3%), hemophiliacs (75%), intravenous drug abusers (40–80%), hemodialysis patients (1–30%), male homosexuals (4%).	Sensitivity of current assays is 86%, specificity 99.5%. Seropositivity for hepatitis C documents previous exposure, not necessarily acute infection. Seronegativity in acute hepatitis does not exclude the diagnosis of hepatitis C, especially in immunosuppressed patients. Testing of donor blood for hepatitis C has significantly reduced the incidence of posttransfusion hepatitis. Am Fam Physician 1999;59:79. Infect Dis Clin North Am 2000;14:633. Clin Liver Dis 2001;5:1105. Transfus Clin Biol 2001;8:200.

Test/Range/Collection	Physiologic Basis	Interpretation	Comments
Hepatitis D antibody, serum (anti-HDV) Negative Marbled $$	This antibody is a marker for acute or persisting infection with the delta agent, a defective RNA virus that can only infect HBsAg-positive patients. Hepatitis B virus (HBV) plus hepatitis D virus (HDV) infection may be more severe than HBV infection alone. Antibody to HDV ordinarily persists for about 6 months following acute infection. Further persistence indicates carrier status.	**Positive in:** Hepatitis D.	Test only indicated in HBsAg-positive patients. Chronic HDV hepatitis occurs in 80–90% of HBsAg carriers who are superinfected with delta, but in less than 5% of those who are co-infected with both viruses simultaneously. Ann Intern Med 1989;110:779. Crit Rev Clin Lab Sci 2000;37:45.
Heterophile aggluti-nation, serum (monospot, Paul-Bunnell test) Negative Marbled $	Infectious mononucleosis is an acute saliva-transmitted infectious disease due to the Epstein-Barr virus (EBV). Heterophile (Paul-Bunnell) antibodies (IgM) appear in 60% of mononucle-osis patients within 1–2 weeks and in 80–90% within the first month. They are not specific for EBV but are found only rarely in other disorders. Titers are substantially diminished by 3 months after primary infection and are not detectable by 6 months.	**Positive in:** Infectious mononucleosis (90–95%). **Negative in:** Heterophile-negative mononucleosis: CMV, heterophile-negative EBV, toxoplasmosis, hepatitis viruses, HIV-1 seroconversion, listerio-sis, tularemia, brucellosis, cat scratch disease, Lyme disease, syphilis, rick-ettsial infections, medications (phenytoin, sulfasalazine, dapsone), collagen-vascular diseases (especially lupus), subacute infective endocarditis.	The three classic signs of infectious mononucleosis are lymphocytosis, a "significant number" (>10–20%) of atypical lymphocytes on Wright-stained peripheral blood smear, and positive heterophile test. If heterophile test is negative in the setting of hematologic and clinical evidence of illness, a repeat test in 1–2 weeks may be positive. EBV serology (anti-VCA and anti-EBNA) may also be indicated, especially in children and teenage patients who may have negative heterophile tests (see EBV antibodies, p 82). Pediatrics 1985;75:1011. Clin Microbiol Rev 1988;1:300. Postgrad Med 2000;107:175. Clin Otolaryngol 2001:26:3.

Histoplasma capsulatum antigen			
***Histoplasma capsulatum* antigen,** urine, serum, CSF (HPA) Negative Marbled (serum) $$ Deliver urine, CSF in a clean plastic or glass container tube.	Heat-stable *H capsulatum* polysaccharide is detected by radioimmunoassay or ELISA using alkaline phosphatase or horseradish peroxidase-conjugated antibodies.	**Increased in:** Disseminated histoplasmosis (90–97% in urine, 50–78% in blood, and approximately 42% in CSF, localized disease (16% in urine), blastomycosis (urine and serum), coccidioidomycosis (CSF).	RIA for *H capsulatum* var *capsulatum* polysaccharide antigen in urine is a useful test in diagnosis of disseminated histoplasmosis and in assessing efficacy of treatment or in detecting relapse, especially in AIDS patients and when serologic tests for antibodies may be negative. Because the test has low sensitivity in localized pulmonary disease, it is not useful for ruling out localized pulmonary histoplasmosis. HPA in bronchoalveolar lavage fluid has 70% sensitivity for the diagnosis of pulmonary histoplasmosis. The antigenuria test's high sensitivity and specificity have dispelled the confusion in interpreting antibody test results. Am Rev Respir Dis 1999;145:1421. Semin Respir Infect 2001;16:131. J Antimicrob Chemother 2002;49(Suppl 1):11. Semin Respir Infect 2002;17:158.

Test/Range/Collection	Physiologic Basis	Interpretation	Comments
	Histoplasma capsulatum precipitins		
Histoplasma capsulatum precipitins, serum Negative Marbled $$	Histoplasmosis is the most common systemic fungal infection and typically starts as a pulmonary infection with influenza-like symptoms. This may heal, progress, or lie dormant with reinfection occurring at a later time. This test screens for presence of histoplasma antibody by detecting precipitin "H" and "M" bands. Positive H band indicates active infection; M band indicates acute or chronic infection or prior skin testing. Presence of both suggests active histoplasmosis.	**Positive in:** Previous, chronic, or acute histoplasma infection, recent histoplasmin skin testing. Cross-reactions at low levels in patients with blastomycosis and coccidioidomycosis.	Histoplasmosis is usually seen in the Mississippi and Ohio River valleys but may appear elsewhere. Test is useful as a screening test or as an adjunct to complement fixation test (see below) in diagnosis of systemic histoplasmosis. Rose NR et al (editors): *Manual of Clinical Laboratory Immunology*, 6th ed. American Society for Microbiology, 2002.
	Histoplasma capsulatum CF antibody		
Histoplasma capsulatum complement fixation (CF) antibody, serum <1:4 titer Marbled $$ Submit paired sera, one specimen collected within 1 week after onset of illness and another 2 weeks later.	Quantitates level of histoplasma antibody. Antibodies in primary pulmonary infections are generally found within 4 weeks after exposure and frequently are present at the time symptoms appear. Two types of CF test are available based on mycelial antigen and yeast phase antigen. The yeast phase test is considerably more sensitive. Latex agglutination (LA) and ELISA tests are also available but are less reliable.	**Increased in:** Previous, chronic, or acute histoplasma infection (75–80%), recent histoplasmin skin testing (20%), other fungal disease, leishmaniasis. Cross-reactions in patients with blastomycosis and coccidioidomycosis.	Elevated CF titers of >1:16 are suggestive of infection. Titers of >1:32 or rising titers are usually indicative of active infection. Histoplasmin skin test is not recommended for diagnosis because it interferes with subsequent serologic tests. About 3.5–12% of clinically normal persons have positive titers, usually less than 1:16. Hosp Pract (Off Ed) Feb 1991;26:41. Rose NR et al (editors): *Manual of Clinical Laboratory Immunology*, 6th ed. American Society for Microbiology, 2002.

		HIV antibody	
HIV antibody, serum Negative Marbled $$	This test detects antibody against the human immunodeficiency virus-1 (HIV-1), the etiologic agent of AIDS. HIV antibody test is considered positive only when a repeatedly reactive enzyme immunoassay (EIA) is confirmed by a Western blot analysis or immunofluorescent antibody test (IFA).	**Positive in:** HIV infection: EIA sensitivity >99% after first 2–4 months of infection, specificity 99%. When combined with confirmatory test, specificity is 99.995%.	A positive p24 antigen test in an HIV antibody-negative individual must be confirmed by a viral neutralization assay. While Western blot test is currently the most sensitive and specific assay for HIV serodiagnosis, it is highly dependent on the proficiency of the laboratory performing the test and on the standardization of the procedure. The CDC recommends that all pregnant women be offered HIV testing. Ann Intern Med 1987;106:671. Arch Pathol Lab Med 1989;113:975. JAMA 1991;266:2861. Infect Dis Clin North Am 1993;7:203. Arch Fam Med 2000;9:924.

		HLA typing	
HLA typing, serum and blood (HLA) Marbled (2 mL) and Yellow (40 mL) $$$$ Specimens must be <24 hours old. Refrigerate serum, but not blood in yellow tubes.	The human leukocyte antigen (HLA) system consists of four closely linked loci (HLA-A, -B, -C, and -DR) located on the short arm of chromosome 6. The traditional technique for HLA typing was the microlymphocyte toxicity test. This is a complement-mediated serologic assay in which antiserum containing specific anti-HLA antibodies is added to peripheral blood lymphocytes. Cell death indicates that the lymphocytes carried the specific targeted antigen.	**Useful in:** Evaluation of transplant candidates and potential donors and for paternity and forensic testing.	While diseases associated with particular HLA antigens have been identified, HLA typing for the diagnosis of these diseases is not generally indicated. DNA-based typing methods have now replaced traditional HLA testing based on serologic assays. Cell.1984:36:1. Curr Opin Nephrol Hypertens 2000;9:683. Hum Immunol 2000;61:92. Semin Hematol 2001;38:194. Arch Pathol Lab Med 2002;126:281.

Test/Range/Collection	Physiologic Basis	Interpretation	Comments
	HLA-B27 typing		
HLA-B27 typing, whole blood Negative Yellow $$$ Specimens must be <24 hours old.	The HLA-B27 allele is found in approximately 8% of the US white population. It occurs less frequently in the African-American population.	There is an increased incidence of spondyloarthritis among patients who are HLA-B27–positive. HLA-B27 is present in 88% of patients with ankylosing spondylitis. It is also associated with the development of Reiter syndrome (80%) following infection with *Shigella* or *Salmonella*.	The best diagnostic test for ankylosing spondylitis is a lumbar spine film and not HLA-B27 typing. HLA-B27 testing is not usually clinically indicated. Br J Rheumatol 1987;36:185. Curr Opin Rheumatol 2001;13:265. Ann Intern Med 2002;136:896. Rheumatology (Oxford) 2002;41:857.
	5-Hydroxyindoleacetic acid		
5-Hydroxy-indoleacetic acid, urine (5-HIAA) 2–8 mg/24 h [10–40 μmol/d] Urine bottle containing hydrochloric acid $$	Serotonin (5-hydroxytryptamine) is a neurotransmitter that is metabolized by monoamine oxidase (MAO) to 5-HIAA and then excreted into the urine. Serotonin is secreted by most carcinoid tumors, which arise from neuroendocrine cells in locations derived from the embryonic gut.	**Increased in:** Metastatic carcinoid tumor (foregut, midgut, and bronchial). Nontropical sprue (slight increase). Diet of bananas, walnuts, avocado, eggplant, pineapple, plums. Drugs: reserpine. **Negative in:** Rectal carcinoids (usually). MAO inhibitors, phenothiazines. Test is often falsely positive because pretest probability is low. Using 5-HIAA/Cr ratio may improve performance.	Because most carcinoid tumors drain into the portal vein and serotonin is rapidly cleared by the liver, the carcinoid syndrome (flushing, bronchial constriction, diarrhea, hypotension, and cardiac valvular lesions) is a late manifestation of carcinoid tumors, appearing only after hepatic metastasis has occurred. Endocrinol Metab Clin North Am 1993;22:823. Clin Chem 1994;40:86. Ann Clin Lab Sci 1998;28:167. Can J Surg 2001;44:25. Med Sci Monit 2001;7:746.

	IgG index	Immunoelectrophoresis
IgG index, serum and CSF 0.29–0.59 ratio Marbled (for serum) and glass/plastic tube (for CSF) $$$ Collect serum and CSF simultaneously.	This test compares CSF IgG and albumin levels to serum levels. An increased ratio allegedly reflects synthesis of IgG within the central nervous system.	**Increased in:** Multiple sclerosis (80–90%), neurosyphilis, subacute sclerosing panencephalitis, other inflammatory and infectious CNS diseases.	Test is reasonably sensitive but not specific for multiple sclerosis. (Compare with Oligoclonal bands, p 135.) J Clin Pathol 1996;49:24. Electromyogr Clin Neurophysiol 2001;41:117. J Neuroimmunol 2002;125:149.
Immunoelectrophoresis, serum (IEP) Negative Marbled $$$	Immunoelectrophoresis is used to identify specific immunoglobulin (Ig) classes. Serum is separated electrophoretically and reacted with antisera of known specificity. Newer technique (immunofixation) is available and easier to interpret.	**Positive in:** Presence of identifiable monoclonal paraprotein: multiple myeloma, Waldenström macroglobulinemia, Franklin disease (heavy chain disease), lymphoma, leukemia, monoclonal gammopathy of undetermined significance. The most common form of myeloma is the IgG type.	Test is indicated to identify an Ig spike seen on serum protein electrophoresis, to differentiate a polyclonal from a monoclonal increase, and to identify the nature of a monoclonal increase. Test is not quantitative and is not sensitive enough to use for the evaluation of immunodeficiency. Order quantitative immunoglobulins for this purpose (see below). Hematol Oncol Clin North Am 1997;11:71. Arch Pathol Lab Med 1999;123:114. Arch Pathol Lab Med 1999;123:126. Clin Chim Acta 2000;302:105.

	Immunoglobulins		
Test/Range/Collection	**Physiologic Basis**	**Interpretation**	**Comments**
Immunoglobulins, serum (Ig) IgA: 78–367 mg/dL IgG: 583–1761 mg/dL IgM: 52–335 mg/dL [IgA: 0.78–3.67 g/L IgG: 5.83–17.6 g/L IgM: 0.52–3.35 g/L] Marbled $$$	IgG makes up about 85% of total serum immunoglobulins and predominates late in immune responses. It is the only immunoglobulin to cross the placenta. IgM antibody predominates early in immune responses. Secretory IgA plays an important role in host defense mechanisms by blocking transport of microbes across mucosal surfaces.	↑**IgG:** *Polyclonal:* Autoimmune diseases (eg, SLE, rheumatoid arthritis), sarcoidosis, chronic liver diseases, some parasitic diseases, chronic or recurrent infections. *Monoclonal:* Multiple myeloma (IgG type), lymphomas, or other malignancies. ↑**IgM:** *Polyclonal:* Isolated infections such as viral hepatitis, infectious mononucleosis, early response to bacterial or parasitic infection. *Monoclonal:* Waldenström macroglobulinemia, lymphoma. ↑**IgA:** *Polyclonal:* Chronic liver disease, chronic infections (especially of the GI and respiratory tracts). *Monoclonal:* Multiple myeloma (IgA). ↓ **IgG:** Immunosuppressive therapy, genetic (SCID, Wiskott-Aldrich syndrome, common variable immunodeficiency). ↓ **IgM:** Immunosuppressive therapy. ↓ **IgA:** Inherited IgA deficiency (ataxia-telangiectasia, combined immunodeficiency disorders).	Quantitative immunoglobulin levels are indicated in the evaluation of immunodeficiency or the quantitation of a paraprotein. IgG deficiency is associated with recurrent and occasionally severe pyogenic infections. The most common form of multiple myeloma is the IgG type. Hematol Oncol Clin North Am 1997;11:71. Am Fam Physician 1999;5:1885. Aust N Z J Med 1999;29:500. Clin Chem 2000;46:1230.

Inhibitor screen, plasma Negative Blue $$ Fill tube completely.	Test is useful for evaluating a prolonged PTT, PT, or thrombin time. (Presence of heparin should first be excluded.) Patient's plasma is mixed with normal plasma and a PTT is performed. If the patient has a factor deficiency, the postmixing PTT will be normal. If an inhibitor is present, it will be prolonged.	**Positive in:** Presence of inhibitor: Antiphospholipid antibodies (lupus anticoagulant [LAC] or anticardiolipin antibodies), factor-specific antibodies. **Negative in:** Factor deficiencies.	LAC prolongs PTT immediately and is the most common inhibitor. Poor sensitivity for lupus anticoagulant owing to relatively high phospholipid levels in this assay system. 1–4 hour incubation period may be needed to detect factor-specific antibodies with low in vitro affinities. About 15% of hemophilia A patients develop inhibitor against factor VIII. Semin Thromb Hemost 1994;20:79. Thromb Haemost 1996;16:146.	**Inhibitor screen**
Insulin antibody, serum Negative Marbled $$$	Insulin antibodies develop in nearly all diabetics treated with insulin. Most antibodies are IgG and do not cause clinical problems. Occasionally, high-affinity antibodies can bind to exogenous insulin and cause insulin resistance.	**Increased in:** Insulin therapy, type I diabetics before treatment (secondary to autoimmune pancreatic B cell destruction).	Insulin antibodies interfere with most assays for insulin. Insulin antibody test is not sensitive or specific for the detection of surreptitious insulin use; use C-peptide level (see p 59). Anti-insulin and islet cell antibodies are poor predictors of IDDM and only roughly correlate with insulin requirements in patients with diabetes. Diabetes 1996;45:1720. Diabetes Care 1996;19:146. Autoimmunity 2000;32:17.	**Insulin antibody**

Test/Range/Collection	Physiologic Basis	Interpretation	Comments
Insulin, immuno- reactive, serum 6–35 μU/mL [42–243 pmol/L] Marbled $$ Fasting sample required. Measure glucose concurrently.	Measures levels of insulin, either endogenous or exogenous.	**Increased in:** Insulin-resistant states (eg, obesity, type II diabetes mellitus, uremia, glucocorticoids, acromegaly), liver disease, surreptitious use of insulin or oral hypoglycemic agents, insulinoma (pancreatic islet cell tumor). **Decreased in:** Type I diabetes mellitus, hypopituitarism.	Measurement of serum insulin level has little clinical value except in the diagnosis of fasting hypoglycemia. An insulin-to-glucose ratio of >0.3 is presumptive evidence of insulinoma. C-peptide should be used as well as serum insulin to distinguish insulinoma from surreptitious insulin use, since C-peptide will be absent with exoge- nous insulin use (see C-peptide, p 59). J Clin Endocrinol Metab 2000;85:3222. Eur J Endocrinol 1998;138:86.
Iron, serum (Fe^{2+}) 50–175 μg/dL [9–31 μmol/L] Marbled $ Avoid hemolysis.	Plasma iron concentration is deter- mined by absorption from the intes- tine; storage in the liver, spleen, bone marrow; rate of break- down or loss of hemoglobin; and rate of synthesis of new hemoglobin.	**Increased in:** Hemosiderosis (eg, multi- ple transfusions, excess iron adminis- tration), hemolytic anemia, pernicious anemia, aplastic or hypoplastic anemia, viral hepatitis, lead poisoning, tha- lassemia, hemochromatosis. Drugs: estrogens, ethanol, oral contraceptives. **Decreased in:** Iron deficiency, nephrotic syndrome, chronic renal failure, many infections, active hematopoiesis, remis- sion of pernicious anemia, hypo- thyroidism, malignancy (carcinoma), postoperative state, kwashiorkor.	Absence of stainable iron on bone mar- row aspirate differentiates iron defi- ciency from other causes of microcytic anemia (eg, thalassemia, sideroblastic anemia, some chronic disease ane- mias), but the procedure is invasive and expensive. Serum iron, iron-binding capacity, and transferrin saturation—or serum ferritin—may obviate the need for bone marrow examination. Serum iron, iron-binding capacity, and transferrin saturation are useful (see p 117) in screening family members for hereditary hemochromatosis. Recent transfusion will confound the test results. Kidney Int 2001;60:300. Med Sci Monit 2001;7:962. Am Fam Physician 2002;65:853. Eur J Gastroenterol Hepatol 2002;14:217.

Test/Specimen/Cost	Description	Increased/Decreased in	Comments / References
Iron-binding capacity, total (TIBC), serum 250–460 µg/dL [45–82 µmol/L] Marbled $$	Iron is transported in plasma complexed to transferrin, which is synthesized in the liver. Total iron-binding capacity is calculated from transferrin levels measured immunologically. Each molecule of transferrin has two iron-binding sites, so its iron-binding capacity is 1.47 mg/g. Normally, transferrin carries an amount of iron representing about 16–60% of its capacity to bind iron (ie, % saturation of iron-binding capacity is 16–60%).	**Increased in:** Iron deficiency anemia, late pregnancy, infancy, hepatitis. Drugs: oral contraceptives. **Decreased in:** Hypoproteinemic states (eg, nephrotic syndrome, starvation, malnutrition, cancer), hyperthyroidism, chronic inflammatory disorders, chronic liver disease, other chronic disease.	Increased % transferrin saturation with iron is seen in iron overload (iron poisoning, hemolytic anemia, sideroblastic anemia, thalassemia, hemochromatosis, pyridoxine deficiency, aplastic anemia). Decreased % transferrin saturation with iron is seen in iron deficiency (usually saturation <16%). Transferrin levels can also be used to assess nutritional status. Recent transfusion will confound the test results. Kidney Int 2001;60:300. Med Sci Monit 2001;7:962.
Lactate dehydrogenase (LDH), serum 88–230 U/L [1.46–3.82 µkat/L] (laboratory-specific) Marbled $ Hemolyzed specimens are unacceptable.	LDH is an enzyme that catalyzes the interconversion of lactate and pyruvate in the presence of NAD/NADH. It is widely distributed in body cells and fluids. Because LDH is highly concentrated in red blood cells (RBCs), spuriously elevated serum levels will occur if RBCs are hemolyzed during specimen collection.	**Increased in:** Tissue necrosis, especially in acute injury of cardiac muscle, RBCs, kidney, skeletal muscle, liver, lung, or skin. Commonly elevated in various carcinomas and in *Pneumocystis carinii* pneumonia (78–94%) and lymphoma in AIDS. Marked elevations occur in hemolytic anemias, vitamin B_{12} deficiency anemia, folate deficiency anemia, polycythemia vera, thrombotic thrombocytopenic purpura (TTP), hepatitis, cirrhosis, obstructive jaundice, renal disease, musculoskeletal disease, CHF. Drugs causing hepatotoxicity (eg, acetaminophen) or hemolysis. **Decreased in:** Drugs: clofibrate, fluoride (low dose).	LDH is elevated after myocardial infarction (for 2–7 days), in liver congestion (eg, in CHF), and in *P carinii* pneumonia. LDH is not a useful liver function test, and it is not specific enough for the diagnosis of hemolytic or megaloblastic anemias. Its main diagnostic use has been in myocardial infarction, when the creatine kinase-MB elevation has passed (see CK-MB, p 76, and Figure 10–7, p 415). LDH isoenzymes are preferred over total serum LDH in late diagnosis of MI, but both tests are now being replaced by cardiac troponin I levels. Am J Clin Oncol 2001;24:547. Eur J Gynaecol 2001;22:228. Leuk Res 2001;25:287. Acta Oncol 2002;41:77.

Test/Range/Collection	Physiologic Basis	Interpretation	Comments
Lactate dehydrogenase isoenzymes, serum (LDH isoenzymes) LDH_1/LDH_2: <0.85 Marbled $$ Hemolyzed specimens are unacceptable.	LDH consists of five isoenzymes separable by electrophoresis. The fraction with the greatest electrophoretic mobility is called LDH_1; the one with the least, LDH_5. LDH_1 is found in high concentrations in heart muscle, RBCs, and kidney cortex; LDH_5 in skeletal muscle and liver.	**Increased in:** LDH_1/LDH_2 >0.85 in myocardial infarction, hemolysis (hemolytic or megaloblastic anemia) or acute renal infarction. LDH_5 is increased in liver disease, congestive heart failure, skeletal muscle injury, and essential thrombocythemia.	The only clinical indication for LDH isoenzyme measurement has been to rule out myocardial infarction in patients presenting more than 24 hours after onset of symptoms (LDH_1/LDH_2 >0.85 is usually present within 12–48 hours). It may also be helpful if CK-MB results cannot be easily interpreted. The test is being replaced by measurement of cardiac troponin I (see CK-MB, p 76). Arch Intern Med 1997;157:1441.
Lactate, venous blood 0.5–2.0 meq/L [mmol/L] Gray $$ Collect on ice in gray-top tube containing fluoride to inhibit in vitro glycolysis and lactic acid production.	Severe tissue anoxia leads to anaerobic glucose metabolism with production of lactic acid.	**Increased in:** Lactic acidosis, ethanol ingestion, sepsis, shock, liver disease, diabetic ketoacidosis, muscular exercise, hypoxia; regional hypoperfusion (bowel ischemia); prolonged use of a tourniquet (spurious elevation); type I glycogen storage disease, fructose 1,6-diphosphatase deficiency (rare), pyruvate dehydrogenase deficiency. **Drugs:** phenformin, metformin, isoniazid toxicity.	Lactic acidosis should be suspected when there is a markedly increased anion gap (>18 meq/L) in the absence of other causes (eg, renal failure, ketosis, ethanol, methanol, or salicylate). Lactic acidosis is characterized by lactate levels >5 mmol/L in association with metabolic acidosis. Tissue hypoperfusion is the most common cause. Blood lactate levels may indicate whether perfusion is being restored by therapy. J Am Coll Surg 2000;190:656. AIDS 2001;15:717. BJOG 2001;108:263. Clin Infect Dis 2001;33:1914. Curr Opin Infect Dis 2002;15:23.

	Lead	Lecithin/sphingomyelin ratio
Lead, whole blood (Pb) Child (<6 yrs): <10μg/dL Child (>6 yrs): <25 μg/dL Adult: <40 μg/dL [Child (<6): <0.48 μmol/L Child (>6): <1.21 μmol/L Adult: <1.93 μmol/L] Navy $$ Use trace metal-free navy blue top tube with heparin.	Lead salts are absorbed through ingestion, inhalation, or the skin. About 5–10% of ingested lead is found in blood, and 95% of this is in erythrocytes. 80–90% is taken up by bone, where it is relatively inactive. Lead poisons enzymes by binding to protein disulfide groups, leading to cell death. Lead levels fluctuate. Several specimens may be needed to rule out lead poisoning.	**Increased in:** Lead poisoning, including abnormal ingestion (especially lead-containing paint, moonshine whiskey), occupational exposures (metal smelters, miners, welders, storage battery workers, auto manufacturers, ship builders, paint manufacturers, printing workers, pottery workers, gasoline refinery workers), retained bullets.	Subtle neurologic impairment may be detectable in children with lead levels of 15 μg/dL and in adults at 30 μg/dL; full-blown symptoms appear at >60 μg/dL. Most chronic lead poisoning leads to a moderate anemia with basophilic stippling of erythrocytes on peripheral blood smear. Acute poisoning is rare and associated with abdominal pain and constipation. Blood lead levels are useful in the diagnosis. Industrial workers' limit: <50 μg/dL. Ann Intern Med 1999;130:7. Ambul Pediatr 2001;1:256. Arch Environ Health 2001;56:312.
Lecithin/sphingomyelin ratio, amniotic fluid (L/S ratio) >2.0 (method-dependent) $$$ Collect in a plastic tube.	This test is used to estimate lung maturity in fetuses at risk for hyaline membrane disease. As fetal pulmonary surfactant matures, there is a rapid rise in amniotic fluid lecithin content. To circumvent the dependency of lecithin concentrations on amniotic fluid volume and analytic recovery of lecithin, the assay examines the lecithin/sphingomyelin ratio.	**Increased in:** Contamination of amniotic fluid by blood, meconium, or vaginal secretions that contain lecithin (false-positives). **Decreased in:** Fetal lung immaturity; 95% of normal fetuses.	Test identifies fetal lung maturity effectively only 60% of the time: ie, 40% of fetuses with an L/S ratio of <2.0 will not develop hyaline membrane disease. Precision of L/S ratio test is poor: results on a single sample may vary by ±25%. Test is not reliable to assess fetal lung maturity in offspring of diabetic mothers. Clin Chem 1994;40:541. Am J Obstet Gynecol 1998;179;1640. J Perinatol 2002;22:21.

Test/Range/Collection	Physiologic Basis	Interpretation	Comments
	***Legionella* antibody**		**Leukocyte alkaline phosphatase**
Legionella antibody, serum <1:32 titer Marbled $$$ Submit paired sera, one collected within 2 weeks of illness and another 2–3 weeks later.	*Legionella pneumophila* is a weakly staining gram-negative bacillus that causes Pontiac fever (acute influenza-like illness) and Legionnaire's disease (a pneumonia that may progress to a severe multisystem illness). It does not grow on routine bacteriologic culture media. Antibodies are detected by indirect immunofluorescent tests to serogroup 1 of *L pneumophila*. There are at least six serogroups of *L pneumophila* and at least 22 species of *Legionella*.	**Increased in:** Legionella infection (80% of patients with pneumonia have a fourfold rise in titer); cross-reactions with other infectious agents (*Yersinia pestis* [plague], *Francisella tularensis* [tularemia], *Bacteroides fragilis, Mycoplasma pneumoniae, Leptospira interrogans,* campylobacter serotypes).	A greater than fourfold rise in titer to >1:128 in specimens gathered more than 3 weeks apart indicates recent infection. A single titer of >1:256 is considered diagnostic. About 50–60% of cases of legionellosis may have a positive direct fluorescent antibody test. Culture can have a sensitivity of 50%. All three methods may increase sensitivity to 90%. This test is species-specific. Polyvalent antiserum is needed to test for all serogroups and species. Clin Infect Dis 1996;23:656. Curr Opin Infect Dis 2001;14:443.
Leukocyte alkaline phosphatase, whole blood (LAP) 40–130 Based on 0–4+ rating of 100 PMNs Green $$ Blood smear from finger stick preferred. If collecting venous blood, make smear as soon as possible.	The test measures the amount of alkaline phosphatase in neutrophils in a semiquantitative fashion. Neutrophilic leukocytes on a peripheral blood smear are stained for alkaline phosphatase activity and then scored on a scale from 0 to 4+ on the basis of the intensity of the dye in their cytoplasm.	**Increased in:** Leukemoid reaction (eg, severe infections), polycythemia vera, myelofibrosis with myeloid metaplasia. **Decreased in:** Chronic myeloid leukemia, paroxysmal nocturnal hemoglobinuria, hypophosphatasia.	Test may be helpful for distinguishing leukemoid reactions (high-normal or increased LAP) from chronic myeloid leukemia (decreased LAP), but it is poorly reproducible. Br J Haematol 1997;96:815. Clin Chim Acta 2000;302:49. J Cancer Res Clin Oncol 2000;126:425.

	Leukocyte count, total	Lipase
Test / Specimen	Leukocyte (white blood cell) count, total, whole blood (WBC count) $3.4-10 \times 10^3/\mu L$ $[\times 10^9/L]$ *Panic:* $<1.5 \times 10^3/\mu L$ Lavender $	Lipase, serum 0–160 U/L $[0-2.66\ \mu kat/L]$ (laboratory-specific) Marbled $$
Description	Measure of the total number of leukocytes in whole blood. Counted on automated instruments using light scattering or electrical impedance after lysis of red blood cells. WBCs are distinguished from platelets by size.	Lipases are responsible for hydrolysis of glycerol esters of long-chain fatty acids to produce fatty acids and glycerol. Lipases are produced in the liver, intestine, tongue, stomach, and many other cells. Assays are highly dependent on the substrate used.
Clinical significance	**Increased in:** Infection, inflammation, hematologic malignancy, leukemia, lymphoma. Drugs: corticosteroids. **Decreased in:** Aplastic anemia (decreased production), B$_{12}$ or folate deficiency (maturation defect), sepsis (decreased survival). Drugs: phenothiazines, chloramphenicol, aminopyrine.	**Increased in:** Acute, recurrent, or chronic pancreatitis, pancreatic pseudocyst, pancreatic malignancy, peritonitis, biliary disease, hepatic disease, diabetes mellitus (especially diabetic ketoacidosis), intestinal disease, gastric malignancy or perforation, cystic fibrosis, inflammatory bowel disease (Crohn disease and ulcerative colitis).
Comments	A spurious increase may be seen when there are a large number of nucleated red cells. WBC count is a poor predictor of severity of disease in the diagnosis of appendicitis. Lab Med 1983;14:509. J Clin Pathol 1996;49:664. Am Surg 1998;64:983.	The sensitivity of lipase in acute pancreatitis is similar to that of amylase; lipase remains elevated longer than amylase. The specificity of lipase and amylase in acute pancreatitis is similar, though both are poor. Test sensitivity is not very good for chronic pancreatitis or pancreatic cancer. Lipase to amylase ratio is not useful in distinguishing alcoholic from non-alcoholic pancreatitis. Clin Chem Lab Med 2000;38:1141. AUST N Z J Surg 2001;71:577. J Clin Gastroenterol 2002;34:459.

	Luteinizing hormone	Lyme disease antibody
Comments	Intact human chorionic gonadotropin (hCG) cross-reacts with LH in most immunoassays so that LH levels appear to be falsely elevated in pregnancy or in individuals with hCG-secreting tumors. Repeated measurement may be required to diagnose gonadotropin deficiencies. Measurement of total testosterone is the test of choice to diagnose polycystic ovary syndrome. Gynecol Endocrinol 2000;14:392. Psychoneuroendocrinology 2001;26:721. Reproduction 2001;121:761.	Test is less sensitive in patients with only a rash. Because culture or direct visualization of the organism is difficult, serologic diagnosis (by ELISA) is indicated, although sensitivity and specificity and standardization of procedure between laboratories need improvement. Cross-reactions may occur with syphilis (should be excluded by RPR and treponemal antibody assays). Arch Intern Med 2001;161:2015. Clin Infect Dis 2001;33:2023. Expert Rev Mol Diagn 2001;1:413. Med Clin North Am 2002;86:311.
Interpretation	**Increased in:** Primary hypogonadism, polycystic ovary syndrome, postmenopause, endometriosis, after depot leuprolide injection. **Decreased in:** Pituitary or hypothalamic failure, anorexia nervosa, bulimia, advanced prostate cancer, severe stress, malnutrition, Kallmann syndrome (gonadotropin deficiency associated with anosmia). Drugs: digoxin, oral contraceptives, phenothiazines.	**Positive in:** Lyme disease, asymptomatic individuals living in endemic areas, immunization with recombinant OspA Lyme disease vaccine, syphilis (*Treponema pallidum*), tick-borne relapsing fever (*Borrelia hermsii*). **Negative** during the first 5 weeks of infection or after antibiotic therapy.
Physiologic Basis	LH is stimulated by the hypothalamic hormone gonadotropin-releasing hormone (GnRH). It is secreted from the anterior pituitary and acts on the gonads. LH is the principal regulator of steroid biosynthesis in the ovary and testis.	Test detects the presence of antibody to *Borrelia burgdorferi*, the etiologic agent in Lyme disease, an inflammatory disorder transmitted by the ticks *Ixodes dammini*, *I pacificus*, and *I scapularis* in the northeastern and midwestern, western, and southeastern United States, respectively. Detects IgM antibody, which develops within 3–6 weeks after the onset of rash or IgG, which develops within 6–8 weeks after the onset of disease. IgG antibody may persist for months.
Test/Range/Collection	**Luteinizing hormone, serum** (LH) Male: 1–10 mIU/mL Female: (mIU/mL) Follicular 1–18 Luteal 0.4–20 Midcycle peak 24–105 Postmenopausal 15–62 (laboratory-specific) Marbled $$	**Lyme disease antibody, serum** ELISA: negative (<1 : 8 titer) Western blot: nonreactive Marbled $

Common Laboratory Tests: Selection and Interpretation

Test / Specimen	Physiologic Basis	Interpretation	Comments
Magnesium, serum (Mg^{2+}) 1.8–3.0 mg/dL [0.75–1.25 mmol/L] *Panic:* <0.5 or >4.5 mg/dL Marbled $	Magnesium is primarily an intracellular cation (second most abundant, 60% found in bone); it is a necessary cofactor in numerous enzyme systems, particularly ATPases. In extracellular fluid, it influences neuromuscular response and irritability. Magnesium concentration is determined by intestinal absorption, renal excretion, and exchange with bone and intracellular fluid.	**Increased in:** Dehydration, tissue trauma, renal failure, hypoadrenocorticism, hypothyroidism. Drugs: aspirin (prolonged use), lithium, magnesium salts, progesterone, triamterene. **Decreased in:** Chronic diarrhea, enteric fistula, starvation, enteric alcoholism, total parenteral nutrition with inadequate replacement, hypoparathyroidism (especially post parathyroid surgery), acute pancreatitis, chronic glomerulonephritis, hyperaldosteronism, diabetic ketoacidosis, CHF, critical illness, Gitelman syndrome (familial hypokalemia–hypomagnesemia–hypocalciuria), hereditary isolated magnesium wasting, induced hypothermia. Drugs: albuterol, amphotericin B, calcium salts, cisplatin, citrates (blood transfusion), cyclosporine, diuretics, ethacrynic acid.	Hypomagnesemia is associated with tetany, weakness, disorientation, and somnolence. A magnesium deficit may exist with little or no apparent change in serum level. There is a progressive reduction in serum magnesium level during normal pregnancy (related to hemodilution). J Nephrol 2001;14:43. Eur J Heart Fail 2002;4:167.
Mean corpuscular hemoglobin, blood (MCH) 26–34 pg Lavender $	MCH indicates the amount of hemoglobin per red blood cell in absolute units. Low MCH can mean hypochromia or microcytosis or both. High MCH is evidence of macrocytosis.	**Increased in:** Macrocytosis, hemochromatosis. **Decreased in:** Microcytosis (iron deficiency, thalassemia), hypochromia (lead poisoning, sideroblastic anemia, anemia of chronic disease).	MCH is calculated from measured values of hemoglobin (Hb) and red cell count (RBC) by the formula: $$MCH = \frac{Hb}{RBC}$$ Obstet Gynecol 1999;93:427. Genet Test 2000;4:103.

Test/Range/Collection	Physiologic Basis	Interpretation	Comments
Mean corpuscular hemoglobin concentration			
Mean corpuscular hemoglobin concentration, blood (MCHC) 31–36 g/dL [310–360 g/L] Lavender $	MCHC describes how fully the erythrocyte volume is filled with hemoglobin and is calculated from measurement of Hb, mean corpuscular volume (MCV), and RBC by the formula: $$MCHC = \dfrac{Hb}{MCV \times RBC}$$	**Increased in:** Marked spherocytosis. Spuriously increased in autoagglutination, hemolysis (with spuriously high Hb or low MCV or RBC), lipemia, cellular dehydration syndromes, xerocytosis. **Decreased in:** Hypochromic anemia (iron deficiency, thalassemia, lead poisoning), sideroblastic anemia, anemia of chronic disease. Spuriously decreased with high white blood cell count, low Hb, or high MCV or RBC.	Lab Med 1983;14:509.

Mean corpuscular volume		
Mean corpuscular volume, blood (MCV) 80–100 fL Lavender $	Average volume of the red cell is measured by automated instrument, electrical impedance, or light scatter.	**Increased in:** Liver disease (alcoholic and nonalcoholic), alcohol abuse, hemochromatosis, megaloblastic anemia (folate, B_{12} deficiencies), reticulocytosis, newborns. Spurious increase in autoagglutination, high white blood cell count. Drugs: methotrexate, phenytoin, zidovudine. **Decreased in:** Iron deficiency, thalassemia; decreased or normal in anemia of chronic disease.	MCV can be normal in combined iron and folate deficiency. In patients with two red cell populations (macrocytic and microcytic), MCV may be normal. MCV is an insensitive test in the evaluation of anemia. Patients with iron deficiency anemia or pernicious anemia commonly have a normal MCV. The MCV can be used as a guide to phlebotomy therapy for hemochromatosis and an indication of iron depletion in frequent blood donors. Alcohol Clin Exp Res 2000;24:1414. Clin Lab Haematol 2000;22:253. Genet Test 2000;4:103. J Lab Clin Med 2001;138:332. Transfusion 2001;41:819.

Test/Range/Collection	Physiologic Basis	Interpretation	Comments
Metanephrines, free (unconjugated), plasma <0.56 pmol/L Marbled $$$	Catecholamines, secreted in excess by pheochromocytomas, are metabolized within tumor cells by the enzyme catechol-O-methyltransferase to metanephrines (normetanephrine and metanephrine), and these can be detected in plasma. Measurement of plasma concentrations of free (unconjugated) metanephrines offers several advantages for the detection of pheochromocytoma: independence of short-term changes in catecholamine secretion in response to change of posture, exercise, or intraoperative stress; good correlation with tumor mass; and only minor interference from drugs. In diagnosis of pheochromocytoma, determination of plasma free metanephrines is more reliable and efficient than other biochemical tests.	**Increased in :** Pheochromocytoma (sensitivity ~100%; specificity 89–94%).	Plasma free metanephrines is now recommended as the first-line biochemical test for the diagnosis of pheochromocytoma. (See Pheochromocytoma algorithm, p 353.) Measurement of free catecholamines in plasma and urine, or of their metabolites, vanillylmandelic acid and total metanephrines (free + conjugated normetanephrine and metanephrine) in urine, suffers from interference from external factors and lower test sensitivity and/or specificity. Sensitivity of plasma free metanephrines (99%) is higher than that of urinary fractionated metanephrines (97%), plasma catecholamines (84%), urinary vanillylmandelic acid (64%). Specificity of plasma free metanephrines (89–94%) compares favorably to urinary vanillylmandelic acid (95%), urinary total metanephrines (93%), urinary catecholamines (88%), plasma catecholamines (81%), and urinary fractionated metanephrines (69%). Curr Hypertens Rep 2002;4:250. JAMA 2002;287:1427. J Clin Endocrinol Metab 2002;87:1955. Wien Klin Wochenschr 2002;114:246.

Metanephrines, urine 0.3–0.9 mg/24 h [1.6–4.9 μmol/24 h] Urine bottle containing hydrochloric acid $$$ Collect 24-hour urine.	Catecholamines, secreted in excess by pheochromocytomas, are metabolized by the enzyme catechol-O-methyltransferase to metanephrines, and these are excreted in the urine.	**Increased in:** Pheochromocytoma (97% sensitivity, 93% specificity), neuroblastoma, ganglioneuroma. Drugs: monoamine oxidase inhibitors.	Plasma metanephrines is now the preferred test (see Pheochromocytoma algorithm, p 353). Because <0.1% of hypertensives have a pheochromocytoma, routine screening of all hypertensives would yield a positive predictive value of <10%. Avoid overutilization of tests. Do not order urine vanillylmandelic acid, urine catecholamines, and plasma metanephrines and catecholamines at the same time. Plasma catecholamine levels are often spuriously increased when drawn in the hospital setting. Mayo Clin Proc 1990;65:88. Ann Intern Med 1995;123:101. Ann Intern Med 1996;125:331.	**Metanephrines**
Methanol, whole blood Negative Green or lavender $$	Methanol is extensively metabolized by alcohol dehydrogenase to formaldehyde and by aldehyde dehydrogenase to formic acid, the major toxic metabolite. Serum methanol levels >20 mg/dL are toxic and levels >40 mg/dL are life-threatening.	**Increased in:** Methanol intoxication.	Methanol intoxication is associated with metabolic acidosis and an osmolal gap. Methanol is commonly ingested in its pure form or in cleaning and copier solutions. Acute ingestion causes an optic neuritis that may result in blindness. Methanol poisoning can be fatal. Fomepizole, a competitive alcohol dehydrogenase inhibitor, can be used to treat methanol poisoning and can obviate the need for hemodialysis. Intensive Care Med 2001;27:1370. N Engl J Med 2001;344:424.	**Methanol**

	Methemoglobin		
Test/Range/Collection	Physiologic Basis	Interpretation	Comments
Methemoglobin, whole blood (MetHb) <0.15 g/dL [<1.5 g/L] Lavender $$ Analyze promptly; do not freeze specimen.	Methemoglobin has its heme iron in the oxidized ferric state and thus cannot combine with and transport oxygen. Methemoglobin can be assayed spectrophotometrically by measuring the decrease in absorbance at 630–635 nm due to the conversion of methemoglobin to cyanmethemoglobin with cyanide.	**Increased in:** Hemoglobin variants (HbM) (rare), methemoglobin reductase deficiency. Oxidant drugs such as sulfonamides (dapsone, sulfasalazine), nitrites (eg, food preservative sodium nitrite) and nitrates, aniline dyes, phenacetin, local anesthetics such as benzocaine, ifosfamide chemotherapy, chloramine toxicity during hemodialysis.	Levels of 1.5 g/dL (10% of total Hb) result in visible cyanosis. Patients with levels of about 35% have headache, weakness, and breathlessness. Levels in excess of 70% are usually fatal. Fetal methemoglobin is accurately measured using newer multiple-wavelength spectrophotometers. J Clin Anesth 2001;13:128. Am J Kidney Dis 2002;39:1307. MMWR Morbid Mortal Wkly Rep 2002;51:639.

Methylmalonic acid		
Methylmalonic acid, serum 0–0.4 µmol/L Marbled $$	Elevation of serum methylmalonic acid in cobalamin deficiency results from impaired conversion of methylmalonyl-CoA to succinyl-CoA, a pathway involving methylmalonyl-CoA mutase as enzyme and adenosylcobalamin as coenzyme.	**Increased in:** Vitamin B_{12} (cobalamin) deficiency (95%), pernicious anemia, renal insufficiency, elderly (5–15%).	Explanation of high frequency (5–15%) of increased serum methylmalonic acid in the elderly with low or normal serum cobalamin is unclear. Only a small number have pernicious anemia confirmed. Normal levels can exclude vitamin B_{12} deficiency in the presence of low unexplained cobalamin levels found in lymphoid disorders. Test is usually normal in HIV patients who may have low vitamin B_{12} levels without cobalamin deficiency, because of low vitamin B_{12} binding protein. In individuals with mildly elevated methylmalonic acid levels (0.40–2.00 µmol/L), vitamin B_{12} treatment normalizes methylmalonic acid level but has no significant effect on hemoglobin, MCV, or anemic, neurologic, or gastroenterologic symptoms, at least in the short term. Clin Chem 2001;47:1396. J Am Geriatr Soc 2002;50:624.

	Metyrapone test (overnight)		
Test/Range/Collection	**Physiologic Basis**	**Interpretation**	**Comments**
Metyrapone test (overnight), plasma or serum 8 AM cortisol: <10 μg/dL [<280 nmol/L] 8 AM 11-deoxycortisol: >7 μg/dL [>202 nmol/L] Marbled, lavender, or green $$$ Give 2.0–2.5 g of metyrapone orally at 12:00 midnight. Draw serum cortisol and 11-deoxycortisol levels at 8:00 AM.	The metyrapone stimulation test assesses both pituitary and adrenal reserve and is mainly used to diagnose secondary adrenal insufficiency (see Adrenocortical Insufficiency algorithm, p 340). Metyrapone is a drug that inhibits adrenal 11 β-hydroxylase and blocks cortisol synthesis. The consequent fall in cortisol increases release of ACTH and hence production of steroids formed proximal to the block (eg, 11-deoxycortisol).	**Decreased in:** An 8 AM 11-deoxycortisol level ≤7 μg/dL indicates primary or secondary adrenal insufficiency.	The overnight metyrapone test assesses the integrity of the entire hypothalamic–pituitary–adrenal axis. It can be useful in assessing the HPA axis post-hypophysectomy, in diagnosing secondary adrenal insufficiency in AIDS patients, or in steroid-treated patients to assess the extent of suppression of the pituitary-adrenal axis. The use of an extended metyrapone test in the differential diagnosis of ACTH-dependent Cushing syndrome (pituitary versus ectopic) has been questioned. Clin Endocrinol (Oxf) 2000;53:309. Am J Med Sci 2001;321:137. Clin Endocrinol (Oxf) 2002;56:533.

β$_2$-Microglobulin		
β$_2$-Microglobulin, serum (β$_2$-M) <0.2 mg/dL [<2.0 mg/L] Marbled $$$	β$_2$-Microglobulin is a portion of the HLA molecule on cell surfaces synthesized by all nucleated cell types and is present in all body fluids. It is increased in many conditions that are accompanied by high cell turnover.	**Increased in:** Any type of inflammation (such as inflammatory bowel disease), autoimmune disorders, lymphoid malignancies, multiple myeloma, viral infections (HIV, CMV). Marked elevation in patients with amyloidosis and renal failure.	Of tests used to predict progression to AIDS in HIV-infected patients, CD4 cell number has the most predictive power, followed closely by β$_2$-microglobulin. Asymptomatic HIV patients with elevated β$_2$-microglobulin levels have a two- to threefold increased chance of disease progression. β$_2$-Microglobulin is of prognostic value in multiple myeloma and Waldenström macroglobulinemia: serum level increases with increasing tumor mass. Am J Gastroenterol 2001;96:2177. Br J Haematol 2001;115:575.

Test/Range/Collection	Physiologic Basis	Interpretation	Comments
Microhemagglutination-*Treponema pallidum*	The MHA-TP test measures specific antibody against *T pallidum* in a patient's serum by agglutination of *T pallidum* antigen-coated erythrocytes. Antibodies to nonpathogenic treponemes are first removed by binding to nonpathogenic treponemal antigens.	**Increased in:** Syphilis: primary (64–87%), secondary (96–100%), late latent (96–100%), tertiary (94–100%); infectious mononucleosis, collagenvascular diseases, hyperglobulinemia and dysglobulinemia.	Test is used to confirm reactive serologic tests for syphilis (RPR or VDRL). Compared to FTA-ABS, MHA-TP is slightly less sensitive in all stages of syphilis and becomes reactive somewhat later in the disease.
serum (MHA-TP)			Because test usually remains positive for long periods of time regardless of therapy, it is not useful in assessing the effectiveness of therapy.
Nonreactive			In one study, 36 months after treatment of syphilis, 13% of patients had nonreactive MHA-TP tests.
Marbled			Ann Intern Med 1986;104:368.
$$			J Infect Dis 1990;162:862.
			Ann Intern Med 1991;114:1005.
			Clin Microbiol Rev 1995;8:1.

*(Header of table: **Microhemagglutination–*Treponema pallidum***)*

Mitochondrial antibody			
Mitochondrial antibody, serum Negative Marbled $$	Antimitochondrial antibodies (particularly those reacting with epitopes on the E2 members of the 2-oxoacid dehydrogenase components of multienzyme complexes, including pyruvate dehydrogenase, branched chain 2-oxo acid dehydrogenase, and oxoglutarate dehydrogenase) are virtually pathognomonic of primary biliary cirrhosis (PBC). Originally demonstrated using immunofluorescence approaches, antimitochondrial antibodies can now be detected using commercially available ELISAs. Although ELISAs are more practical, they are slightly less sensitive than immunofluorescence techniques. In AMA–negative patients suspected of PBC, antimitochondrial autoantibodies can be detected using recombinant autoantigens.	**Increased in:** Primary biliary cirrhosis (85–95%), chronic active hepatitis (25–28%); lower titers in viral hepatitis, infectious mononucleosis, neoplasms, cryptogenic cirrhosis (25–30%).	Primarily used to distinguish PBC (antibody present) from extrahepatic biliary obstruction (antibody absent). AMA subtype profiles do not predict prognosis in patients with PBC. J Clin Pathol 2000;53:813. Hepatology 2001;34:243. Scand J Clin Lab Invest Suppl 2001:53. Am J Gastroenterol 2002;97:999.

	Neutrophil cytoplasmic antibodies		
Test/Range/Collection	**Physiologic Basis**	**Interpretation**	**Comments**
Neutrophil cytoplasmic antibodies, serum (ANCA) Negative Marbled $$$	Measurement of autoantibodies in serum against cytoplasmic constituents of neutrophils. (See also Autoantibodies table, p 366.) Dual testing by standard indirect immunofluorescence for serum cytoplasmic ANCA (cANCA) and perinuclear ANCA (pANCA) and target antigen-specific assays (myeloperoxidase-ANCA or proteinase 3-ANCA) is often recommended.	**Positive in:** Wegener granulomatosis, systemic vasculitis, pauci-immune crescentic glomerulonephritis, paraneoplastic vasculitis, Churg-Strauss angiitis, microscopic polyangiitis, drug-induced vasculitis, ulcerative colitis.	In the patient with systemic vasculitis, elevated ANCA levels imply active disease and high likelihood of recurrence. However, ANCA levels can be persistently elevated and should be used in conjunction with other clinical indices in treatment decisions. For ANCA-associated vasculitis, ANCA sensitivity, specificity, positive predictive value, and negative predictive value vary with method and population studied. J Rheumatol 2001;28:1584. QJM 2001;94:615. Rheum Dis Clin North Am 2001;27:799. Am Fam Physician 2002;65:1615. Arch Intern Med 2002;162:1509. Clin Immunol 2002;103:196.

		Nuclear antibody	Oligoclonal bands
Nuclear antibody, serum (ANA) <1:20 Marbled $$	Heterogeneous antibodies to nuclear antigens (DNA and RNA), histone and nonhistone proteins). Nuclear antibody is measured in serum by layering the patient's serum over human epithelial cells and detecting the antibody with fluorescein-conjugated polyvalent antihuman immunoglobulin.	Elevated in: Patients over age 65 (35–75%, usually in low titers), systemic lupus erythematosus (98%), drug-induced lupus (100%), Sjögren syndrome (80%), rheumatoid arthritis (30–50%), scleroderma (60%), mixed connective tissue disease (100%), Felty syndrome, mononucleosis, hepatic or biliary cirrhosis, hepatitis, leukemia, myasthenia gravis, dermatomyositis, polymyositis, chronic renal failure.	A negative ANA test does not completely rule out SLE, but alternative diagnoses should be considered. Pattern of ANA staining may give some clues to diagnoses, but because the pattern also changes with serum dilution, it is not routinely reported. Only the rim (peripheral) pattern is highly specific (for SLE). Not useful as a screening test. Should be used only when there is clinical evidence of a connective tissue disease. Curr Opin Rheumatol 2000;12:364. Am J Clin Pathol 2002;117:316.
Oligoclonal bands, serum and CSF (OCBs) Negative Marbled and glass or plastic tube for CSF $$ Collect serum and CSF simultaneously.	Electrophoretic examination of IgG found in CSF may show oligoclonal bands not found in serum. This suggests local production in CSF of limited species of IgG. The pathogenesis of OCBs in MS is still obscure.	Positive in: Multiple sclerosis (sensitivity 81–95%; specificity 43%; positive predictive value 30%; negative predictive value 88%), CNS syphilis, subacute sclerosing panencephalitis, progressive multifocal leukoencephalopathy, Guillain-Barré syndrome, other CNS inflammatory diseases.	Test is indicated only when multiple sclerosis is suspected clinically. Test interpretation is very subjective. IgG index is a more reliable test analytically, but neither test is specific for multiple sclerosis. Quantification of OCBs in CSF is an insensitive prognostic indicator and should not be used to influence treatment decisions. Arch Neurol 2001;58:2044. Mult Scler 2001;7:359. J Neurol 2002;249:375.

Test/Range/Collection	Physiologic Basis	Interpretation	Comments
Osmolality, serum (Osm) 285–293 mosm/kg H_2O [mmol/kg H_2O] *Panic:* <240 or >320 mosm/kg H_2O Marbled $$	Test measures the osmotic pressure of serum by the freezing point depression method. Plasma and urine osmolality are more useful indicators of degree of hydration than BUN, hematocrit, or serum proteins. Serum osmolality can be estimated by the following formula: $$Osm = 2(Na^+) + \frac{BUN}{2.8} + \frac{Glucose}{18}$$ where Na^+ is in meq/L and BUN and glucose are in mg/dL.	**Increased in:** Diabetic ketoacidosis, nonketotic hyperosmolar hyperglycemic coma, hypernatremia secondary to dehydration (diarrhea, severe burns, vomiting, fever, hyperventilation, inadequate water intake, central or nephrogenic diabetes insipidus, or osmotic diuresis), hypernatremia with normal hydration (hypothalamic disorders, defective osmostat), hypernatremia with overhydration (iatrogenic or accidental excessive NaCl or $NaHCO_3$ intake), alcohol or other toxic ingestion (see Comments), hypercalcemia; tube feedings. Drugs: corticosteroids, mannitol, glycerin. **Decreased in:** Pregnancy (third trimester); hyponatremia with hypovolemia (adrenal insufficiency, renal losses, diarrhea, vomiting, severe burns, peritonitis, pancreatitis), hyponatremia with normovolemia (CHF, cirrhosis, nephrotic syndrome, SIADH, postoperative state). Drugs: chlorthalidone, cyclophosphamide, thiazides.	If the difference between calculated and measured serum osmolality is greater than 10 mosm/kg H_2O, suspect the presence of a low-molecular-weight toxin (alcohol, methanol, isopropyl alcohol, ethylene glycol, acetone, ethyl ether, paraldehyde, or mannitol), ethanol being the most common. (See p 383 for further explanation.) Every 100 mg/dL of ethanol increases serum osmolality by 22 mosm/kg H_2O. While the osmolal gap may overestimate the blood alcohol level, a normal serum osmolality excludes ethanol intoxication. Measurement of serum osmolality is an important first step in the laboratory evaluation of the hyponatremic patient. The simultaneous measurement of plasma ADH (vasopressin) and plasma osmolality in a dehydration test is the most powerful diagnostic tool in the differential diagnosis of polyuria/polydipsia. Clin Endocrinol (Oxf) 2001;54:665. CMAJ 2002:166:1056.

Test	Description	Interpretation	Comments
Osmolality, urine (Urine Osm) Random: 100–900 mosm/kg H$_2$O [mmol/kg H$_2$O] Urine container $$	Test measures renal tubular concentrating ability.	**Increased in:** Hypovolemia. Drugs: anesthetic agents (during surgery), carbamazepine, chlorpropamide, cyclophosphamide, metolazone, vincristine. **Decreased in:** Diabetes insipidus, primary polydipsia, exercise, starvation. Drugs: acetohexamide, demeclocycline, glyburide, lithium, tolazamide.	In the hypoosmolar state (serum osmolality <280 mOsm/kg), urine osmolality is used to determine whether water excretion is normal or impaired. A urine osmolality value of <100 mOsm/kg indicates complete and appropriate suppression of antidiuretic hormone secretion. With average fluid intake, normal random urine osmolality is 100–900 mosm/kg H$_2$O. After 12-hour fluid restriction, normal random urine osmolality is >850 mosm/kg H$_2$O. CMAJ 2002;166:1056.
Oxygen, partial pressure, whole blood (Po$_2$) $$$ 83–108 mm Hg [11.04–14.36 kPa] Heparinized syringe Collect arterial blood in a heparinized syringe. Send to laboratory immediately on ice.	Test measures the partial pressure of oxygen (oxygen tension) in arterial blood. Partial pressure of oxygen is critical since it determines (along with hemoglobin and blood supply) tissue oxygen supply.	**Increased in:** Oxygen therapy. **Decreased in:** Ventilation/perfusion mismatching (asthma, COPD, atelectasis, pulmonary embolism, pneumonia, interstitial lung disease, airway obstruction by foreign body, shock); alveolar hypoventilation (kyphoscoliosis, neuromuscular disease, head injury, stroke); right-to-left shunt (congenital heart disease). Drugs: barbiturates, opioids.	% saturation of hemoglobin (So$_2$) represents the oxygen content divided by the oxygen carrying capacity of hemoglobin. % saturation on blood gas reports is calculated, not measured. It is calculated from Po$_2$ and pH using reference oxyhemoglobin dissociation curves for normal adult hemoglobin (lacking methemoglobin, carboxyhemoglobin, etc). At Po$_2$ <60 mm Hg, the oxygen saturation (and content) cannot be reliably estimated from the Po$_2$. Therefore, oximetry should be used to determine % saturation directly. Am J Clin Pathol 1995;(1 Suppl):579. Obstet Gynecol Surv 1998;53:645. Anesthesiol Clin North Am 2001;19:885.

	p24 Antigen		
Test/Range/Collection	**Physiologic Basis**	**Interpretation**	**Comments**
p24 antigen Negative Marbled, green, or yellow $$$	Human immunodeficiency virus (HIV-1) p24 antigen is present prior to the onset of antibody production in some cases of recent HIV infection. Because HIV antibodies are absent in the very early phase of HIV infection, HIV transmission by viremic but antibody negative individuals is possible. p24 antigen testing by enzyme immunoassay (EIA) permits earlier detection of HIV infection. Combined p24 antigen testing and HIV antibody testing reduces the diagnostic "window" period between the time of HIV infection and the detection of antibodies. p24 antigen testing has also been used as a sensitive, precise and inexpensive marker for disease progression and treatment failure.	**Increased in:** Human immunodeficiency virus (HIV-1) infection.	The sensitivity and specificity of p24 antigen EIA for detecting preseroconversion HIV infection are 79% and 99%, respectively. In contrast, sensitivity and specificity of HIV-1 RNA by branched chain DNA were 100% and 95%; HIV-1 RNA by PCR 100% and 97%; HIV-1 RNA by transcription-mediated amplification testing, 100% and 98%. Thus, p24 antigen is more specific than HIV-1 RNA testing but less sensitive. AIDS Patients Care STDS 1997;11:429. Int J Antimicrob Agents 2000;16:441. J Virol Methods 2000;90:153. AIDS 2002;16:1119.

Parathyroid hormone			
Parathyroid hormone, serum (PTH) Intact PTH: 11–54 pg/mL [1.2–5.7 pmol/L] (laboratory-specific) Marbled $$$$ Fasting sample preferred; simultaneous measurement of serum calcium and phosphorus is also required.	PTH is secreted from the parathyroid glands. It mobilizes calcium from bone, increases distal renal tubular reabsorption of calcium, decreases proximal renal tubular reabsorption of phosphorus, and stimulates 1,25-hydroxy vitamin D synthesis from 25-hydroxy vitamin D by renal 1α-hydroxylase. The "intact" PTH molecule (84 amino acids) has a circulating half-life of about 5 minutes. Carboxyl terminal and mid-molecule fragments make up 90% of circulating PTH. They are biologically inactive, cleared by the kidney, and have half-lives of about 1–2 hours. The amino terminal fragment is biologically active and has a half-life of 1–2 minutes. Measurement of PTH by immunoassay depends on the specificity of the antibodies used.	**Increased in:** Primary hyperparathyroidism, secondary hyperparathyroidism due to renal disease, vitamin D deficiency. Drugs: lithium, furosemide, propofol, phosphates. **Decreased in:** Hypoparathyroidism, sarcoidosis, hyperthyroidism, hypomagnesemia, malignancy with hypercalcemia, nonparathyroid hypercalcemia.	PTH results must always be evaluated in light of concurrent serum calcium levels. PTH tests differ in sensitivity and specificity from assay to assay and from laboratory to laboratory. Carboxyl terminal antibody measures intact, carboxyl terminal and midmolecule fragments. It is 85% sensitive and 95% specific for primary hyperparathyroidism. Amino terminal antibody measures intact and amino terminal fragments. It is about 75% sensitive for hyperparathyroidism. Intact PTH assays are preferred because they detect PTH suppression in nonparathyroid hypercalcemia. Sensitivity of immunometric assays is 85–90% for primary hyperparathyroidism. Intraoperative quick PTH monitoring in patients undergoing parathyroidectomy can be used to confirm cure and predict long-term operative success in most cases. A low intraoperative PTH level during thyroid surgery is a predictor of postoperative hypocalcemia resulting from parathyroid gland ischemia. J Clin Endocrinol Metab 2001;86:3086. Arch Surg 2002;137:186. Arch Surg 2002;137:659. Surgery 2002;131:515.

	Parathyroid hormone-related protein		
Test/Range/Collection	**Physiologic Basis**	**Interpretation**	**Comments**
Parathyroid hormone-related protein (PTHrP), plasma Assay-specific (pmol/L or undetectable) Tube containing anti-coagulant and protease inhibitors; specimen drawn without a tourniquet. $$	Parathyroid hormone-related protein (PTHrP) is a 139- to 173-amino acid protein with amino terminal homology to PTH. The homology explains the ability of PTHrP to bind to the PTH receptor and have PTH-like effects on bone and kidney. PTHrP induces increased plasma calcium, decreased plasma phosphorus, and increased urinary cAMP. PTHrP is found in keratinocytes, fibroblasts, placenta, brain, pituitary gland, adrenal gland, stomach, liver, testicular Leydig cells, and mammary glands. Its physiologic role in these diverse sites is unknown. PTHrP is secreted by solid malignant tumors (lung, breast, kidney; other squamous tumors) and produces humoral hypercalcemia of malignancy. PTHrP can act as an oncoprotein to regulate the growth and proliferation of many common malignancies. PTHrP analysis is by immunoradiometric assay (IRMA). Assay of choice is amino terminal-specific IRMA. Two-site IRMA assays require sample collection in protease inhibitors because serum proteases destroy immunoreactivity.	**Increased in:** Humoral hypercalcemia of malignancy (80% of solid tumors).	Assays directed at the amino terminal portion of PTHrP are not influenced by renal failure. Increases in PTHrP concentrations are readily detectable with most current assays in the majority of patients with humoral hypercalcemia of malignancy. About 20% of patients with malignancy and hypercalcemia will have low PTHrP levels because their hypercalcemia is caused by local osteolytic processes. Cancer 1994;73:2223. Endocrinol Metab Clin North Am 2000;29:629.

Partial thromboplastin time			
Partial thromboplastin time, activated, plasma (PTT) 25–35 seconds (range varies) *Panic:* ≥60 seconds (off heparin) Blue $$ Fill tube adequately. Do not contaminate specimen with heparin.	Patient's plasma is activated to clot in vitro by mixing it with phospholipid and an activator substance. Test screens the intrinsic coagulation pathway and adequacy of all coagulation factors except XIII and VII. PTT is usually abnormal if any factor level drops below 30–40% of normal.	**Increased in:** Deficiency of any individual coagulation factor except XIII and VII; presence of nonspecific inhibitors (eg, lupus anticoagulant), specific factor inhibitors, von Willebrand disease (PTT may also be normal), hemophilia A and B, disseminated intravascular coagulation (DIC). Drugs: heparin, warfarin. **Decreased in:** Hypercoagulable states, DIC.	PTT is the best test to monitor adequacy of heparin therapy, but it does not reliably predict the risk of bleeding. Test is not always abnormal in von Willebrand disease. Test may be normal in chronic DIC. A very common cause of PTT prolongation is the spurious presence of heparin in the plasma sample. Sensitivity and degree of prolongation of PTT depend on particular reagents used. Therapeutic levels of heparin are best achieved using a weight-based dosing nomogram with dose adjustment based on the PTT at 6 hours. Br J Haematol 2000;111:1230. Thromb Haemost 2000;84:1012. Acad Emerg Med 2002;9:567. Am J Hematol 2002;70:195.

Test/Range/Collection	Physiologic Basis	Interpretation	Comments
pH, whole blood Arterial: 7.35–7.45 Venous: 7.31–7.41 Heparinized syringe $$$ Specimen must be collected in heparinized syringe and immediately transported on ice to lab without exposure to air.	pH assesses the acid-base status of blood, an extremely useful measure of integrated cardiorespiratory function. The essential relationship between pH, P_{CO_2}, and bicarbonate (HCO_3^-) is expressed by the Henderson–Hasselbalch equation (at 37°C): $$pH = 6.1 + \log\left(\frac{HCO_3^-}{P_{CO_2} \times 0.03}\right)$$ Arteriovenous pH difference is 0.01–0.03 but is greater in patients with CHF and shock.	**Increased in:** *Respiratory alkalosis:* hyperventilation (eg, anxiety), sepsis, liver disease, fever, early salicylate poisoning, and excessive artificial ventilation. *Metabolic alkalosis:* Loss of gastric HCl (eg, vomiting), potassium depletion, excessive alkali administration (eg, bicarbonate, antacids), diuretics, volume depletion. **Decreased in:** *Respiratory acidosis:* decreased alveolar ventilation (eg, COPD, respiratory depressants), neuromuscular diseases (eg, myasthenia). *Metabolic acidosis* (bicarbonate deficit): increased formation of acids (eg, ketosis [diabetes mellitus, alcohol, starvation], lactic acidosis); decreased H^+ excretion (eg, renal failure, renal tubular acidosis, Fanconi syndrome); increased acid intake (eg, ion-exchange resins, salicylates, ammonium chloride, ethylene glycol, methanol); and increased loss of alkaline body fluids (eg, diarrhea, fistulas, aspiration of gastrointestinal contents, biliary drainage).	The pH of a standing sample decreases because of cellular metabolism. The correction of pH (measured at 37°C), based on the patient's temperature, is not clinically useful. Crit Care Nurs 1996;16:89. Crit Care 2000;4:6. Anesthesiol Clin North Am 2001;19:885.

Phosphorus		
Phosphorus, serum 2.5–4.5 mg/dL [0.8–1.45 mmol/L] *Panic:* <1.0 mg/dL Marbled $ Avoid hemolysis.	The plasma concentration of inorganic phosphate is determined by parathyroid gland function, action of vitamin D, intestinal absorption, renal function, bone metabolism, and nutrition.	**Increased in:** Renal failure, calcific uremic arteriolopathy (calciphylaxis), tumor lysis syndrome, massive blood transfusion, hypoparathyroidism, sarcoidosis, neoplasms, adrenal insufficiency, acromegaly, hypervitaminosis D, osteolytic metastases to bone, leukemia, milk-alkali syndrome, healing bone fractures, pseudohypoparathyroidism, diabetes mellitus with ketosis, malignant hyperpyrexia, cirrhosis, lactic acidosis, respiratory acidosis. Drugs: phosphate infusions or enemas, anabolic steroids, ergocalciferol, furosemide, hydrochlorothiazide, clonidine, verapamil, potassium supplements, and others. **Decreased in:** Hyperparathyroidism, hypovitaminosis D (rickets, osteomalacia), malabsorption (steatorrhea), malnutrition, starvation or cachexia, refeeding syndrome, bone marrow transplantation, renal phosphate wasting due to autosomal-dominant or X-linked dominant hypophosphatemic rickets, GH deficiency, chronic alcoholism, severe diarrhea, vomiting, nasogastric suction, severe hypercalcemia (any cause), acute gout, osteoblastic metastases to bone, severe burns (diuretic phase), respiratory alkalosis, hyperalimentation with inadequate phosphate repletion, carbohydrate administration (eg, intravenous $D_{50}W$ glucose bolus), renal tubular acidosis and other renal tubular defects, diabetic ketoacidosis (during recovery), acid-base disturbances, hypokalemia, pregnancy, hypothyroidism, hemodialysis. Drugs: acetazolamide, phosphate-binding antacids, anticonvulsants, β-adrenergic agonists, catecholamines, estrogens, isoniazid, oral contraceptives, prolonged use of thiazides, glucose infusion, insulin therapy, salicylates (toxicity).	Thrombocytosis may cause spurious elevation of serum phosphate, but plasma phosphate levels are normal. Endocrinol Metab Clin North Am 2000;29:569. Endocrinol Metab Clin North Am 2000;29:591. Kidney Int 2001;60:2079. Semin Hematol 2001;38(4 Suppl 10):4. Semin Dial 2002;15:172.

	Platelet aggregation		
Test/Range/Collection	**Physiologic Basis**	**Interpretation**	**Comments**
Platelet aggregation, whole blood Aggregation by adenosine diphosphate (ADP), collagen, epinephrine, thrombin, ristocetin, and arachidonic acid Drawn by lab $$$$ Whole blood in citrate is drawn into a plastic tube. Platelet-rich plasma (PRP) is obtained by centrifuging at $100 \times g$ for 10–15 minutes.	Platelet aggregometry can provide information concerning possible qualitative platelet defects. Aggregation is measured as an increase in light transmission through stirred PRP when a specific agonist is added. Test examines platelet aggregation response to various agonists (eg, ADP, collagen, epinephrine, thrombin, ristocetin, arachidonic acid). Newer lumiaggregation measures aggregation and simultaneous platelet ATP release—the so-called platelet release reaction.	**Abnormal in:** Acquired defects in the platelet release reaction (eg, drugs, following cardiopulmonary bypass, uremia, paraproteinemias, myeloproliferative disorders), congenital release abnormalities, Glanzmann thrombasthenia (absent aggregation to ADP, collagen, epinephrine), essential athrombia (similar to Glanzmann disease except clot retraction is normal), storage pool disease (no secondary wave with ADP, epinephrine, and decreased aggregation with collagen), cyclooxygenase and thromboxane synthetase deficiencies (rare hereditary aspirin-like defects), von Willebrand disease (normal aggregation with all factors except ristocetin). Drugs: aspirin (absent aggregation curves to ADP and epinephrine, collagen, arachidonate), interferon-alpha-2b therapy.	Acquired platelet dysfunction is more common than the hereditary form. Hereditary storage pool disease is common enough to be suspected in a child with easy or spontaneous bruising. Test should not be done if the patient has taken aspirin within the previous 10 days. Direct PRP aggregation by ristocetin (1.5 mg/mL) may be normal or abnormal in von Willebrand disease (vWD). Because this test has limited sensitivity for detection of vWD, it is no longer used for that purpose (see instead Bleeding time, p 55, and von Willebrand factor protein, p 186). Best Pract Res Clin Haematol 2001;14:299. J Cell Mol Med 2001;5:79. Cancer 2002;94:780.

Platelet count		
Platelet count, whole blood (Plt) 150–450 × 10³/μL [× 10⁹/L] ***Panic:*** <25 × 10³/μL Lavender $	Platelets are released from megakaryocytes in bone marrow and are important for normal hemostasis. Platelet counting is done by flow cytometry with size discrimination based on electrical impedance or electro-optical systems.	**Increased in:** Myeloproliferative disorders: polycythemia vera, chronic myeloid leukemia, essential thrombocythemia, myelofibrosis; after bleeding, postsplenectomy, reactive thrombocytosis secondary to inflammatory diseases, iron deficiency, malignancies, alkalosis. **Decreased in:** Decreased production: bone marrow suppression or replacement, chemotherapeutic agents, drugs (eg, ethanol). Increased destruction or removal: splenomegaly, DIC, platelet antibodies (idiopathic thrombocytopenic purpura, posttransfusion purpura, neonatal isoimmune thrombocytopenia, drugs [eg, quinidine, cephalosporins, clopidogrel, heparin-induced thrombocytopenia]).	Thrombocytosis is caused by three major pathophysiologic mechanisms: (1) reactive or secondary thrombocytosis, (2) familial thrombocytosis, and (3) clonal thrombocytosis, including essential thrombocythemia and related myeloproliferative disorders. Acta Haematol 2001;106:33. Blood Rev 2001;15:121. Blood Rev 2001;15:159. Curr Opin Hematol 2001;8:294. Oncology 2001;15:989. Rev Clin Exp Hematol 2001;5:166. Chest 2002;122:37. Semin Oncol 2002;29(3 Suppl 10):16. Vasc Endovascular Surg 2002;36:163.

Platelet-associated IgG

Test/Range/Collection	Physiologic Basis	Interpretation	Comments
Platelet-associated IgG, whole blood Negative Yellow $$$$ 17 mL of blood is needed.	Immune thrombocytopenia is due to platelet destruction by circulating glycoprotein-specific antibodies and is found in various disorders. Methods for the detection of platelet-associated IgG are generally sensitive but non-specific, whereas glycoprotein-specific assays are highly specific but less sensitive. Antibody screening involves direct testing of a patient's platelets to demonstrate platelet-associated IgG (which may be directed against specific platelet antigens or may represent immune complexes nonspecifically absorbed to the platelet surface) in idiopathic (autoimmune) thrombocytopenic purpura (ITP). It also involves indirect testing of the patient's serum against a panel of reagent platelets to detect circulating antiplatelet antibodies. In alloimmune thrombocytopenia, the patient's direct test is negative and the patient's serum reacts with reagent platelets. Antibody specificity can be identified, and platelets lacking the involved antigen can be transfused.	**Positive in:** Some autoimmune thrombocytopenias (eg, ITP) (90–95%), autoimmune thyroid disease (51%).	In ITP, the direct antiplatelet antibody test may be useful to confirm the diagnosis and monitor subsequent response to therapy. It is also useful in diagnosing posttransfusion purpura and suspected neonatal isoimmune thrombocytopenia. Platelet-associated IgG is also useful for patients with thrombocytopenia or as part of a platelet cross-match prior to transfusion of patients who have repeatedly failed to respond to random donor platelet transfusions. Br J Haematol 1997;96:204 Thromb Haemost 2000;84:779. Horm Res 2001;56:172.

Porphobilinogen			
Porphobilinogen, urine (PBG) Negative $$ Protect from light.	Porphyrias are characterized clinically by neurologic and cutaneous manifestations and chemically by overproduction of porphyrin and other precursors of heme production. PBG is a water-soluble precursor of heme whose urinary excretion is increased in symptomatic hepatic porphyrias. PBG is detected qualitatively by a color reaction with Ehrlich reagent and confirmed by extraction into chloroform (Watson–Schwartz test).	**Positive in:** Acute intermittent porphyria, variegate porphyria, coproporphyria, lead poisoning (rare). **Negative in:** 20–30% of patients with hepatic porphyria between attacks.	Positive qualitative urinary PBG tests should be followed up by quantitative measurements. Many labs report frequent false positives with the Watson–Schwartz test. A screening PBG test is insensitive, and a negative test does not rule out porphyria between attacks or the carrier state. Specific porphyrias can be better defined by quantitative measurement of urine PBG and by measurement of erythrocyte uroporphyrinogen-I-synthetase. Semin Liver Dis 1998;18:57 J Clin Pathol 2001;54:500. Int J Clin Pract 2002;56:272.

	Potassium		
Test/Range/Collection	Physiologic Basis	Interpretation	Comments
Potassium, serum (K⁺) 3.5–5.0 meq/L [mmol/L] *Panic:* <3.0 or >6.0 meq/L Marbled $ Avoid hemolysis.	Potassium is predominantly an intracellular cation whose plasma level is regulated by renal excretion. Plasma potassium concentration determines neuromuscular irritability. Elevated or depressed potassium concentrations interfere with muscle contraction.	**Increased in:** Massive hemolysis, severe tissue damage, rhabdomyolysis, acidosis, dehydration, acute or chronic renal failure, Addison disease, renal tubular acidosis type IV (hyporeninemic hypoaldosteronism), hyperkalemic familial periodic paralysis, exercise (transient). Drugs: potassium salts, potassium-sparing diuretics (eg, spironolactone, triamterene), nonsteroidal anti-inflammatory drugs, β-blockers, ACE inhibitors, high-dose trimethoprim-sulfamethoxazole. **Decreased in:** Low potassium intake, prolonged vomiting or diarrhea, renal tubular acidosis types I and II, hyperaldosteronism, Cushing syndrome, osmotic diuresis (eg, hyperglycemia), alkalosis, familial periodic paralysis, trauma (transient), subarachnoid hemorrhage genetic hypokalemic salt-losing tubulopathies such as Gitelman syndrome (familial hypokalemia-hypocalciuria-hypomagnesemia). Drugs: adrenergic agents (isoproterenol), diuretics.	Spurious hyperkalemia can occur with hemolysis of sample, delayed separation of serum from erythrocytes, prolonged fist clenching during blood drawing, and prolonged tourniquet placement. Very high white blood cell or platelet counts may cause spurious elevation of serum potassium, but plasma potassium levels are normal. Am J Med 2000;109:307. Crit Care Clin 2001;17:503. J Nephrol 2001;14:43. Postgrad Med J 2001;77:759. Am J Med 2002;112:183. Neurology 2002;59:134.

Procalcitonin			
Procalcitonin, serum >0.5 ng/mL Marbled $$$$	Procalcitonin is a 14-kDa protein encoded by the *Calc-1* gene along with calcitonin and katacalcin. It is reported to be selectively induced by severe bacterial infections, such as the systemic inflammatory response syndrome (SIRS), sepsis, or multiorgan dysfunction syndrome. Procalcitonin expression is only slightly induced, if at all, by viral infections, autoimmune disorders, neoplastic diseases, myocardial infarction, and surgical trauma. An elevated plasma procalcitonin level is found in nonleukopenic patients with severe bacterial infections and sepsis, and appears to have greater specificity and sensitivity than acute phase proteins such as C-reactive protein or nonspecific indicators such as leukocyte count.	**Increased in:** Severe bacterial infections (eg, pneumonia, meningitis) and systemic infections (SIRS, sepsis, septic shock).	Rapid determination of the plasma procalcitonin level can be useful in triage decisions in the emergency department and in treatment decisions in the critical care unit. Procalcitonin level has reduced sensitivity and specificity for sepsis in severely leukopenic (WBC $<1.0 \times 10^9$/L) and immunosuppressed patients. However, the test retains its utility in patients with renal failure. Am J Respir Crit Care Med 2001;164:396. Ann Clin Biochem 2001;38:483. Br J Haematol 2001;115:53. Eur J Anaesthesiol 2001;18:79. Am J Emerg Med 2002;20:202. Clin Infect Dis 2002;34:895. Crit Care Med 2002;30:757.

			Prolactin
Test/Range/Collection	**Physiologic Basis**	**Interpretation**	**Comments**
Prolactin, serum (PRL) <20 ng/mL [μg/L] Marbled $$$	Prolactin is a polypeptide hormone secreted by the anterior pituitary. It functions in the initiation and maintenance of lactation in the postpartum period. PRL secretion is inhibited by hypothalamic secretion of dopamine. Prolactin levels increase with renal failure, hypothyroidism, and drugs that are dopamine antagonists.	**Increased in:** Sleep, nursing, nipple stimulation, exercise, hypoglycemia, stress, hypothyroidism, pituitary tumors (prolactinomas and others), hypothalamic/pituitary stalk lesions, renal failure. HIV infection (21%), CHF, SLE, advanced multiple myeloma, Rathke cleft cyst. Drugs: phenothiazines, haloperidol, risperidone, reserpine, methyldopa, estrogens, opiates, cimetidine. **Decreased in:** Drugs: levodopa.	Serum PRL is used primarily in work-up of suspected pituitary tumor (60% of pituitary adenomas secrete PRL). Clinical presentation is usually amenorrhea and galactorrhea in women and impotence in men. (See Amenorrhea algorithm, p 341.) Only 4% of impotence is caused by hyperprolactinemia, and hyperprolactinemia is rare in the absence of low serum testosterone. Many patients with hyperprolactinemia (8–26%, depending on the population studied) have in fact normal amounts of circulating prolactin but falsely high values in commercial assays. This is caused by macromolecular prolactin (macroprolactin), a complex of prolactin with IgG antibodies leading to apparent hyperprolactinemia. Macroprolactinemia is a cause of hyperprolactinemia in patients with maintained fertility. PRL levels usually remain stable over time. Endocrinol Metab Clin North Am 2001;30:585. Eur J Clin Invest 2002;32:74. HIV Clin Trials 2002;3:133. J Clin Endocrinol Metab 2002;87:581. J Clin Psychiatry 2002;63(Suppl 4):56.

Prostate-specific antigen		
Prostate-specific antigen, serum (PSA) 0–4 ng/mL [µg/L] Marbled $$$	Prostate-specific antigen is a glycoprotein produced by cells of the prostatic ductal epithelium and is present in the serum of all men. It is absent from the serum of women.	**Increased in:** Prostate carcinoma (sensitivity ~44%; specificity ~94% at a 4.0 ng/mL cutoff), benign prostatic hypertrophy (BPH), following prostate examination. **Negative in:** Metastatic prostate carcinoma treated with antiandrogen therapy, postprostatectomy.
		PSA is used both for the early detection of prostate cancer and as a tumor marker to asses response and monitor recurrence of treated prostate cancer. Randomized trials of the benefits and risks of PSA testing for prostate cancer screening are underway. Decrease in mortality rates resulting from use for cancer screening is unproved, and the risks of early therapy are significant. The PSA nadir (the lowest PSA level achieved after therapeutic intervention) appears to correlate with the likelihood of remaining disease-free. Three consecutive PSA rises are interpreted as an indicator of treatment (biochemical) failure. PSA is often increased in BPH, and the predictive value of a positive test in healthy older men is low. PSA replaces the acid phosphatase test. J Urol 2001;166:2189. Int J Cancer 2002;97:237. Semin Oncol 2002;29:264.

	Protein C		
Test/Range/Collection	**Physiologic Basis**	**Interpretation**	**Comments**
Protein C, plasma 71–176% Blue $$$	Protein C is a vitamin K-dependent proenzyme synthesized in the liver. Following its activation by thrombin, it exerts an anticoagulant effect through inactivation of factors Va and VIIIa using protein S as cofactor. Tests to assay quantitative (antigenic) or functional activity are available. Deficiency is inherited in an autosomal dominant fashion with incomplete penetrance or is acquired. Deficient patients may present with a hypercoagulable state, with recurrent thrombophlebitis or pulmonary emboli.	**Decreased in:** Congenital deficiency, liver disease, cirrhosis (13–25%), warfarin use (28–60%), vitamin K deficiency, DIC.	Homozygous deficiency of protein C (<1% activity) is associated with fatal neonatal purpura fulminans and massive venous thrombosis. Heterozygous patients (one in 200–300 of the population, with levels 25–50% of normal) may be at risk for venous thrombosis. Low protein C levels account for ~2.5% of venous thromboembolic events in some populations. In one study, patients with APC levels <5th percentile of controls (<0.69 ng/mL) had a 4.2-fold increased risk of a single venous thromboembolism and a 6.9-fold increased risk of a recurrent thromboembolic episode compared with controls. Patients with APC levels <10th percentile of controls (<0.77 ng/mL) increased these risks 3.4-fold and 5.1-fold, respectively. Interpretation of an abnormally low protein C must be tempered by the clinical setting. Anticoagulant therapy, DIC, and liver disease must not be present. There is overlap between lower limits of normal values and values found in heterozygotes. Kindred with dysfunctional protein C of normal quantity have been identified. Emerg Med Clin North Am 2001;19:839. Thromb Haemost 2001;86:1368. Arterioscler Thromb Vasc Biol 2002;22:1018.

Protein electrophoresis		
Protein electro-phoresis, serum Adults: Albumin: 3.3–5.7 g/dL α_1: 0.1–0.4 g/dL α_2: 0.3–0.9 g/dL β: 0.7–1.5 g/dL γ: 0.5–1.4 g/dL Marbled $$	Electrophoresis of serum will separate serum proteins into albumin, α_1, α_2, β, and γ fractions. Albumin is the principal serum protein (see Albumin, p 43). The term *globulin* generally refers to the nonalbumin fraction of serum protein. The α_1 fraction contains α_1-antiprotease (90%), α_1-lipoprotein, and α_1-acid glycoprotein. The α_2 fraction contains α_2-macroglobulin, haptoglobin, and ceruloplasmin. The β fraction contains transferrin, hemopexin, complement C3, and β-lipoproteins. The γ fraction contains immunoglobulins G, A, D, E, and M.	↑ α_1: inflammatory states (α_1-antiprotease), pregnancy. ↑α_2: nephrotic syndrome, inflammatory states, oral contraceptives, steroid therapy, hyperthyroidism. ↑ β: hyperlipidemia, hemoglobinemia, iron deficiency anemia. ↑ γ polyclonal gammopathies (liver disease, cirrhosis [associated with β–γ "bridging"], chronic infections, autoimmune disease); monoclonal gammopathies (multiple myeloma, Waldenström macroglobulinemia, lymphoid malignancies, monoclonal gammopathy of undetermined significance). →↓ α_1: α_1-antiprotease deficiency. →↓ α_2: in vivo hemolysis, liver disease. →↓ β: hypo-β-lipoproteinemias. →↓ γ: immune deficiency.	Presence of "spikes" in α_2, β_2, or γ regions necessitates the use of immunoelectrophoresis to verify the presence of a monoclonal gammopathy (see Immunoelectrophoresis, p 113). If Bence Jones proteins (light chains) are suspected, urine protein electrophoresis needs to be done. Test is insensitive for detection of decreased levels of immunoglobulins and α_1-antiprotease. Specific quantitation is required (see Immunoglobulins, p 114 and α_1-Antiprotease, p 51). If plasma is used, fibrinogen will be detected in the β–γ region. The "acute-phase protein pattern" seen with acute illness, surgery, infarction or trauma is characterized by an ↑α_2 (haptoglobin) and ↑α_1 (α_1-antiprotease). Arch Pathol Lab Med 1999;123:114. Blood 2001;98:1332.

Test/Range/Collection	Physiologic Basis	Interpretation	Comments
Protein S (antigen), plasma 76–178% Blue $$$	Protein S is a vitamin K-dependent glycoprotein, synthesized in the liver. It acts as a cofactor for protein C in producing its anticoagulant effect. 60% of protein S is protein-bound; only free protein S has anticoagulant function. Deficiency is associated with recurrent venous thrombosis before the age of 40.	**Decreased in:** Congenital protein S deficiency, liver disease, warfarin therapy, disseminated intravascular coagulation, vitamin K deficiency, nephrotic syndrome.	This test measures antigen and not biologic activity. Protein S can also be measured in a functional activity assay. Thromb Haemost 1997;78:351. Ann Intern Med 1998;128:8. Thromb Haemost 1998;79:802. Emerg Med Clin North Am 2001;19:839.
Protein, total, plasma or serum 6.0–8.0 g/dL [60–80 g/L] Marbled $ Avoid prolonged venous stasis during collection.	Plasma protein concentration is determined by nutritional state, hepatic function, renal function, hydration, and various disease states. Plasma protein concentration determines the colloidal osmotic pressure.	**Increased in:** Polyclonal or monoclonal gammopathies, marked dehydration. Drugs: anabolic steroids, androgens, corticosteroids, epinephrine. **Decreased in:** Protein-losing enteropathies, acute burns, nephrotic syndrome, severe dietary protein deficiency, chronic liver disease, malabsorption syndrome, agammaglobulinemia.	Serum total protein consists primarily of albumin and globulin. Serum globulin level is calculated as total protein minus albumin. Hypoproteinemia usually indicates hypoalbuminemia, because albumin is the major serum protein. Ann Thorac Surg 1999;67:236.

		Prothrombin time
Prothrombin time, whole blood (PT) 11–15 seconds ***Panic:*** ≥ 30 seconds Blue $ Fill tube completely.	PT screens the extrinsic pathway of the coagulation system. It is performed by adding calcium and tissue thromboplastin to a sample of citrated, platelet-poor plasma and measuring the time required for fibrin clot formation. It is most sensitive to deficiencies in the vitamin K-dependent clotting factors II, VII, IX, and X. It is also sensitive to deficiencies of factor V. It is insensitive to fibrinogen deficiency and not affected by heparin. PT is also used to monitor warfarin therapy. In liver disease, the PT reflects the hepatic capacity for protein synthesis. PT responds rapidly to altered hepatic function because the serum half-lives of factors II and VII are short (hours).	**Increased in:** Liver disease, vitamin K deficiency, intravascular coagulation, circulating anticoagulant, massive transfusion. Drugs: warfarin.	Routine preoperative measurement of PT is unnecessary unless there is clinical history of a bleeding disorder. Efforts to standardize and report the prothrombin time as an International Normalized Ratio (INR) depend on assigning reagents an International Sensitivity Index (ISI) so that: $$INR = \left(\frac{PT \text{ patient}}{PT \text{ normal}} \right)^{ISI}$$ However, assignment of incorrect ISI by reagent manufacturers has caused a greater lack of standardization. Bleeding has been reported to be three times more common in patients with INRs of 3.0–4.5 than in patients with INRs of 2.0–3.0. PT is quite insensitive to individual decreases in factors VII, IX, and X to 50% of normal but is much more sensitive to mild deficiencies in two or more factors. Thus, patients starting warfarin therapy or with liver disease may have elevated PT with no significant in vivo coagulation defects. Clin Lab Sci 2000;13:229. Acad Emerg Med 2002;9:567. Lancet 2002;359:47.

	Q fever antibody		
Test/Range/Collection	**Physiologic Basis**	**Interpretation**	**Comments**
Q fever antibody, serum <1:8 titer Marbled $$$ Submit paired sera, one collected within 1 week of illness and another 2–3 weeks later. Avoid hemolysis.	*Coxiella burnetii* is a rickettsial organism that is the causative organism for Q fever. Most likely mode of transmission is inhalation of aerosols from exposure to common reservoirs, sheep and cattle. Antibodies to the organism can be detected by the presence of agglutinins, by complement fixation (CF), by immunofluorescent antibody testing (IFA), or by ELISA. Agglutinin titers are found 5–8 days after infection. IgM can be detected at 7 days (IFA, ELISA) and may persist for up to 32 weeks (ELISA). IgG (IFA, ELISA) appears after 7 days and peaks at 3–4 weeks. Diagnosis of Q fever is usually confirmed by serologic findings of antiphase II antigen IgM titers of ≥1:50 and IgG titers of ≥ 1:200. The finding of elevated levels of both IgM and IgA by ELISA has both high sensitivity and high specificity for acute Q fever. In chronic Q fever, phase I antibodies, especially IgG and IgA, are predominant.	**Increased in:** Acute or chronic Q fever (CF antibodies are present by the second week in 65% of cases and by the fourth week in 90%; acute and convalescent titers [IFA or ELISA] detect infection with 89–100% sensitivity and 100% specificity), and recent vaccination for Q fever.	Clinical presentation is similar to that of severe influenza. Typically, there is no rash. Tests are usually performed in large reference labs or public health centers. Occasionally, titers do not rise for 4–6 weeks, especially if antimicrobial therapy has been given. Patients with Q fever have a high prevalence of antiphospholipid antibody (81%), especially as measured by lupus anticoagulant test or measurement of antibodies to cardiolipin. These tests may be useful in diagnosing patients presenting with fever alone. Recent Q fever vaccination causes a rise in antibody titers similar to that seen with acute infection. Antibodies to Q fever do not cross-react with other rickettsial antibodies. Clin Diag Lab Immunol 1997;4:384. Chest 1998;114:808. J Clin Microbiol 1998;36:1823. Clin Diag Lab Immunol 1999;6:173. Clin Lab 2000;46:239.

	Physiology/Method	Increased in	Comments
Rapid plasma reagin, serum (RPR) Nonreactive Marbled $	Measures nontreponemal antibodies that are produced when *Treponema pallidum* interacts with host tissue. The card test is a flocculation test performed by using a cardiolipin-lecithin-cholesterol carbon-containing antigen reagent mixed on a card with the patient's serum. A positive test (presence of antibodies) is indicated when black carbon clumps produced by flocculation are seen by the naked eye.	**Increased in:** Syphilis: primary (78%), secondary (97%), symptomatic late (74%). Biologic false positives occur in a wide variety of conditions, including leprosy, malaria, intravenous drug abuse, aging, infectious mononucleosis, HIV infection (≤15%), autoimmune diseases (SLE, rheumatoid arthritis), pregnancy.	RPR is used as a screening test and in suspected primary and secondary syphilis. Because the test lacks specificity (false-positive rates 5-20%), positive tests should be confirmed with the FTA-ABS or MHA-TP test (see pp 90 and 132, respectively). RPR titers can be used to follow serologic response to treatment. (See Syphilis test table, Table 9-20, p 393.) Ann Intern Med 1991;114:1005. J Clin Microbiol 1995;33:1829. Sex Trans Dis 1998;25:569. J Emerg Med 2000;18:361.
Red cell volume, whole blood (RCV) Male: 24-32 Female: 22-28 mL/kg Yellow Lavender (for Hct) $$$ A sample of the patient's whole blood is labeled with radioactive ^{51}Cr (which is taken up into red cells) and reinjected into the patient. Blood is sampled 10 and 60 minutes later to measure radioactivity.	Test measures absolute volume of red cells based on hemodilution of a known quantity of radioactivity in the circulation. Test can distinguish between absolute polycythemia (increased hematocrit [Hct], increased RCV) and relative polycythemia (hemoconcentration) (increased Hct, normal RCV). Alternative techniques can be used to measure RCV without exposing the patient to radiation, including use of biotin-, ^{53}Cr-, and sodium fluorescein-labeled red cells.	**Increased in:** Polycythemia vera, secondary polycythemia due to tissue hypoxemia (pulmonary disease, congenital heart disease, carboxyhemoglobinemia [cigarette smoking], methemoglobinemia), or neoplasms (renal cell carcinoma, hepatoma, large uterine leiomyomas), high altitude, pregnancy. Correction of RBC volume for degree of body fat increases accuracy.	Test is clinically indicated (but not always required) in the diagnosis of polycythemia vera. Mayo Clin Proc 1991;66:102. J Soc Gynecol Investig 1997;4:254. Transfusion 1999;39:149. Anesth Analg 1998;87:1234. Am J Clin Pathol 2000;114:922.

		Renin activity	
Test/Range/Collection	**Physiologic Basis**	**Interpretation**	**Comments**
Renin activity, plasma (PRA) *High-sodium diet* (75–150 meq Na⁺/d): supine, 0.2–2.3; standing, 1.3–4.0 ng/mL/h *Low-sodium diet* (30–75 meq Na⁺/d): standing, 4.0–7.7 ng/mL/h Lavender $$	The renal juxtaglomerular apparatus generates renin, an enzyme that converts angiotensinogen to angiotensin I. The inactive angiotensin I is then converted to angiotensin II, which is a potent vasopressor. Renin activity is measured by the ability of patient's plasma to generate angiotensin I from substrate (angiotensinogen). Normal values depend on the patient's hydration, posture, and salt intake.	**Increased in:** Dehydration, some hypertensive states (eg, renal artery stenosis); edematous states (cirrhosis, nephrotic syndrome, CHF); hypokalemic states (gastrointestinal sodium and potassium loss, Bartter syndrome); adrenal insufficiency, chronic renal failure, left ventricular hypertrophy. Drugs: ACE inhibitors, estrogen, hydralazine, nifedipine, minoxidil, oral contraceptives. **Decreased in:** Hyporeninemic hypoaldosteronism, some hypertensive states (eg, primary aldosteronism, severe preeclampsia). Drugs: β-blockers, aspirin, clonidine, prazosin, reserpine, methyldopa, indomethacin.	PRA alone is not a satisfactory screening test for hyperaldosteronism because suppressed PRA has only 64% sensitivity and 83% specificity for primary hyperaldosteronism. However, when plasma aldosterone and PRA testing are combined, the sensitivity for primary hyperaldosteronism increases to 95% (see Aldosterone, plasma, p 44). Test is also useful in evaluation of hypoaldosteronism (low-sodium diet, patient standing). Measurement of peripheral vein renin activity is not useful in classification of hypertensive patients or in diagnosis of renal artery stenosis. J Hum Hypertens 2002;16:153.

	Reptilase clotting time	Reticulocyte count
Reptilase clotting time, plasma 13–19 seconds Blue $$	Reptilase is an enzyme derived from the venom of *Bothrops atrox* or *Bothrops jararaca*, South American pit vipers. Reptilase cleaves a fibrinopeptide from fibrinogen directly, bypassing the heparin–antithrombin system, and produces a fibrin clot. The reptilase time will be normal in heparin toxicity, even when the thrombin time is infinite.	**Increased in:** Hypofibrinogenemia, dysfibrinogenemia, afibrinogenemia, and DIC. **Normal in:** Presence of heparin.	When the thrombin time is prolonged, the reptilase time is useful in distinguishing the presence of an anti-thrombin (normal reptilase time) from hypo- or dysfibrinogenemia (prolonged reptilase time). The reptilase time is normal when heparin is the cause of a prolonged thrombin time. The reptilase time is only slightly prolonged by fibrin degradation products. Arch Pathol Lab Med 2002;126:499.
Reticulocyte count, whole blood $33–137 \times 10^3/\mu L$ $[\times 10^9/L]$ Lavender $	Reticulocytes are immature red blood cells that contain cytoplasmic mRNA.	**Increased in:** Hemolytic anemia, blood loss; recovery from iron, B_{12}, or folate deficiency or drug-induced anemia. **Decreased in:** Iron deficiency anemia, aplastic anemia, anemia of chronic disease, megaloblastic anemia, sideroblastic anemia, bone marrow suppression.	This test is indicated in the evaluation of anemia to distinguish hypoproliferative from hemolytic anemia or blood loss. The old method of measuring reticulocytes (manual staining and counting) has been replaced by automated methods (eg, flow cytometry), which are more precise. Method-specific reference ranges must be used. Am J Clin Pathol 1994;102:623. Clin Lab Haematol 1996;18(Suppl 1):1 Clin Lab Med 2002;22:63.

	Rh grouping		
Test/Range/Collection	**Physiologic Basis**	**Interpretation**	**Comments**
Rh grouping, red cells (Rh) Red $ Proper identification of specimen is critical.	The Rhesus blood group system is second in importance only to the ABO system. Anti-Rh antibodies are the leading cause of hemolytic disease of the newborn and may also cause hemolytic transfusion reactions. Although there are other Rhesus antigens, only tests for the D antigen are performed routinely in pretransfusion testing because the D antigen is the most immunogenic. The terms Rh-positive and -negative refer to the presence or absence of the red cell antigen, D, on the cell surface. Persons whose red cells lack D do not regularly have anti-D in their serum. Formation of anti-D almost always results from exposure through transfusion or pregnancy to red cells possessing the D antigen.	Sixty percent of US whites are Rh(D)-positive, 40% negative; 72% of African-Americans are Rh(D)-positive, 28% negative; 95% of Asian-Americans are Rh(D)-positive, 5% negative.	Of D⁻ persons receiving a single D⁺ unit, 50–75% will develop anti-D. The blood of all donors and recipients is therefore routinely tested for D, so that D⁻ recipients can be given D⁻ blood. Donor bloods must also be tested for a weak form of D antigen, called Dᵘ, and must be labeled D⁺ if the Dᵘ test is positive. Recipient blood need not be tested for Dᵘ. *Current Opin Hematol* 2001;8:397. *Technical Manual of the American Association of Blood Banks,* 14th ed. American Association of Blood Banks, 2002.

	Rheumatoid factor		**Ribonucleoprotein antibody**
Rheumatoid factor, serum (RF) Negative (<1 : 16) Marbled $	Rheumatoid factor consists of heterogeneous autoantibodies usually of the IgM class that react against the Fc region of human IgG.	**Positive in:** Rheumatoid arthritis (75–90%), Sjögren syndrome (80–90%), scleroderma, dermatomyositis, SLE (30%), sarcoidosis, Waldenström macroglobulinemia. Drugs: methyldopa, others. Low-titer RF can be found in healthy older patients (20%), in 1–4% of normal individuals, and in a variety of acute immune responses (eg, viral infections, including infectious mononucleosis and viral hepatitis), chronic bacterial infections (tuberculosis, leprosy, subacute infective endocarditis), and chronic active hepatitis.	Rheumatoid factor can be useful in differentiating rheumatoid arthritis from other chronic inflammatory arthritides. However, a positive RF test is only one of several criteria needed to make the diagnosis of rheumatoid arthritis. (See also Autoantibodies table, p 366.) RF must be ordered selectively because its predictive value is low (34%) if it is used as a screening test. The test has poor positive predictive value because of its lack of specificity. The subset of patients with seronegative rheumatic disease limits its sensitivity and negative predictive value. Arch Intern Med 1992;152:2417. Scand J Rheumatol 2001;30:87.
Ribonucleoprotein antibody, serum (RNP) Negative Marbled $$	This is an antibody to a ribonucleoprotein-extractable nuclear antigen.	**Increased in:** Scleroderma (20–30% sensitivity, low specificity), mixed connective tissue disease (MCTD) (95–100% sensitivity, low specificity), SLE (38–44%), Sjögren syndrome, rheumatoid arthritis (10%), discoid lupus (20–30%). Anti-RNP is present in 2.7% of patients with positive ANA.	A negative test essentially excludes MCTD. (See also Autoantibodies table, p 366.) Rheum Dis Clin North Am 1992;18:283. Rheum Dis Clin North Am 1992;18:311. Rheum Dis Clin North Am 1994;20:29. Arthr Rheum 2000;43:689. Ann Rheum Dis 2001;60:1131.

Test/Range/Collection	Physiologic Basis	Interpretation	Comments
Rubella antibody, serum <1:8 titer Marbled $ For diagnosis of a recent infection, submit paired sera, one collected within 1 week of illness and another 2–4 weeks later.	Rubella (German measles) is a viral infection that causes fever, malaise, coryza, lymphadenopathy, fine maculopapular rash, and congenital birth defects when infection occurs in utero. Antibodies to rubella can be detected by hemagglutination inhibition (HI), complement fixation (CF), indirect hemagglutination (IHA), ELISA, or latex agglutination (LA). Tests can detect IgG and IgM antibody. Titers usually appear as rash fades (1 week) and peak at 10–14 days for HI and 2–3 weeks for other techniques. Baseline titers may remain elevated for life.	**Increased in:** Recent rubella infection, congenital rubella infection, previous rubella infection or vaccination (immunity). Spuriously increased IgM antibody occurs in the presence of rheumatoid factor or by cross-reacting antibodies to other viral infections or autoimmune illnesses.	Rubella titers of ≤1:8 indicate susceptibility and need for immunization to prevent infection during pregnancy. Titers of >1:32 indicate immunity from prior infection or vaccination. The recent resurgence of congenital rubella can largely be prevented with improved rubella testing and vaccination programs. Rev Infect Dis 1985;7(Suppl 1):S108. Am J Clin Pathol 1996;106:170. J Infect Dis 1997;175:749. BMJ 2002;325:147.

Russell's viper venom clotting time		
Russell's viper venom clotting time (dilute), plasma (RVVT) 24–37 seconds Blue $$	Russell viper venom is extracted from a pit viper (*Vipera russelli*), which is common in Southeast Asia (especially Burma) and causes a rapidly fatal syndrome of consumptive coagulopathy with hemorrhage, shock, rhabdomyolysis, and renal failure. Approximately 70% of the protein content of the venom is phospholipase A$_2$, which activates factor X in the presence of phospholipid, bypassing factor VII. RVVT is a phospholipid-dependent coagulation test used in detection of antiphospholipid antibodies (so-called lupus anticoagulants). It should be noted that the anticoagulant detected in vitro may be associated with thrombosis (and not bleeding) in vivo.	**Increased in:** Circulating lupus anticoagulants (LAC) (sensitivity 96%; specificity 50–70%), severe fibrinogen deficiency (<50 mg/dL), deficiencies in prothrombin, factor V, factor X, and heparin therapy. **Normal in:** Factor VII deficiency and all intrinsic pathway factor deficiencies.	The LAC may be associated with a prolonged PTT and a positive inhibitor screen (mixing study). If heparin is not present, a dilute Russell viper venom test may be indicated to confirm that the inhibitor is an LAC. Because specific factor inhibitors against factors VIII and IX are associated with clinically significant bleeding and require specific treatment, they must not be missed. The LAC is associated with an increased risk of thrombosis (venous > arterial), recurrent spontaneous abortion, and the primary antiphospholipid syndrome of arterial thrombosis. J Autoimmun 2000;15:173.

	Salicylate	Scleroderma-associated antibody
Test/Range/Collection	**Salicylate, serum (aspirin)** 20–30 mg/dL [200–300 mg/L] *Panic:* >35 mg/dL Marbled $$	**Scleroderma-associated antibody (Scl-70 antibody), serum** Negative Marbled $$
Physiologic Basis	At high concentrations, salicylate stimulates hyperventilation, uncouples oxidative phosphorylation, and impairs glucose and fatty acid metabolism. Salicylate toxicity is thus marked by respiratory alkalosis and metabolic acidosis.	This antibody reacts with a cellular antigen (DNA topoisomerase 1) that is responsible for the relaxation of supercoiled DNA.
Interpretation	**Increased in:** Acute or chronic salicylate intoxication.	**Increased in:** Scleroderma (15–20% sensitivity, high specificity).
Comments	The potential toxicity of salicylate levels after acute ingestion can be determined by using the salicylate nomogram, p 419. Nomograms have become less valid with the increasing popularity of enteric-coated slow-release aspirin preparations. Pediatrics 1960;26:800. Ann Pharmacother 1996;30:935. Am J Emerg Med 1996;14:443.	Predictive value of a positive test is >95% for scleroderma. Test has prognostic significance for severe digital ischemia in patients with Raynaud disease and scleroderma. (See also Autoantibodies table, p 366.) Am Fam Physician 2002;15;65:1073. Dermatology 2002;204:29.

Semen analysis		
Semen analysis, ejaculate Sperm count: >20 × 10⁶/mL [10⁹/L] Motility score: >60% motile Volume: 2–5 mL Normal morphology: >60% $$ Semen is collected in a urine container after masturbation following 3 days of abstinence from ejaculation. Specimen must be examined promptly.	Sperm are viewed under the microscope for motility and morphology. Infertility can be associated with low counts or with sperm of abnormal morphology or decreased motility. **Decreased in:** Primary or secondary testicular failure, cryptorchidism, following vasectomy, drugs.	A low sperm count should be confirmed by sending two other appropriately collected semen specimens for evaluation. Functional and computer-assisted sperm analyses increase diagnostic accuracy but are not yet widely available. Endocrinol Metab Clin North Am 1994;23:725. J Androl 1996;17:718. Int J Androl 1997;20:201. Fertil Steril 1997;67:1156. Hum Fertil (Camb)1999;2:25. Int J Androl 2002;25:306.

Note: Sperm count uses $>20 \times 10^6$/mL [10^9/L].

Test/Range/Collection	Physiologic Basis	Interpretation	Comments
Smith (anti-Sm) antibody, serum Negative Marbled $$	This antibody to Smith antigen (an extractable nuclear antigen) is a marker antibody for SLE.	**Positive in:** SLE (30–40% sensitivity, high specificity).	A positive test substantially increases posttest probability of SLE. Test rarely needed for the diagnosis of SLE. (See also Autoantibodies table, p 366.) Clin Rheumatol 1990;9:346. Rheum Dis Clin North Am 1992;18:311. Clin Rheumatol 1993;12:350. Arthritis Rheum 1996;39:1055. J Rheumatol 1998;25:1743. Arthr Rheum 2000;43:689. Ann Rheum Dis 2001;60:1131.
Smooth muscle antibodies, serum Negative Marbled $$	Antibodies against smooth muscle proteins are found in patients with chronic active hepatitis and primary biliary cirrhosis.	**Positive in:** Autoimmune chronic active hepatitis (40–70%, predominantly IgG antibodies), lower titers in primary biliary cirrhosis (50%, predominantly IgM antibodies), viral hepatitis, infectious mononucleosis, cryptogenic cirrhosis (28%), HIV infection, vitiligo (25%), endometriosis, Behçet disease (<2% of normal individuals).	The presence of high titers of smooth muscle antibodies (>1:80) is useful in distinguishing autoimmune chronic active hepatitis from other forms of hepatitis. Gut 1980;21:878. Br J Obstet Gynaecol 1991;98:680. J Clin Pathol 1991;44:64. J Dermatol 1993;20:679. Arthr Rheum 2000;43:689. Ann Rheum Dis 2001;60:1131.

	Sodium	Somatomedin C

Sodium, serum (Na⁺)

135—145 meq/L [mmol/L]
Panic: <125 or >155 meq/L

Marbled
$

Sodium is the predominant extracellular cation. The serum sodium level is primarily determined by the volume status of the individual. Hyponatremia can be divided into hypovolemia, euvolemia, and hypervolemia categories. (See Hyponatremia algorithm, p 350.)

Increased in: Dehydration (excessive sweating, severe vomiting or diarrhea), polyuria (diabetes mellitus, diabetes insipidus), hyperaldosteronism, inadequate water intake (coma, hypothalamic disease). Drugs: steroids, licorice, oral contraceptives.
Decreased in: CHF, vomiting, diarrhea, excessive sweating (with replacement of water but not salt), salt-losing nephropathy, adrenal insufficiency, nephrotic syndrome, water intoxication, SIADH. Drugs: thiazides, diuretics, ACE inhibitors, chlorpropamide, carbamazepine, antidepressants (selective serotonin reuptake inhibitors), antipsychotics.

Spurious hyponatremia may be produced by severe lipemia or hyperproteinemia if sodium analysis involves a dilution step.
The serum sodium falls about 1.6 meq/L for each 100 mg/dL increase in blood glucose.
Hyponatremia in a normovolemic patient with urine osmolality higher than plasma osmolality suggests the possibility of SIADH, myxedema, hypopituitarism, or reset osmostat.
Treatment of disorders of sodium balance relies on clinical assessment of the patient's extracellular fluid volume rather than the serum sodium.
Sodium is commonly measured by ion-selective electrode.
N Engl J Med 2000;342:1493.
CMAJ 2002;1666:1056.

Somatomedin C, plasma (also known as insulin-like growth factor I or IGF-I)

123–463 ng/mL (age- and sex-dependent)

Lavender
$$$$

Somatomedin C is a growth hormone-dependent plasma peptide produced by the liver. It is believed to mediate the growth-promoting effect of growth hormone (GH). It has an anabolic, insulin-like action on fat and muscle and stimulates collagen and protein synthesis. Its level is relatively constant throughout the day.

Increased in: Acromegaly (level correlates with disease activity better than GH level).
Decreased in: Pituitary dwarfism, Laron dwarfism (end-organ resistance to GH), fasting for 5–6 days, poor nutrition, hypothyroidism, cirrhosis. Values may be normal in GH-deficient patients with hyperprolactinemia or craniopharyngioma.

IGF-I is a sensitive test for acromegaly. Normal IGF-I levels rule out active acromegaly.
IGF-I can be decreased in adult growth hormone deficiency, but it is not a sensitive test.
J Clin Endocrinol Metab 2001;86:3001.

Test/Range/Collection	Physiologic Basis	Interpretation	Comments
		SS-A/Ro antibody	**SS-B/La antibody**
SS-A/Ro antibody, serum Negative Marbled $$	Antibodies to Ro (SSA) cellular ribonucleoprotein complexes are found in connective tissue diseases such as Sjögren syndrome (SS), SLE, rheumatoid arthritis (RA), and vasculitis.	**Increased in:** Sjögren syndrome (60–70% sensitivity, low specificity), SLE (30–40%), RA (10%), subacute cutaneous lupus, vasculitis.	Useful in counseling women of child-bearing age with known connective tissue disease, because a positive test is associated with a small but real risk of neonatal SLE and congenital heart block. The few (< 10%) patients with SLE who do not have a positive ANA commonly have antibodies to SS-A. (See also Autoantibodies table, p 366.) Medicine 1995;74:109. J Rheumatol 1996;23:1897. J Am Acad Dermatol 1996;35 (2 Part 1):147. J Autoimmun 1998;11:29. Br J Dermatol 1998;138:114. Clin Exper Rheumatol 1999;17:63,130.
SS-B/La antibody, serum Negative Marbled $$	Antibodies to La (SSB) cellular ribonucleoprotein complexes are found in Sjögren syndrome and appear to be relatively more specific for Sjögren syndrome than are anti-bodies to SSA. They are quantitated by immunoassay.	**Increased in:** Sjögren syndrome (50% sensitivity, higher specificity than anti-SSA), SLE (10%).	Direct pathogenicity and usefulness of autoantibody test in predicting dis-ease exacerbation not proved. (See also Autoantibodies table, p 366.) Arthritis Rheum 1996;39:1055. Ann Rheum Dis 1997;156:272. J Autoimmun 1998;11:29. Clin Exper Rheumatol 1999;17:130.

	T-cell receptor gene rearrangement	**Testosterone**
Test / Specimen / Cost	T-cell receptor gene rearrangement Whole blood, bone marrow, or frozen tissue Lavender $$$$	Testosterone, serum Males: 3.0–10.0 Females: 0.3–0.7 ng/mL [Males: 10–35 Females: 1.0–2.4 nmol/L] Marbled $$$
Physiologic Characteristics	In general, the percentage of T lymphocytes with identical T-cell receptors is very low; in malignancies, however, the clonal expansion of one population of cells with identical T-cell receptor gene rearrangement. Southern blot is used to identify a monoclonal population.	Testosterone is the principal male sex hormone, produced by the Leydig cells of the testes. Dehydroepiandrosterone (DHEA) is produced in the adrenal cortex, testes, and ovaries and is the main precursor for serum testosterone in women. In normal males after puberty, the testosterone level is twice as high as all androgens in females. In serum, it is largely bound to albumin (38%) and to a specific steroid hormone–binding globulin (SHBG) (60%), but it is the free hormone (2%) that is physiologically active. The total testosterone level measures both bound and free testosterone in the serum (by immunoassay).
Interpretation	Positive test results may be seen in T-cell neoplasms such as T-cell lymphocytic leukemia and cutaneous or nodal T-cell lymphomas.	**Increased in:** Idiopathic sexual precocity (in boys, levels may be in adult range), adrenal hyperplasia (boys), adrenocortical tumors, trophoblastic disease during pregnancy, idiopathic hirsutism, virilizing ovarian tumors, arrhenoblastoma, virilizing luteoma, testicular feminization (normal or moderately elevated), cirrhosis (through elevated SHBG), hyperthyroidism. Drugs: anticonvulsants, barbiturates, estrogens, oral contraceptives (through increased SHBG). **Decreased in:** Hypogonadism (primary and secondary), orchidectomy, Klinefelter syndrome, uremia, hemodialysis, hepatic insufficiency, ethanol [men]). Drugs: digoxin, spironolactone, acarbose.
Comments	Samples with >10% of cells showing a given T-cell rearrangement are considered positive. However, a large monoclonal population is not absolutely diagnostic of malignancy. Presence of clonal cells in peripheral blood is an independent marker of poor prognosis. Ann J Hematol 1996;52:171. Mol Pathol 1997;50:77. Arch Dermatol 1998;134:15. J Am Acad Dermatol 1998;39 (4 Part 1):554. Leukemia 1998;12:1081. J Invest Dermatol 2000;114:117.	Initial testing for hypogonadism should use total serum testosterone. Levels below 3.0 ng/mL should be treated. Free testosterone should be measured in symptomatic patients with normal total testosterone levels. In men, there is a small diurnal variation in serum testosterone with a 20% elevation in levels in the evenings. Endocrinol Metab Clin North Am 1992;21:921. Endocrinol Metab Clin North Am 1994;23:709. Fertil Steril 1998;69:286. Arch Androl 1998;40:153. Ann Intern Med 1999;130(4 Part 1):270. Am J Med 2001;110:563.

Test/Range/Collection	Physiologic Basis	Interpretation	Comments
Thrombin time, plasma 24–35 seconds (laboratory-specific) Blue $	Prolongation of the thrombin time indicates a defect in conversion of fibrinogen to fibrin.	**Increased in:** Low fibrinogen (<50 mg/dL), abnormal fibrinogen (dysfibrinogenemia), increased fibrin degradation products (eg, disseminated intravascular coagulation), heparin, fibrinolytic agents (streptokinase, urokinase, tissue plasminogen activator), primary systemic amyloidosis (40%).	Thrombin time can be used to monitor fibrinolytic therapy and to screen for dysfibrinogenemia or circulating anticoagulants. Arch Pathol Lab Med 2002;126:499.
Thyroglobulin, serum 3–42 ng/mL [µg/L] Marbled $$$	Thyroglobulin is a large protein specific to the thyroid gland from which thyroxine is synthesized and cleaved. Highly sensitive immunoradiometric assays (IRMAs) have minimal interference from autoantibodies.	**Increased in:** Hyperthyroidism, subacute thyroiditis, untreated thyroid carcinomas (except medullary carcinoma): follicular cancer (sensitivity 72%, specificity 72%), Hürthle cell cancer (sensitivity 56%, specificity 84%). **Decreased in:** Factitious hyperthyroidism, presence of thyroglobulin autoantibodies, after (>25 days) total thyroidectomy.	Thyroglobulin is useful to follow patients after treatment of non-medullary thyroid carcinomas. Levels fall after successful therapy and rise when metastases develop. Sensitivity of the test is increased if patients are off thyroid replacement for 6 weeks prior to testing or if given T_3 (Cytomel) for the first 4 weeks, then no medication for the last 2 weeks. Athyrotic patients on T_4 (levothyroxine) should have values <5 ng/mL and those off T_4 should have values <10 ng/mL. Endocrinol Metab Clin North Am 2001;30:429.

Thyroglobulin antibody, serum <1 : 10 (highly method-dependent) Marbled $$	Antibodies against thyroglobulin are produced in autoimmune diseases of the thyroid and other organs. Ten percent of the normal population have slightly elevated titers (especially women and the elderly).	**Increased in:** Hashimoto thyroiditis (>90%), thyroid carcinoma (45%), thyrotoxicosis, pernicious anemia (50%), SLE (20%), subacute thyroiditis, Graves disease. **Not Increased in:** Multinodular goiter, thyroid adenomas, and some carcinomas.	The thyroperoxidase antibody test is more sensitive than the thyroglobulin antibody test in autoimmune thyroid disease. There is little indication for this test. (See Thyroperoxidase Antibody, below.) Endocrinol Metab Clin North Am 2001;30:315. Scand J Clin Lab Invest Suppl 2001;235:45.	**Thyroglobulin antibody**
Thyroperoxidase antibody (TPO), serum Negative Marbled $$	TPO is a membrane-bound glycoprotein. This enzyme mediates the oxidation of iodide ions and incorporation of iodine into tyrosine residues of thyroglobulin. Its synthesis is stimulated by thyroid-stimulating hormone (TSH). TPO is the major antigen involved in thyroid antibody-dependent cell-mediated cytotoxicity. Antithyroperoxidase antibody assays are performed by ELISA or radioimmunoassay.	**Increased in:** Hashimoto thyroiditis (>99%), idiopathic myxedema (>99%), Graves disease (75–85%), Addison disease (50%), and Riedel thyroiditis. Low titers are present in approximately 10% of normal individuals and patients with nonimmune thyroid disease.	Thyroperoxidase antibody is an antibody to the main autoantigenic component of microsomes and is a more sensitive and specific test than hemagglutination assays for microsomal antibodies in the diagnosis of autoimmune thyroid disease. Thyroperoxidase antibody testing alone is almost always sufficient to detect autoimmune thyroid disease. Endocrinol Metab Clin North Am 2001;30:315.	**Thyroperoxidase antibody**

Test/Range/Collection	Physiologic Basis	Interpretation	Comments
Thyroid-stimulating hormone, serum (TSH; thyrotropin) 0.4–6 µU/mL [mU/L] Marbled $$	TSH is an anterior pituitary hormone that stimulates the thyroid gland to produce thyroid hormones. Secretion is stimulated by thyrotropin-releasing hormone from the hypothalamus. There is negative feedback on TSH secretion by circulating thyroid hormone.	**Increased in:** Hypothyroidism. Mild increases in recovery phase of acute illness. **Decreased in:** Hyperthyroidism, acute medical or surgical illness, pituitary hypothyroidism. Drugs: dopamine, high-dose corticosteroids.	Newer sensitive assays can detect low enough levels of TSH to be useful in the diagnosis of hyperthyroidism as well as hypothyroidism and in distinguishing hyperthyroidism from sub-normal TSH values occasionally found in euthyroid sick patients. (See also Thyroid function table, p 395.) Test is useful for following patients taking thyroid medication. Neonatal and cord blood levels are 2–4 times higher than adult levels. Clin Chem 1996;42:140. Clin Chem 1997;43:2428. J R Soc Med 1997;90:547. Lancet 2001;357:619.

Thyroid-stimulating hormone receptor antibody		Thyroxine, total
Thyroid-stimulating hormone receptor antibody, serum (TSH-R [stim] Ab) < 130% basal activity of adenylyl cyclase Marbled $$$$	Test detects heterogeneous IgG antibodies directed against the TSH receptor on thyroid cells. Frequently, they cause excess release of hormone from the thyroid. Test measures antibodies indirectly by their stimulation of adenylyl cyclase to produce cAMP.	**Increased in:** Graves disease.	Although TSH-R [stim] Ab is a marker of Graves disease, the test is not necessary for the diagnosis in most cases. Test is very rarely indicated but may be helpful in (1) pregnant women with a history of Graves disease, because TSH-R [stim] Ab may have some predictive value for neonatal thyrotoxicosis; (2) patients presenting with exophthalmos who are euthyroid, to confirm Graves disease. Use of the test to predict relapse of hyperthyroidism at the end of a course of antithyroid drugs is controversial. Endocrinol Metab Clin North Am 2000;29:339.
Thyroxine, total, serum (T$_4$) 5.0–11.0 µg/dL [64–142 nmol/L] Marbled $	Total T$_4$ is a measure of thyroid gland secretion of T$_4$, bound and free, and thus is influenced by serum thyroid hormone binding activity.	**Increased in:** Hyperthyroidism, increased thyroid-binding globulin (TBG) (eg, pregnancy, drug). Drugs: amiodarone, high-dose β-blockers (especially propranolol). **Decreased in:** Hypothyroidism, low TBG due to illness or drugs, congenital absence of TBG. Drugs: phenytoin, carbamazepine, androgens.	Total T$_4$ should be interpreted with the TBG level or as part of a free thyroxine index. Lancet 2001;357:619.

Test/Range/Collection	Physiologic Basis	Interpretation	Comments
Thyroxine, free, serum (FT₄) Varies with method Marbled $$	FT₄ (if done by equilibrium dialysis or ultrafiltration method) is a more direct measure of the free T₄ hormone concentration (biologically available hormone) than the free T₄ index. FT₄ done by a two-step immunoassay is similar to the free thyroxine index. The presence of rheumatoid factor or drug treatment with furosemide, intravenous heparin, and subcutaneous low-molecular-weight heparin may interfere with newer assays for free thyroxine.	**Increased in:** Hyperthyroidism, nonthyroidal illness, especially psychiatric. Drugs: amiodarone, β-blockers (high dose). **Decreased in:** Hypothyroidism, nonthyroidal illness. Drugs: phenytoin.	FT_4I is functionally equivalent to the FT_4I (see below). The free thyroxine and sensitive TSH assays have similar sensitivities for detecting clinical hyperthyroidism and hypothyroidism. The TSH assay detects subclinical dysfunction and monitors thyroxine treatment better; the free thyroxine test detects central hypothyroidism and monitors rapidly changing function better. Arch Intern Med 1996;156:2333. Clin Chem 1996;42:146. Arch Intern Med 1998;158:266. Lancet 2001;357:619.
Thyroxine index, free, serum (FT₄I) 6.5–12.5 Marbled $$	Free thyroxine index is expressed as total $T_4 \times T_3$ (or T_4) resin uptake and provides an estimate of the level of free T_4, since the T_3 (or T_4) resin uptake (ie, thyroid hormone binding ratio) is an indirect estimate of the TBG concentration (TBG binds 70% of circulating thyroid hormone). The unbound form of circulating T_4, normally 0.03% of total serum T_4, determines the amount of T_4 available to cells.	**Increased in:** Hyperthyroidism, nonthyroidal illness, especially psychiatric. Drugs: amiodarone, β-blockers (high dose). **Decreased in:** Hypothyroidism, nonthyroidal illness. Drugs: phenytoin.	Test is useful in patients with clinically suspected hyper- or hypothyroidism, in elderly patients admitted to geriatric units, or in women over 40 with one or more somatic complaints. (See Thyroid function table, p 395.) Screening for thyroid disease is not indicated in younger women, men, or patients admitted with acute medical or psychiatric illnesses because transient abnormalities are indistinguishable from true thyroid disease. FT_4I is functionally equivalent to the FT_4 (see above). Lancet 2001;357:619.

Toxoplasma antibody		
Toxoplasma antibody, serum or CSF (Toxo) IgG: <1:16 IgM: Infant <1:2 Adult <1:8 titer Marbled or CSF $$$ Submit paired sera, one collected within 1 week of illness and another 2–3 weeks later.	*Toxoplasma gondii* is an obligate intracellular protozoan that causes human infection via ingestion, transplacental transfer, blood products, or organ transplantation. Cats are the definitive hosts of *T gondii* and pass oocysts in their feces. Human infection occurs through ingestion of sporulated oocysts or via the transplacental route. In the immunodeficient host, acute infection may progress to lethal meningoencephalitis, pneumonitis, or myocarditis. In acute primary infection, IgM antibodies develop 1–2 weeks after onset of illness, peak in 6–8 weeks, and then decline. IgG antibodies develop on a similar time-course but persist for years. In adult infection, the disease usually represents a reactivation, not a primary infection. Therefore, the IgM test is less useful. Approximately 30% of all US adults have antibodies to *T gondii*.	**Increased in:** Acute or congenital toxoplasmosis (IgM), previous toxoplasma exposure (IgG), and false-positive (IgM) reactions (SLE, HIV infection, rheumatoid arthritis).	Single IgG titers of >1:256 are considered diagnostic of active infection; titers of >1:128 are suspicious. Titers of 1:16–1:64 may merely represent past exposure. If titers subsequently rise, they probably represent early disease. IgM titer >1:16 is very important in the diagnosis of congenital toxoplasmosis. High titer IgG antibody results should prompt an IgM test. IgM, however, is generally not found in adult AIDS patients because the disease usually represents a reactivation. Some recommend ordering baseline toxoplasma IgG titers in all asymptomatic HIV-positive patients because a rising toxoplasma titer can help diagnose CNS toxoplasmosis in the future. Culture of the *T gondii* organism is difficult, and most laboratories are not equipped for the procedure. (See also Brain abscess, p 199.) J Clin Lab Anal 1997;11:214. J Clin Microbiol 1997;35:174. Br J Biomed Sci 2002;59:4. J Infect Dis 2002;185(Suppl 1):S73. Trans R Soc Trop Med Hyg 2002;96(Suppl 1):S205.

	Test/Range/Collection	Physiologic Basis	Interpretation	Comments
Triglycerides	**Triglycerides,** serum (TG) <165 mg/dL [<1.65 g/L] Marbled $ Fasting specimen required.	Dietary fat is hydrolyzed in the small intestine, absorbed and resynthesized by mucosal cells, and secreted into lacteals as chylomicrons. Triglycerides in the chylomicrons are cleared from the blood by tissue lipoprotein lipase. Endogenous triglyceride production occurs in the liver. These triglycerides are transported in association with β-lipoproteins in very low density lipoproteins (VLDL).	**Increased in:** Hypothyroidism, diabetes mellitus, nephrotic syndrome, chronic alcoholism (fatty liver), biliary tract obstruction, stress, familial lipoprotein lipase deficiency, familial dysbetalipoproteinemia, familial combined hyperlipidemia, obesity, viral hepatitis, cirrhosis, pancreatitis, chronic renal failure, gout, pregnancy, glycogen storage diseases types I, III, and VI, anorexia nervosa, dietary excess. Drugs: β-blockers, cholestyramine, corticosteroids, diazepam, diuretics, estrogens, oral contraceptives. **Decreased in:** Tangier disease (α-lipoprotein deficiency), hypo- and abetalipoproteinemia, malnutrition, malabsorption, parenchymal liver disease, hyperthyroidism, intestinal lymphangiectasia. Drugs: ascorbic acid, clofibrate, nicotinic acid, gemfibrozil.	If serum is clear, the serum triglyceride level is generally <350 mg/dL. Despite extensive research, it remains unclear whether triglycerides are an independent risk factor for coronary artery disease. Triglycerides >1000 mg/dL can be seen when a primary lipid disorder is exacerbated by alcohol or fat intake or by corticosteroid or estrogen therapy. Am J Cardiol 2000;86:943. Arch Intern Med 2000;160:1937.
Triiodothyronine	**Triiodothyronine,** total, serum (T_3) 95–190 ng/dL [1.5–2.9 nmol/L] Marbled $$	T_3 reflects the metabolically active form of thyroid hormone and is influenced by thyroid hormone-binding activity.	**Increased in:** Hyperthyroidism (some), increased thyroid-binding globulin. **Decreased in:** Hypothyroidism, nonthyroidal illness, decreased thyroid-binding globulin. Drugs: amiodarone.	T_3 may be increased in approximately 5% of hyperthyroid patients in whom T_4 is normal (T_3 toxicosis). Therefore, test is indicated when hyperthyroidism is suspected and T_4 value is normal. Test is of no value in the diagnosis of hypothyroidism. Lancet 2001;357:619.

Troponin-I, cardiac		
Troponin-I, cardiac, serum (cTnI) < 1.5 ng/mL Marbled $$	Troponin is the contractile regulatory protein of striated muscle. It contains three subunits: T, C, and I. Subunit I consists of three forms, which are found in slow-twitch skeletal muscle, fast-twitch skeletal muscle, and cardiac muscle, respectively. Troponin I is predominantly a structural protein and is released into the circulation after cellular necrosis. Cardiac troponin I is expressed only in cardiac muscle, throughout development and despite pathology, and thus its presence in serum can distinguish between myocardial injury and skeletal muscle injury. cTnI is measured by immunoassay using monoclonal antibodies.	**Increased in:** Myocardial infarction (sensitivity 50% at 4 hours, 97% at 6 hours; specificity 95%), cardiac trauma, cardiac surgery, myocardial damage following PTCA, defibrillations and other cardiac interventions, nonischemic dilated cardiomyopathy. Slight elevations noted in patients with recent aggravated unstable angina, muscular disorders, CNS disorders, HIV infection, chronic renal failure, cirrhosis, sepsis, lung diseases, and endocrine disorders. **Not Increased in:** Skeletal muscle disease (myopathy, myositis, dystrophy), noncardiac trauma or surgery, rhabdomyolysis, severe muscular exertion, chronic renal failure.	Cardiac troponin I is a more specific marker for myocardial infarction than CK–MB with roughly equivalent sensitivity early in the course of infarction (4–36 hours). Sensitivity and specificity for peak concentrations of cTnI (100%; 96%) are equivalent to or better than those for CK–MB (88%; 93%) and total CK (73%; 85%). cTnI appears in serum approximately 4 hours after onset of chest pain, peaks at 8–12 hours, and persists for 5–7 days. This prolonged persistence gives it much greater sensitivity than CK–MB for diagnosis of myocardial infarction beyond the first 36–48 hours. Minor elevations of cardiac troponin I should be interpreted with caution, particularly in patients suffering from acute illnesses who do not have chest pain or prior myocardial infarction. Am Heart J 1999;137:332. Am J Emerg Med 1999;17:225 Ann Clin Biochem 2001;38(Pt 5):423. Cardiol Rev 2002;10:306.

	Tularemia agglutinins	Type and cross-match
Test/Range/Collection	**Tularemia agglutinins,** serum <1:80 titer Marbled $$	**Type and cross-match,** serum and red cells (type and cross) Red $$ Specimen label must be signed by the person drawing the blood. A second "check" specimen is needed at some hospitals.
Physiologic Basis	*Francisella tularensis* is an organism of wild rodents (rabbits and hares) that infects humans (eg, trappers and skinners) via contact with animal tissues, by the bite of certain ticks and flies, and by consumption of undercooked meat or contaminated water. Agglutinating antibodies appear in 10–14 days and peak in 5–10 weeks. A four-fold rise in titers is typically needed to prove acute infection. Titers decrease over years.	A type and cross-match involves ABO and Rh grouping (see pp 41 and 160, respectively), antibody screen (see p 50), and cross-match. (Compare with Type and Screen, below.) A major cross-match involves testing recipient serum against donor cells. It uses antihuman globulin to detect recipient's antibodies on donor red cells. If the recipient's serum contains a clinically significant alloantibody by antibody screen, a cross-match is required.
Interpretation	**Increased in:** Tularemia; cross-reaction with brucella antigens and proteus OX-19 antigen (but at lower titers).	
Comments	Single titers of >1:160 are indicative of infection. Maximum titers are >1:1280. A history of exposure to rabbits, ticks, dogs, cats, or skunks is suggestive of—but is not a requirement for—the diagnosis. Most common presentation is a single area of painful lymphadenopathy with low-grade fever. Initial treatment should be empiric. Culture of the organism is difficult, requiring special media, and hazardous to laboratory personnel. Serologic tests are the mainstay of diagnosis. Clin Microbiol Rev 2002;15:631.	A type and screen is adequate preparation for operative procedures unlikely to require transfusion. Unnecessary type and cross-match orders reduce blood availability and add to costs. In addition, a preordering system should be in place, indicating the number of units of blood likely to be needed for each operative procedure. J Trauma 2001;50:878. *Technical Manual of the American Association of Blood Banks,* 14th ed. American Association of Blood Banks, 2002.

Type and screen		
Type and screen, serum and red cells Red or lavender $$ Specimen label must be signed by the person drawing the blood. A second "check" specimen is needed at some hospitals.	Type and screen includes ABO and Rh grouping (see pp 41 and 160, respectively) and antibody screen (see p 50). (Compare with type and cross-match, above.)	A negative antibody screen implies that a recipient can receive un-cross-matched type-specific blood with minimal risk. If the recipient's serum contains a clinically significant alloantibody by antibody screen, a cross-match is required.	Type and screen is indicated for patients undergoing operative procedures unlikely to require transfusion. However, in the absence of preoperative indications, routine preoperative blood type and screen testing is not cost-effective and may be eliminated for some procedures, such as laparoscopic cholecystectomy, expected vaginal delivery, and vaginal hysterectomy. Am J Obstet Gynecol 1996;175:1201. Obstet Gynecol 1998;94(4 Part 1):493. Surg Endosc 1999;13:146. Br J Anaesth 2002;89:221. *Technical Manual of the American Association of Blood Banks,* 14th ed. American Association of Blood Banks, 2002.

Test/Range/Collection	Physiologic Basis	Interpretation	Comments
Uric acid, serum Males: 2.4–7.4 Females 1.4–5.8 mg/dL [Males: 140–440 Females: 80–350 μmol/L] Marbled $	Uric acid is an end product of nucleo-protein metabolism and is excreted by the kidney. An increase in serum uric acid concentration occurs with increased nucleoprotein synthesis or catabolism (blood dyscrasias, therapy of leukemia) or decreased renal uric acid excretion (eg, thiazide diuretic therapy or renal failure).	**Increased in:** Renal failure, gout, myelo-proliferative disorders (leukemia, lymphoma, myeloma, polycythemia vera), psoriasis, glycogen storage disease (type I), Lesch-Nyhan syndrome (X-linked hypoxanthine-guanine phosphoribosyltransferase deficiency), lead nephropathy, hypertensive diseases of pregnancy, menopause. Drugs: antimetabolite and chemotherapeutic agents, diuretics, ethanol, nicotinic acid, salicylates (low dose), theophylline. **Decreased in:** SIADH, xanthine oxidase deficiency, low-purine diet, Fanconi syndrome, neoplastic disease (various, causing increased renal excretion), liver disease. Drugs: salicylates (high dose), allopurinol (xanthine oxidase inhibitor).	Sex, age, and renal function affect uric acid levels. The incidence of hyperuricemia is greater in some ethnic groups (eg, Filipinos) than others (whites). Whether uric acid level is an independent risk factor for heart disease is controversial. Curr Hypertens Rep 2001;3:184. Curr Hypertens Rep 2001;3:190. Curr Opin Rheumatol 2002;14:281.

	Vanillylmandelic acid	VDRL test, serum
Vanillylmandelic acid, urine (VMA) 2–7 mg/24 h [10–35 μmol/d] Urine bottle containing hydrochloric acid $$ Collect 24-hour urine.	Catecholamines secreted in excess by pheochromocytomas are metabolized by the enzymes monoamine oxidase and catechol-O-methyltransferase to VMA, which is excreted in urine.	**Increased in:** Pheochromocytoma (64% sensitivity, 95% specificity), neuroblastoma, ganglioneuroma, generalized anxiety. **Decreased in:** Drugs: monoamine oxidase inhibitors.	A plasma free metanephrine level (p 126) is the recommended test for the diagnosis of pheochromocytoma. (See also Pheochromocytoma algorithm, p 353.) <0.1% of hypertensive patients have a pheochromocytoma. JAMA 2002;287:1427.
Venereal Disease Research Laboratory test, serum (VDRL) Nonreactive Marbled $	This syphilis test measures nontreponemal antibodies that are produced when *Treponema pallidum* interacts with host tissues. The VDRL usually becomes reactive at a titer of >1:32 within 1–3 weeks after the genital chancre appears.	**Increased in:** Syphilis: primary (59–87%), secondary (100%), late latent (79–91%), tertiary (37–94%); collagen-vascular diseases (rheumatoid arthritis, SLE), infections (mononucleosis, leprosy, malaria), pregnancy, drug abuse.	VDRL is used as a syphilis screening test and in suspected cases of primary and secondary syphilis. Positive tests should be confirmed with an FTA-ABS or MHA-TP test (see pp 90 and 132, respectively). The VDRL has similar sensitivity and specificity to the RPR (see Syphilis test table, p 393). Ann Intern Med 1986;104:368. Ann Intern Med 1991;114:1005. Sex Trans Dis 1998;26:12. J Emerg Med 2000;18:361.

	VDRL test, CSF		
Test/Range/Collection	Physiologic Basis	Interpretation	Comments
Venereal Disease Research Laboratory test, CSF (VDRL) Nonreactive $$ Deliver in a clean plastic or glass tube.	The CSF VDRL test measures nontreponemal antibodies that develop in the CSF when *Treponema pallidum* interacts with the central nervous system.	**Increased in:** Tertiary neurosyphilis (10–27%).	The quantitative VDRL is the test of choice for CNS syphilis. Because the sensitivity of CSF VDRL is very low, a negative test does not rule out neurosyphilis. Clinical features, CSF white cell count, and CSF protein should be used together to make the diagnosis (see CSF profiles, p 368). Because the specificity of the CSF VDRL test is high, a positive test confirms the presence of neurosyphilis. Patients being screened for neurosyphilis with CSF VDRL testing should have a positive serum RPR, VDRL, FTA-ABS, MHA-TP test or other evidence of infection. Repeat testing may be indicated in HIV-infected patients in whom neurosyphilis is suspected. When the CSF VDRL is negative but suspicion of CNS syphilis is high, other commonly used laboratory tests (CSF FTA ABS, serum FTA-ABS, CSF *Treponema pallidum* hemagglutination [TPHA], serum TPHA, and CSF cells) can, in combination, identify 87% of patients with neurosyphilis with 94% specificity. Gen Hosp Psychiatry 1995;17:305. Sex Trans Dis 1996;23:392. Int J Psychiatr Med 1998;28:333. Psychosomatics 2001;42:453.

Vitamin B₁₂		
Vitamin B₁₂, serum 140–820 pg/mL [100–600 pmol/L] Marbled $$ $$ Serum vitamin B₁₂ specimens should be frozen if not analyzed immediately.	Vitamin B₁₂ is a necessary cofactor for three important biochemical processes; conversion of methylmalonyl-CoA to succinyl-CoA and methylation of homocysteine to methionine and demethylation of methyltetrahydrofolate to tetrahydrofolate (THF). Consequent deficiency of folate coenzymes derived from THF is probably the crucial lesion caused by B₁₂ deficiency. All vitamin B₁₂ comes from ingestion of foods of animal origin. Vitamin B₁₂ in serum is protein bound, 70% to transcobalamin I (TC I) and 30% to transcobalamin II (TC II). The B₁₂ bound to TC II is physiologically active; that bound to TC I is not.	**Increased in:** Leukemia (acute myelocytic, chronic myelocytic, chronic lymphocytic, monocytic), marked leukocytosis, polycythemia vera. (Increased B₁₂ levels are not diagnostically useful.) **Decreased in:** Pernicious anemia, gastrectomy, gastric carcinoma, malabsorption (sprue, celiac disease, steatorrhea, regional enteritis, fistulas, bowel resection, *Diphyllobothrium latum* [fish tapeworm] infestation, small bowel bacterial overgrowth), pregnancy, dietary deficiency, HIV infection (with or without malabsorption), chronic high-flux hemodialysis, Alzheimer disease, drugs (eg, omeprazole, metformin, carbamazepine). Using a cutoff of 150 pmol/L, this test has sensitivity 90%, specificity 60% for B₁₂ deficiency.	Differentiation among the causes of vitamin B₁₂ deficiency can be accomplished by a vitamin B₁₂ absorption (Schilling) test (see below). The commonly available competitive protein binding assay measures total B₁₂. It is insensitive to significant decreases in physiologically significant B₁₂ bound to TC II. Low B₁₂ levels warrant treatment; intermediate levels should be followed with serum methylmalonic acid test (p 129). Neuropsychiatric disorders caused by low serum B₁₂ level can occur in the absence of anemia or macrocytosis. Clin Chem 2000;46:1744.

Vitamin B$_{12}$ absorption test			
Test/Range/Collection	Physiologic Basis	Interpretation	Comments
Vitamin B$_{12}$ absorption test, 24-hour urine (Schilling test) Excretion of >8% of administered dose \$\$\$\$ Stage I: 0.5–1.0 µCi of ^{52}Co–B$_{12}$ is given orally, followed by 1.0 mg of unlabeled B$_{12}$ IM 2 hours later. A 24-hour urine is collected. Stage II: After 5 days, test is repeated with 60 mg active hog intrinsic factor added to the oral labeled B$_{12}$.	Absorption of vitamin B$_{12}$ is dependent on two factors: adequate intrinsic factor produced by the stomach antrum and normal ileal absorption. Lack of either can lead to B$_{12}$ deficiency.	**Decreased in:** Ileal disease or resection, bacterial overgrowth, B$_{12}$ deficiency (because megaloblastosis of the intestinal wall leads to decreased B$_{12}$ absorption, pernicious anemia (<2.5% excretion of administered dose), postgastrectomy, chronic pancreatitis, cystic fibrosis, giardiasis, Crohn disease.	Schilling test is no longer an integral part of diagnosing and treating vitamin B$_{12}$ deficiency. J Intern Med 1997;241:47.

	Physiology	Increased/Decreased in	Interpretation
Vitamin D₃, 25-hydroxy, serum or plasma (25[OH]D₃) 10–50 ng/mL [25–125 nmol/L] Marbled or green $$$	The vitamin D system functions to maintain serum calcium levels. Vitamin D is a fat-soluble steroid hormone. Two molecular forms exist: D₃ (cholecalciferol), synthesized in the epidermis, and D₂ (ergocalciferol), derived from plant sources. To become active, both need to be further metabolized. Two sequential hydroxylations occur: in the liver to 25(OH)D₃ and then, in the kidney, to 1,25[OH]₂D₃. Plasma levels increase with sun exposure.	**Increased in:** Heavy milk drinkers (up to 64 ng/mL), vitamin D intoxication, sun exposure. **Decreased in:** Dietary deficiency, malabsorption (rickets, osteomalacia), biliary and portal cirrhosis, nephrotic syndrome, lack of sun exposure, osteoarthritis, age. Drugs: phenytoin, phenobarbital.	**Vitamin D₃, 25-hydroxy** Measurement of 25(OH)D₃ is the best indicator of both vitamin D deficiency and toxicity. It is indicated in hypocalcemic disorders associated with increased PTH levels, in children with rickets and in adults with osteomalacia. In hypercalcemic disorders, 25(OH)D₃ is useful in disorders associated with decreased PTH levels, or possible vitamin D overdose (hypervitaminosis D). Vitamin D toxicity is manifested by hypercalcemia, hyperphosphatemia, soft tissue calcification, and renal failure. *Clin Lab Med* 2000;20:569.
Vitamin D₃, 1,25-dihydroxy, serum or plasma (1,25[OH]₂D₃) 20–76 pg/mL Marbled or green $$$$	1,25-Dihydroxy vitamin D₃ is the most potent form of vitamin D. The main actions of vitamin D are the acceleration of calcium and phosphate absorption in the intestine and stimulation of bone resorption.	**Increased in:** Primary hyperparathyroidism, idiopathic hypercalciuria, sarcoidosis, some lymphomas, 1,25(OH)₂D₃-resistant rickets, normal growth (children), pregnancy, lactation, vitamin D toxicity. **Decreased in:** Chronic renal failure, anephric patients, hypoparathyroidism, pseudohypoparathyroidism, 1 α-hydroxylase deficiency, postmenopausal osteoporosis.	**Vitamin D₃, 1,25-dihydroxy** Test is rarely needed. Measurement of 1,25(OH)₂D₃ is only useful in distinguishing 1 α-hydroxylase deficiency from 1,25(OH)₂D₃-resistant rickets or in monitoring vitamin D status of patients with chronic renal failure. Test is not useful for assessment of vitamin D intoxication because of efficient feedback regulation of 1,25(OH)₂D₃ synthesis. *Clin Lab Med* 2000;20:569.

Test/Range/Collection	Physiologic Basis	Interpretation	Comments
von Willebrand factor protein (immunologic), plasma (vWF) 44–158% units Blue $$$	vWF is produced by endothelial cells, circulates in the plasma complexed to factor VIII coagulant protein, and mediates platelet adhesion. vWF is a marker of endothelial injury. Both quantitative and qualitative changes can cause disease. vWF can be measured as protein antigen (immunologic measure) or by ristocetin cofactor activity (functional assay).	**Increased in:** Inflammatory states (acute phase reactant). **Decreased in:** von Willebrand disease.	In von Willebrand disease, the platelet count and morphology are generally normal and the bleeding time is usually prolonged (markedly prolonged by aspirin). Variant forms associated with mild thrombocytopenia and angiodysplasia are described. The PTT may not be prolonged if factor VIII coagulant level is >30%. Diagnosis is suggested by bleeding symptoms and family history. Laboratory diagnosis of von Willebrand disease has become more difficult because of the identification of numerous variant forms. In the classic type I disease, vWF antigen is decreased. Thromb Haemost 2000;84:160. Rev Clin Exp Hematol 2001;5:335.
		von Willebrand factor protein	

D-Xylose absorption test		
D-Xylose absorption test, urine >5 g per 5-hour urine (>20% excreted in 5 hours) $$$ Fasting patient is given D-xylose, 25 g in two glasses of water, followed by four glasses of water over the next 2 hours. Urine is collected for 5 hours and refrigerated.	Xylose is normally easily absorbed from the small intestine. Measuring xylose in serum or its excretion in urine after ingestion evaluates the carbohydrate absorption ability of the proximal small intestine.	**Decreased in:** Intestinal malabsorption, small intestinal bacterial overgrowth, renal insufficiency, small intestinal HIV enteropathy, cryptosporidiosis, cytotoxic therapy-related malabsorption.	Test can be helpful in distinguishing intestinal malabsorption (decreased D-xylose absorption) from pancreatic insufficiency (normal D-xylose absorption). Urinary xylose excretion may be spuriously decreased in renal failure, thus limiting the specificity and usefulness of the test. In this case, a serum xylose level (gray-top tube) obtained 1 hour after administration of a 25-g dose of D-xylose can be used to evaluate xylose absorption. The normal level should be >29 mg/dL (1.9 mmol/L). Dig Dis Sci 1991;36:188. J Acquir Immune Defic Syndr 1992;5:1047. Gastroenterology 1995;108:1075. Dig Dis Sci 1997;42:2599. J Clin Oncol 1997;15:2254. J Clin Gastroenterol 2001;33:36.

4

Therapeutic Drug Monitoring: Principles and Test Interpretation

Diana Nicoll, MD, PhD, MPA

UNDERLYING ASSUMPTIONS

The basic assumptions underlying therapeutic drug monitoring (Table 4–1) are that drug metabolism varies from patient to patient and that the plasma level of a drug is more closely related to the drug's therapeutic effect or toxicity than is the dosage.

INDICATIONS FOR DRUG MONITORING

Drugs with a **narrow therapeutic index** (where therapeutic drug levels do not differ greatly from levels associated with serious toxicity) should be monitored. *Example:* Lithium.

Patients who have **impaired clearance of a drug with a narrow therapeutic index** are candidates for drug monitoring. The clearance mechanism of the drug involved must be known. *Example:* Patients with renal failure have decreased clearance of gentamicin and therefore are at a higher risk for gentamicin toxicity.

Drugs whose **toxicity is difficult to distinguish from a patient's underlying disease** may require monitoring. *Example:* Theophylline in patients with chronic obstructive pulmonary disease.

Drugs whose efficacy is **difficult to establish clinically** may require monitoring of plasma levels. *Example:* Phenytoin.

SITUATIONS IN WHICH DRUG MONITORING MAY NOT BE USEFUL

Drugs that can be given in extremely high doses before toxicity is apparent are not candidates for monitoring. *Example:* Penicillin.

If there are better means of assessing drug effects, drug level monitoring may not be appropriate. *Example:* Warfarin is monitored by prothrombin time and International Normalized Ratio (INR) determinations, not by serum levels.

Drug level monitoring to assess compliance is limited by the inability to distinguish noncompliance from rapid metabolism without direct inpatient scrutiny of drug administration.

Drug toxicity cannot be diagnosed with drug levels alone; it is a clinical diagnosis. Drug levels within the usual therapeutic range do not rule out drug toxicity in a given patient. *Example:* Digoxin, where other physiologic variables (eg, hypokalemia) affect drug toxicity.

In summary, therapeutic drug monitoring may be useful to guide dosage adjustment of certain drugs in certain patients. Patient compliance is essential if drug monitoring data are to be correctly interpreted.

OTHER INFORMATION REQUIRED FOR EFFECTIVE DRUG MONITORING

Reliability of the Analytic Method

The analytic **sensitivity** of the drug monitoring method must be adequate. For some drugs, plasma levels are in the nanogram per milliliter range. *Example:* Tricyclic antidepressants, digoxin.

The **specificity** of the method must be known, because the drug's metabolites or other drugs may interfere. Interference by metabolites—which may or may not be pharmacologically active—is of particular concern in immunologic assay methods using antibodies to the parent drug.

The **precision** of the method must be known to assess whether changes in levels are caused by method imprecision or by clinical changes.

Reliability of the Therapeutic Range

Establishing the therapeutic range for a drug requires a reliable clinical assessment of its therapeutic and toxic effects, together with plasma drug level measurements by a particular analytic method. In practice, as newer, more specific analytic methods are introduced, the therapeutic ranges for those methods are estimated by comparing the old and new methodologies—without clinical correlation.

Pharmacokinetic Parameters

Five pharmacokinetic parameters that are important in therapeutic drug monitoring include:

1. *Bioavailability.* The bioavailability of a drug depends in part on its formulation. A drug that is significantly metabolized as it first passes through the liver exhibits a marked "first-pass effect," reducing the effective oral absorption of the drug. A reduction in this first-pass effect (eg, because of decreased hepatic blood flow in heart failure) could cause a clinically significant increase in effective oral drug absorption.

2. *Volume of distribution and distribution phases.* The volume of distribution of a drug determines the plasma concentration reached after a loading dose. The distribution phase is the time taken for a drug to distribute from the plasma to the periphery. Drug levels drawn before completion of a long distribution phase may not reflect levels of pharmacologically active drug at sites of action. *Examples:* Digoxin, lithium.

3. *Clearance.* Clearance is either renal or nonrenal (usually hepatic). Whereas changes in renal clearance can be predicted on the basis of serum creatinine or creatinine clearance, there is no routine liver function test for assessment of hepatic drug metabolism. For most therapeutic drugs measured, clearance is independent of plasma drug concentration, so that a change in dose is reflected in a similar change in plasma level. If, however, clearance is dose dependent, dosage adjustments produce disproportionately large changes in plasma levels and must be made cautiously. *Example:* Phenytoin.

4. *Half-life.* The half-life of a drug depends on its volume of distribution and its clearance and determines the time taken to reach a steady state level. In three or four half-lives, the drug level will be 87.5–93.75% of the way to steady state. Patients with decreased drug clearance and therefore increased drug half-lives will take longer to reach a higher steady-state level. In general, because non–steady-state drug levels are potentially misleading and can be difficult to interpret, it is recommended that most clinical monitoring be done at steady state.

5. *Protein binding of drugs.* All routine drug level analysis involves assessment of both protein-bound and free drug. However, pharmacologic activity depends on only the free drug level. Changes in protein binding (eg, in uremia or hypoalbuminemia) may significantly affect interpretation of reported levels for drugs that are highly protein-bound. *Example:* Phenytoin. In such cases, where the ratio of free to total measured drug level is increased, the usual therapeutic range based on total drug level will not apply.

Drug Interactions

For patients receiving several medications, the possibility of drug interactions affecting drug elimination must be considered. *Example:* Quinidine, verapamil, and amiodarone decrease digoxin clearance.

Time to Draw Levels

In general, the specimen should be drawn after steady state is reached (at least three or four half-lives after a dosage adjustment) and just before the next dose (trough level).

Peak and trough levels may be indicated to evaluate the dosage of drugs whose half-lives are much shorter than the dosing interval. *Example:* Gentamicin.

Reference

Winter M: *Basic Clinical Pharmacokinetics,* 3rd ed. Applied Therapeutics, 1994.

TABLE 4–1. THERAPEUTIC DRUG MONITORING.

Drug	Effective Concentrations	Half-Life (hours)	Dosage Adjustment	Comments
Amikacin	Peak: 10–30 µg/mL Trough: <10 µg/mL	2–3 ↑ in uremia	↓ in renal dysfunction	Concomitant kanamycin or tobramycin therapy may give falsely elevated amikacin results by immunoassay.
Amitriptyline	95–250 ng/mL	9–46		Drug is highly protein bound. Patient-specific decrease in protein binding may invalidate quoted range of effective concentration.
Carbamazepine	4–12 mg/mL	15		Induces its own metabolism. Metabolite 10,11-epoxide exhibits 13% cross-reactivity by immunoassay. Toxicity: diplopia, drowsiness, nausea, vomiting, and ataxia.
Cyclosporine	150–400 ng/mL (µg/L) whole blood	6–12	Need to know specimen and methodology used	Cyclosporine is lipid soluble (20% bound to leukocytes; 40% to erythrocytes; 40% in plasma, highly bound to lipoproteins). Binding is temperature dependent, so whole blood is preferred to plasma or serum as specimen. High-performance liquid chromatography or monoclonal fluorescence polarization immunoassay measures cyclosporine reliably. Polyclonal fluorescence polarization immunoassays cross-react with metabolites, so the therapeutic range used with those assays is higher. Anticonvulsants and rifampin increase metabolism. Erythromycin, ketoconazole, and calcium channel blockers decrease metabolism.
Desipramine	100–250 ng/mL	13–23		Drug is highly protein bound. Patient-specific decrease in protein binding may invalidate quoted range of effective concentration.

(continued)

TABLE 4-1 (CONTINUED).

Drug	Effective Concentrations	Half-Life (hours)	Dosage Adjustment	Comments
Digoxin	0.8–2.0 ng/mL	42 ↑ in uremia, CHF, hypothyroidism; ↓ in hyperthyroidism	↓ in renal dysfunction, CHF, hypothyroidism; ↑ in hyperthyroidism	Bioavailability of digoxin tablets is 50–90%. Specimen must not be drawn within 6 hours of dose. Dialysis does not remove a significant amount. Hypokalemia potentiates toxicity. Digitalis toxicity is a clinical and *not* a laboratory diagnosis. Digibind (digoxin-specific antibody) therapy of digoxin overdose can interfere with measurement of digoxin levels depending on the digoxin assay. Elimination is reduced by quinidine, verapamil, and amiodarone.
Ethosuximide	40–100 mg/L	Child: 30 Adult: 50		Levels used primarily to assess compliance. Toxicity is rare and does not correlate well with plasma concentrations.
Gentamicin	Peak: 4–8 μg/mL Trough: <2 μg/mL	2–5 ↑ in uremia (7.3 on dialysis)	↓ in renal dysfunction	Draw peak specimen 30 minutes after end of infusion. Draw trough just before next dose. In uremic patients, carbenicillin may reduce gentamicin half-life from 46 to 22 hours. If a once-daily regimen (5 mg/kg) is used to maximize bacterial killing by optimizing the peak concentration/MIC ratio and to reduce the potential for toxicity, dosage should be reduced if trough concentration is >1 μg/mL (1 mg/L). Measurement of peak concentrations is not recommended with this regimen.
Imipramine	180–350 ng/mL	10–16		Drug is highly protein bound. Patient-specific decrease in protein binding may invalidate quoted range of effective concentration.
Lidocaine	1–5 μg/mL	1.8 ↔ in uremia, CHF; ↑ in cirrhosis	↓ in CHF, liver disease	Levels increased with cimetidine therapy. CNS toxicity common in the elderly.

Lithium	0.7–1.5 mmol/L			Thiazides and loop diuretics may increase serum lithium levels.
Methotrexate		22 ↑ in uremia	↓ in renal dysfunction	
Methotrexate		8.4 ↑ in uremia	↓ in renal dysfunction	7-Hydroxymethotrexate cross-reacts 1.5% in immunoassay. To minimize toxicity, leucovorin should be continued if methotrexate level is >0.1 μmol/L at 48 hours after start of therapy. Methotrexate >1 μmol/L at >48 hours requires an increase in leucovorin rescue therapy.
Nortriptyline	50–140 ng/mL	18–44		Drug is highly protein bound. Patient-specific decrease in protein binding may invalidate quoted range of effective concentration.
Phenobarbital	10–40 μg/mL	86 ↑ in cirrhosis	↓ in liver disease	Metabolized principally by the hepatic microsomal enzyme system. Many drug–drug interactions.
Phenytoin	10–20 μg/mL ↓ in uremia, hypoalbuminemia	Dose dependent		Metabolite cross-reacts 10% in immunoassay. Metabolism is capacity limited. Increase dose cautiously when level approaches therapeutic range, because new steady-state level may be disproportionately higher. Drug is very highly protein bound, and when protein binding is decreased in uremia and hypoalbuminemia, the usual therapeutic range does not apply. In this situation, use a reference range of 5–10 μg/mL.
Primidone	5–10 μg/mL	8		Phenobarbital cross-reacts 0.5%. Metabolized to phenobarbital. Primidone/phenobarbital ratio >1:2 suggests poor compliance.
Procainamide	4–8 μg/mL	3 ↑ in uremia	↓ in renal dysfunction	Thirty percent of patients with plasma levels of 12–16 μg/mL have ECG changes; 40% of patients with plasma levels of >16 μg/mL have severe toxicity. Metabolite N-acetylprocainamide is active.

(continued)

TABLE 4–1 (CONTINUED).

Drug	Effective Concentrations	Half-Life (hours)	Dosage Adjustment	Comments
Quinidine	1–4 µg/L	7 ↔ in CHF; ↑ in liver disease	↓ in liver disease, CHF	Effective concentration is lower in chronic liver disease and nephrosis where binding is decreased.
Salicylate	150–300 µg/mL (15–30 mg/dL)	Dose dependent		See Figure 10–11, p 419, for nomogram of salicylate toxicity.
Theophylline	5–20 µg/mL	9	↓ in CHF, cirrhosis, and with cimetidine	Caffeine cross-reacts 10%. Elimination is increased 1.5–2 times in smokers. 1,3-Dimethyl uric acid metabolite increased in uremia and because of cross-reactivity may cause an apparent slight increase in serum theophylline.
Tobramycin	Peak: 5–10 µg/mL Trough: <2 µg/mL	2–3 ↑ in uremia	↓ in renal dysfunction	Tobramycin, kanamycin, and amikacin may cross-react in immunoassay. If a once-daily regimen is used to maximize bacterial killing by optimizing the peak concentration/MIC ratio and to reduce the potential for toxicity, dosage should be reduced if trough concentration is >1 µg/mL (1 mg/L). Measurement of peak concentrations is not recommended with this regimen.
Valproic acid	55–100 µg/mL	13–19		Ninety-five percent protein-bound. Reduced binding in uremia and cirrhosis.
Vancomycin	Trough: 5–15 µg/mL	6 ↑ in uremia	↓ in renal dysfunction	Toxicity in uremic patients leads to irreversible deafness. Keep peak level <30–40 µg/mL to avoid toxicity.

↔ = unchanged; ↑ = increased; ↓ = decreased; CHF = congestive heart failure

5

Microbiology: Test Selection

Jane Jang, BS, MT (ASCP) SM

HOW TO USE THIS SECTION

This section displays information about clinically important infectious diseases in tabular form. Included in these tables are the *Organisms* involved in the disease/syndrome listed; *Specimens/Diagnostic Tests* that are useful in the evaluation; and *Comments* regarding the tests and diagnoses discussed. Topics are listed by body area/organ system: Central Nervous System, Eye, Ear, Sinus, Upper Airway, Lung, Heart and Vessels, Abdomen, Genitourinary, Bone, Joint, Muscle, Skin, and Blood.

Organisms

This column lists organisms that are known to cause the stated illness. Scientific names are abbreviated according to common usage (eg, *Streptococcus pneumoniae* as *S pneumoniae* or pneumococcus). Specific age or risk groups are listed in order of increasing age or frequency (eg, Infant, Child, Adult, HIV).

When bacteria are listed, Gram stain characteristics follow the organism name in parentheses—eg, "*S pneumoniae* (GPDC)." The following abbreviations are used:

GPC	Gram-positive cocci	**GNC**	Gram-negative cocci
GPDC	Gram-positive diplococci	**GNDC**	Gram-negative diplococci
GPCB	Gram-positive coccobacilli	**GNCB**	Gram-negative coccobacilli
GPR	Gram-positive rods	**GNR**	Gram-negative rods
GVCB	Gram-variable coccobacilli	**AFB**	Acid-fast bacilli

When known, the frequency of the specific organism's involvement in the disease process is also provided in parentheses—eg, "*S pneumoniae* (GPDC) (50%)."

Specimen Collection/Diagnostic Tests

This column describes the collection of specimens, laboratory processing, useful radiographic procedures, and other diagnostic tests. Culture or test sensitivities with respect to the diagnosis in question are placed in parentheses immediately following the test when known—eg, "Gram stain (60%)." Pertinent serologic tests are also listed. Keep in mind that few infections can be identified by definitive diagnostic tests and that clinical judgment is critical to making difficult diagnoses when test results are equivocal.

Comments

This column includes general information about the utility of the tests and may include information about patient management. Appropriate general references are also listed.

Syndrome Name/Body Area

In the last two columns the syndrome name and body area are placed perpendicular to the rest of the table to allow for quick referencing.

CENTRAL NERVOUS SYSTEM		
Brain abscess		
Organism	**Specimen/Diagnostic Tests**	**Comments**
Brain abscess		
Usually polymicrobial	Blood for bacterial and fungal cultures.	Occurs in patients with otitis media and sinusitis.
	Brain abscess aspirate for Gram stain (82%), bacterial (88%), AFB, fungal cultures, and cytology.	Also seen in patients with cyanotic congenital heart disease and right-to-left shunting (eg, tetralogy of
Child: anaerobes (40%), *S aureus* (GPC), *S pneumoniae* (GPDC), *S pyogenes* (GPC in chains),	Lumbar puncture is dangerous and contraindicated.	Fallot) or arteriovenous vascular abnormalities of the lung (eg, Osler-Weber-Rendu).
viridans streptococci (GPC in chains), less common, Entero-	Sources of infection in the ears, sinuses, lungs, or bloodstream should be sought for culture when	Majority of toxoplasmosis abscesses are multiple and are seen on MRI in the basal ganglia, parietal
bacteriaceae (GNR), *P aeruginosa* (GNR), *H influenzae* (GNCB),	abscess is found.	and frontal lobes.
N meningitidis (GNDC).	CT scan and MRI are the most valuable imaging procedures and can guide biopsy if a specimen is	^{99m}Technetium brain scan is a very sensitive test for abscess and the test of choice where CT and MRI
Adults: Viridans and anaerobic streptococci (GPC in chains)	needed. (See CT scan, MRI of head, p 247.)	are unavailable.
(60–70%), bacteroides (GNR) (20–40%), Enterobacteriaceae	Serum toxoplasma antibody in HIV-infected patients may not be positive at outset of presumptive ther-	Pediatr Rev 1999;20:215.
(GNR) (23–33%), *S aureus* (GPC) (10–15%), *N meningi-*	apy. If negative or if no response to empiric ther- apy, biopsy may be needed to rule out lymphoma,	Infect Dis Clin North Am 2001;15:2.
tidis, Group B Streptococcus, listeria spp., other anaerobes,	fungal infection, or tuberculosis. Biopsy material should be sent for toxoplasma antigen (DFA).	Infect Dis Clin North Am 2001;15:4.
including fusobacterium (GNR) and actinomyces (GPR),	Detection of toxoplasma DNA in blood or CSF sam- ples by PCR techniques is now available from spe-	
T solium (cysticerci).	cialized or reference laboratories. A positive PCR result must be interpreted in the context of the clin-	
Immunocompromised: *T gondii*, *C neoformans*, nocardia (GPR),	ical presentation. Active or recent infection is indi- cated by a positive IgM antibody test.	
Listeria, mycobacteria (AFB), fungi, cytomegalovirus (CMV),	(See also toxoplasma antibody, p 175.)	
herpes simplex (HSV), varicella- zoster (VZV), *E histolytica*.		
Posttraumatic: *S aureus* (GPC), Enterobacteriaceae (GNR),		
coagulase-negative staphylococci (GPC), *P acnes* (GPR).		

	CENTRAL NERVOUS SYSTEM
	Encephalitis

Organism	Specimen/Diagnostic Tests	Comments
Encephalitis Arboviruses (California group, St. Louis, eastern and western equine, and West Nile virus in summer and fall), enteroviruses (coxsackie, echo, polio), HSV, *B henselae*, lymphocytic choriomeningitis, mumps, tick-borne encephalitis virus, postinfectious (following influenza in winter and spring, human herpes virus 6 [HHV-6], measles, mumps, rubella, VZV), rabies, Creutzfeldt-Jakob. Postvaccination: Rabies, pertussis. Immunocompromised: CMV, toxoplasmosis, papovavirus (PML).	CSF for pressure (elevated), cell count (WBCs elevated but variable [10–2000/μL], mostly lymphocytes), protein (elevated, especially IgG fraction), glucose (normal), RBCs (especially in herpesvirus). Repeat examination of CSF after 24 hours often useful. (See CSF [enteroviruses, HSV-2, mumps] profiles, p 368.) CSF cultures for viruses and bacteria (low yield). CSF PCR in reference laboratories for CMV (33%), HSV (98%), VZV, enterovirus and West Nile virus. Identification of HSV DNA in CSF by PCR techniques is now the definitive diagnostic test. Throat swab for enterovirus, mumps. Stool culture for enterovirus, which is frequently shed for weeks (especially in children). Urine culture for mumps. Culture of both skin biopsy from hairline and saliva for rabies. Single serum for bartonella (cat-scratch disease) IgM and IgG. Paired sera for arboviruses, mumps, or rabies should be drawn acutely and after 1–3 weeks of illness. Serologic tests are often of academic interest only. Not indicated for herpes simplex. Urine PCR and/or serum PCR are options for enteroviruses diagnoses.	CT scan with contrast or MRI with gadolinium showing temporal lobe lesions suggests herpes simplex. Polyradiculopathy is highly suggestive of CMV in AIDS. Postgrad Med 1998;103:123. Ann Intern Med 1998;128:922. J Neurosurg 1998;89:640. J Child Neurol 1999;14:1. J Clin Microbiol 1999;37:2127. MMWR (Morb Mortal Wkly Rep) 2000;49:714.

CENTRAL NERVOUS SYSTEM		
Aseptic meningitis		
Aseptic meningitis Acute: Enteroviruses (coxsackie, echo, polio) (90%), mumps, HSV, HIV (primary HIV sero-conversion), VZV, lymphocytic choriomeningitis virus (rare). Recurrent: HSV-2 (Mollaret syndrome).	CSF for pressure (elevated), cell count (WBCs 10–100/μL, PMNs early, lymphocytes later), protein (normal or slightly elevated), and glucose (normal). On repeat CSF after 24–48 hours, an increase in lymphocytes is seen. (See CSF profiles, p 368.) CSF viral culture can be negative despite active viral infection. Enteroviruses can be isolated from the CSF in the first few days after onset (positive in 40–80%) but only rarely after the first week. Detection of enteroviral RNA in CSF by PCR from specialized or reference laboratories. Urine viral culture for mumps. Vesicle direct fluorescent antibody (DFA) or culture for HSV or VZV. Paired sera for viral titers: poliovirus, mumps, and VZV. Not practical for other organisms unless actual isolate known and then only useful epidemiologically. Detection of VZV or HSV in CSF by PCR.	Aseptic meningitis is acute meningeal irritation in the absence of pyogenic bacteria or fungi. Diagnosis is usually made by the examination of the CSF and by ruling out other infectious causes (eg, toxoplasmosis, Lyme disease, syphilis, tuberculosis). Consider nonsteroidal anti-inflammatory drugs as a noninfectious cause. Enteroviral aseptic meningitis is rare after age 40. Patients with deficiency of the complement regulatory protein factor I may have recurrent aseptic meningitis. J Clin Microbiol 1997;35:691. Clin Microbiol Rev 1998;11:202. Acta Neurol Scand 1998;98:209. Am Fam Physician 1999;159:2761. Neurol Clin 1999;17:691. Semin Neurol 2000;20:277.

	CENTRAL NERVOUS SYSTEM
	Bacterial meningitis

Organism	Specimen/Diagnostic Tests	Comments
Bacterial meningitis Neonate: *E coli* (GNR), group B or D streptococci (GPC), *L monocytogenes* (GPR). Infant: Group B streptococci, *S pneumoniae* (GPC), *N meningitidis* (GNDC), *Listeria monocytogenes* (GPR), *H influenzae* (GNCB). Child: *S pneumoniae*, *N meningitidis*, *H influenzae*. Adult: *S pneumoniae*, *N meningitidis*, *L monocytogenes*. Postneurosurgical: *S aureus* (GPC), *S pneumoniae*, *P acnes* (GPR), coagulase-negative staphylococci (GPC), pseudomonas (GNR), *E coli* (GNR), other Enterobacteriaceae, Acinetobacter (GNR). Alcoholic patients and the elderly: In addition to the adult organisms, Enterobacteriaceae, pseudomonas, *H influenzae*.	CSF for pressure (>180 mm H_2O), cell count (WBCs 1000–100,000/μL, >50% PMNs), protein (150–500 mg/dL), glucose (<40% of serum). (See CSF profiles, p 368.) CSF for Gram stain of cytocentrifuged material (positive in 70–80%). CSF culture for bacteria. Blood culture positive in 40–60% of patients with pneumococcal, meningococcal, and *H influenzae* meningitis. CSF antigen tests are no longer considered useful because of their low sensitivity and false-positive results.	The first priority in the care of the patient with suspected acute meningitis is therapy, then diagnosis. Antibiotics should be started within 30 minutes of presentation. The death rate for meningitis is about 50% for pneumococcal, less for others. With recurrent *N meningitidis* meningitis, suspect a terminal complement component deficiency. With other recurrent bacterial meningitides, suspect a CSF leak. For *S pneumoniae*, there is an increase in prevalence of penicillin resistance and multidrug resistance (ie, cephalosporins, macrolides, carbapenems, TMP-SMX). Medicine (Baltimore) 1998;77:313. Postgrad Med 1998;103:102. Clin Infect Dis 1999; 26:69. Infect Dis Clin North Am 1999;13:711. Infect Dis Clin North Am 1999;13:579. Neurol Clin 1999;17:691. Medicine (Baltimore) 2000; 79:360. N Engl J Med 2000: 343:1917. Infect Dis Clin North Am 2001;15:1047.

CENTRAL NERVOUS SYSTEM		
Fungal meningitis		
Fungal meningitis *C neoformans* (spherical, budding yeast), *C immitis* (spherules), *H capsulatum*. Immunocompromised: Aspergillus sp.- *P boydii*, candida sp., sporothrix, blastomyces.	CSF for pressure (normal or elevated), cell count (WBCs 50–1000/μL, mostly lymphocytes), protein (elevated), and glucose (decreased). Serum cryptococcal antigen (CrAg) for *C neoformans* (99%). For other fungi, collect at least 5 mL of CSF for fungal culture. Initial cultures are positive in 40% of coccidioides cases and 27–65% of histoplasma cases. Repeat cultures are frequently needed. Culture of bone marrow, skin lesions, or other involved organs should also be performed if clinically indicated. CSF India ink preparation for cryptococcus is not recommended because it is positive in only 50% of cases. Serum coccidioidal serology is a concentrated serum immunodiffusion test for the organism (75–95%). CSF serologic testing is rarely necessary. (See Coccidioides serology, p 71.) Complement fixation test for histoplasma is available from public health department laboratories (see p 110). Histoplasma antigen can be detected in urine, blood, or CSF in 61% of cases of histoplasma meningitis.	The clinical presentation of fungal meningitis in immunocompromised patients is that of an indolent chronic meningitis. Prior to AIDS, cryptococcal meningitis was seen both in patients with cellular immunologic deficiencies and in patients who lacked obvious defects (about 50% of cases). Cryptococcus is the most common cause of meningitis in AIDS patients and may present with normal CSF findings. Titer of CSF CrAg can be used to monitor therapeutic success (falling titer) or failure (unchanged or rising titer) or to predict relapse during suppressive therapy (rising titer). Scand J Infect Dis 1998;30:485. Neurol Clin 1999;17:691.

	CENTRAL NERVOUS SYSTEM
	Spirochetal meningitis/neurologic diseases

Organism	Specimen/Diagnostic Tests	Comments
Spirochetal meningitis/ neurologic diseases *B burgdorferi* (neuroborreliosis), *T pallidum* (neurosyphilis), leptospira, other borreliae.	**Neuroborreliosis:** CSF for pressure (normal or elevated), cell count (WBCs elevated, mostly lymphocytes), protein (may be elevated), and glucose (normal). Serum and CSF for serologic testing. False-positive serologic tests may occur. Western blots should be used to confirm borderline or positive results. CSF serology for anti-*B burgdorferi* IgM (90%). Culture and PCR less specific. For Lyme disease serologies, see p 122. **Acute syphilitic meningitis:** CSF for pressure (elevated), cell count (WBCs 25–2000/μL, mostly lymphocytes), protein (elevated), and glucose (normal or low). (See CSF profiles, p 368.) Serum VDRL. (See VDRL, serum, p 181.) CSF VDRL is the preferred test (see p 182), but is only 66% sensitive for acute syphilitic meningitis. **Neurosyphilis:** CSF for pressure (normal), cell count (WBCs normal or slightly increased, mostly lymphocytes), protein (normal or elevated), glucose (normal), and CSF VDRL. Serum VDRL, FTA-ABS, or MHA-TP should be done. **Leptospirosis:** CSF cell count (WBCs <500/μL, mostly monocytes), protein (slightly elevated), and glucose (normal). Urine for dark-field examination of sediment. Blood and CSF dark-field examination only positive in acute phase prior to meningitis. Serum for serology for IgM.	Neurosyphilis is a late stage of infection and can present with meningovascular (hemiparesis, seizures, aphasia), parenchymal (general paresis, tabes dorsalis), or asymptomatic (latent) disease. Because there is no single highly sensitive or specific test for neurosyphilis, the diagnosis must depend on a combination of clinical and laboratory data. Therapy of suspected neurosyphilis should not be withheld on the basis of a negative CSF VDRL if clinical suspicion is high. In HIV neurosyphilis, treatment failures may be common. Lyme disease can present as a lymphocytic meningitis, facial palsy, or painful radiculitis. Leptospirosis follows exposure to rats. Clin Infect Dis 1998;26:151. J Clin Microbiol 1998;36:3138. J Emerg Med 1998;16:851. J Neurol Sci 1998;153:182. Semin Neurol 1998;18:185. Neurol Clin 1999;17:651.

CENTRAL NERVOUS SYSTEM		
Organism	**Specimen/Diagnostic Test**	**Comments/References**
Parasitic meningoencephalitis *T gondii, E chaffeensis* (human monocytic ehrlichiosis) (HME) and other species of human granulocytic ehrlichiosis (HGE). *E histolytica, N fowleri, T solium* (cysticerci), Acanthamoeba (GAE), Balamuthia spp. (GAE), Angiostrongylus.	CSF for pressure (normal or elevated), cell count (WBCs 100–1000/µL, chiefly monocytes, lymphocytes), protein (elevated), glucose (normal to low). Serology as for brain abscesses. **Toxoplasmosis:** CSF, wet mount, culture, PCR, neuroimaging. **Ehrlichiosis:** White blood cell count low (1300–4000/µL), platelets low (50,000–140,000/µL), hepatic aminotransferases (tenfold above normal). Buffy coat for Giemsa (1% in HME, 18–80% in HGE), PCR of blood available (50–90% depending on prior therapy). Serum IgG and IgM usually not positive until the third week. **Naegleria:** CSF wet mount, culture, and Giemsa stain. Serological tests not helpful. **Cysticercosis:** Characteristic findings on CT and MRI are diagnostic. Serology is less sensitive.	Naegleria follows exposure to warm fresh water. Ehrlichia follows exposure to horses and ticks. Infect Dis Clin North Am 1998;12:123. Neurol Clin 1999;17:691. Semin Pediatr Neurol 1999;6:267.
Tuberculous meningitis *M tuberculosis* (MTb), *M avium* (AFB)	CSF for pressure (elevated), cell count (WBCs 100–500/µL, PMNs early, lymphocytes later), protein (elevated), glucose (decreased). (See CSF profiles, p 368.) CSF for AFB stain. Stain is positive in only 30%. Cytocentrifugation and repeat smears increase yield. CSF for AFB culture (positive in <70%). Repeated sampling of the CSF during the first week of therapy is recommended; ideally, 3 or 4 specimens of 5–10 mL each should be obtained (87% yield with 4 specimens). PCR available but not yet validated. DNA probes are available for rapid confirmation from mycobacterial growth.	Tuberculous meningitis is usually secondary to rupture of a subependymal tubercle rather than blood-borne invasion. Because CSF stain and culture are not sensitive for tuberculosis, diagnosis and treatment should be based on a combination of clinical and microbiologic data. Evidence of inactive or active extrameningeal tuberculosis, especially pulmonary, is seen in 75% of patients. Acta Neurol Belg 1995;95:80. Radiol Clin North Am 1995;33:733. Surg Neurol 1995;44:378. Neurol Clin 1999;17:691. MMWR Recomm Rep 2000;49(RR-6):1.

	EYE	
	Conjunctivitis	
Organism	**Specimen/Diagnostic Tests**	**Comments**
Conjunctivitis Neonate (ophthalmia neonatorum): *C trachomatis, N gonorrhoeae* (GNDC), HSV Children and adults: adenovirus, staphylococci (GPC), HSV, *H influenzae* (GNCB), *S pneumoniae* (GPDC), *S pyogenes* (GPC), VZV, *N gonorrhoeae* (GNDC), *M lacunata* (GNCB), *M catarrhalis,* bartonella sp. (Parinaud oculoglandular syndrome). Adult inclusion conjunctivitis/trachoma: *C trachomatis.* Acute hemorrhagic conjunctivitis (acute epidemic keratoconjunctivitis): enterovirus, coxsackievirus.	Conjunctival Gram stain is especially useful if gonococcal infection is suspected. Bacterial culture for severe cases (routine bacterial culture) or suspected gonococcal infection. Conjunctival scrapings or smears by direct immunofluorescent monoclonal antibody staining for *C trachomatis.* Cell culture for chlamydia. Detection of chlamydial DNA on ocular swabs by PCR techniques. Ocular HSV and VZV PCR available in reference laboratories.	The causes of conjunctivitis change with the season. Adenovirus occurs mainly in the fall, *H influenzae* in the winter. Gonococcal conjunctivitis is an ophthalmologic emergency. Cultures are usually unnecessary unless chlamydia or gonorrhea is suspected or the case is severe. Consider noninfectious causes (eg, allergy, contact lens deposits, trauma). Clin Infect Dis 1995;21:479. Postgrad Med 1997;101:185. Am Fam Physician 1998;57:735. Ophthalmol Clin North Am 1999;12. *Diagnostic Microbiology,* 11th ed. Mosby. 2002.

EYE	
Keratitis	**Endophthalmitis**
Corneal scrapings for Gram stain, KOH, and culture. Routine bacterial culture is used for most bacterial causes, viral culture for herpes, and special media for acanthamoeba (can be detected with trichrome or Giemsa stain of smears). Treatment depends on Gram stain appearance and culture. Corneal biopsy may be needed if initial cultures are negative. Ocular viral DFA for HSV and VZV.	Culture material from anterior chamber, vitreous cavity, and wound abscess for bacteria, mycobacteria, and fungi. Traumatic and postoperative cases should have aqueous and vitreous aspiration for culture and smear (56%). Conjunctival cultures are inadequate and misleading.
Prompt ophthalmologic consultation is mandatory. Acanthamoeba infection occurs in soft contact (extended-wear) lens wearers and may resemble HSV infection on fluorescein examination (dendritic ["branching"] ulcer). Bacterial keratitis is usually caused by contact lens use or trauma. Fungal keratitis is usually caused by trauma. Am Fam Physician 1998;57:735. CLAO J 1998;24:52. Cornea 1998;17:3. Int Ophthalmol Clin 1998;38:115. Int Ophthalmol Clin 1998;38:107. Clin Microbiol Rev 1999;12:445. Cornea 1999;18:144. *Diagnostic Microbiology*, 11th ed. Mosby, 2002.	Endophthalmitis is an inflammatory process of the ocular cavity and adjacent structures. Rapid diagnosis is critical, because vision may be compromised. Bacterial endophthalmitis usually occurs as a consequence of ocular surgery. Prophylactic antibiotic use is of unproved benefit, though topical antibiotics are widely used. Also consider retinitis in immunocompromised patients, caused by CMV, HSV, VZV, and toxoplasma (retinochoroiditis), which is diagnosed by retinal examination. Curr Opin Ophthalmol 1998;9:66. Surv Ophthalmol 1998;43:193. Clin Infect Dis 2000;30:662. Clin Microbiol Rev 2002;15:111. *Diagnostic Microbiology*, 11th ed. Mosby, 2002.

Keratitis

Bacteria: *P aeruginosa* (GNR), staphylococci (GPC), *S pneumoniae* (GPDC), moraxella sp.

Virus: HSV (dendritic pattern on fluorescein slit-lamp examination), VZV.

Contact lens: Acanthamoeba, Enterobacteriaceae (GNR).

Fungus: Candida, fusarium, aspergillus, rhodotorula, other filamentous fungi.

Parasite: *O volvulus* (river blindness), microsporidia (HIV).

Endophthalmitis

Spontaneous or postoperative: coagulase-negative staphylococci (70%) (GPC), *S aureus* (GPC), viridans group streptococci (GPC in chains), *S pneumoniae* (GPDC), other gram-positive organisms, gram-negative rods.

Trauma: Bacillus sp. (GPR), fungi.

Postfiltering bleb: Viridans group streptococcus (57%), *S pneumoniae* (GPDC), *H influenzae* (GNCB).

IV drug abuse: Add *B cereus*.

	EAR
	Otitis media

Organism	Specimen/Diagnostic Tests	Comments
Otitis media	Tympanocentesis aspirate for Gram stain and bacterial culture in the patient who has a toxic appearance. Otherwise, microbiologic studies of effusions are so consistent that empiric treatment is acceptable. CSF examination if clinically indicated. Nasopharyngeal swab may be substituted for tympanocentesis. Blood culture in the toxic patient.	Peak incidence of otitis media occurs in the first 3 years of life, especially between 6 and 24 months of age. In neonates, predisposing factors include cleft palate, hypotonia, mental retardation (Down syndrome). Tympanocentesis is indicated if the patient fails to improve after 48 hours or develops fever. It may hasten resolution and decrease sterile effusion. Persistent middle ear effusion may require placement of ventilating or tympanostomy tubes. Bullous myringitis suggests mycoplasma. Emerging antibiotic resistance should be considered in choice of empiric antibiotic therapy. *Pediatr Infect Dis J* 1998;17:1105. *Pediatr Infect Dis J* 1999;18:1. *Pediatr Infect Dis J* 2000;19:531. *Microbiology*, 3rd ed. Saunders, 2001. *Diagnostic Microbiology*, 11th ed. Mosby, 2002.
Infant, child, and adult: *S pneumoniae* (35%) (GPDC), *H influenzae* (20%) (GNCB), *M catarrhalis* (8%) (GNDC), *S aureus* (GPC), *S pyogenes* (GPC in chains), *M pneumoniae*, *C pneumoniae*, "sterile," anaerobes, viruses (ie, RSV, influenza, rhinoviruses, adenoviruses) (15%).		
Neonate: Same as above plus Enterobacteriaceae (GNR), group B streptococcus (GPC).		
Endotracheal intubation: Pseudomonas sp. (GNR), klebsiella (GNR), Enterobacteriaceae (GNR).		
Chronic: *S aureus* (GPC), *P aeruginosa* (GNR), anaerobes, *M tuberculosis* (AFB).		

EAR		
Otitis externa		
Otitis externa Acute localized: *S aureus* (GPC), anaerobes (32%), *S pyogenes* (GPC in chains). "Swimmer's ear": Pseudomonas sp. (GNR), Enterobacteriaceae (GNR), vibrio (GNR), fungi (rare). Chronic: Usually secondary to seborrhea or eczema. Diabetes mellitus, AIDS ("malignant otitis externa"): *P aeruginosa* (GNR), aspergillus sp. Furuncle of external canal: *S aureus*.	Ear drainage for Gram stain and bacterial culture, especially in malignant otitis externa. CT or MRI can aid in diagnosis by demonstrating cortical bone erosion or meningeal enhancement.	Infection of the external auditory canal is similar to infection of skin and soft tissue elsewhere. If malignant otitis externa is present, exclusion of associated osteomyelitis and surgical drainage may be required. Nurse Pract 1998;23:125. Aust Fam Physician 1999;28:217. Curr Infect Dis Rep 2000;2:160. *Diagnostic Microbiology*, 11th ed. Mosby, 2002.

	SINUS	
	Sinusitis	
Organism	**Specimen/Diagnostic Tests**	**Comments**
Sinusitis Acute: *S pneumoniae* (GPC) (31%), *H influenzae* (GNCB) (21%), *M catarrhalis* (GNDC), *S pyogenes* (2–5%) (GPC), anaerobes (2–5%), viruses (adenovirus, influenza, parainfluenza), *S aureus* (GPC) (rare). Chronic (child): Viridans and anaerobic streptococci (GPC in chains) (23%), *S aureus* (19%), *S pneumoniae*, *H influenzae*, *M catarrhalis*, *P aeruginosa* (GNR) in cystic fibrosis. Chronic (adult): Coagulase-negative staphylococci (GPC) (36%), *S aureus* (GPC) (25%), viridans streptococci (GPC in chains) (8%), corynebacteria (GPR) (5%), anaerobes (6%), including bacteroides sp., prevotella sp. (GNR), peptostreptococcus (GPC), fusobacterium sp. (GNR). Hospitalized with nasogastric tube or nasotracheal intubation: Enterobacteriaceae (GNR), pseudomonas sp. (GNR). Fungal: Zygomycetes (rhizopus), aspergillus, *P boydii*. Immunocompromised: *P aeruginosa* (GNR), CMV, aspergillus sp. and other filamentous fungi plus microsporidia, *Cryptosporidium parvum*, acanthamoeba in HIV-infected patients.	Nasal aspirate for bacterial culture is not usually helpful due to respiratory flora contamination of aerobes and anaerobes. Maxillary sinus aspirate for bacterial culture may be helpful in severe or atypical cases.	Diagnosis and treatment of sinusitis is usually based on clinical and radiologic features. Microbiologic studies can be helpful in severe or atypical cases. Sinus CT scan (or MRI) is better than plain x-ray for diagnosing sinusitis, particularly if sphenoid sinusitis is suspected. However, sinus CT scans should be interpreted cautiously, because abnormalities are also seen in patients with the common cold. Acute and chronic sinusitis occur frequently in HIV-infected patients, may be recurrent or refractory, and may involve multiple sinuses (especially when the CD4 cell count is <200/µL). Acute sinusitis often results from bacterial superinfection following viral upper respiratory infection. Ann Otol Rhinol Laryngol 1998;107:942. Otolaryngol Head Neck Surg 1999;121:639. Ann Otol Rhinol Laryngol 2000;182(Suppl):2.

UPPER AIRWAY		
	Pharyngitis	**Laryngitis**
Organisms	Exudative: *S pyogenes* (GPC) (15–30%), viruses (rhinovirus, coronavirus, adenovirus) (30%), group C and G streptococci (GPC), Epstein-Barr virus (mononucleosis), *N gonorrhoeae* (GNDC), *Arcanobacterium hemolyticum* (GPR). Membranous: *C diphtheriae* (GPR), *C pseudodiphtheriticum* (GPR), Epstein-Barr virus.	Virus (90%) (influenza, rhinovirus, adenovirus, parainfluenza, Epstein-Barr virus), *S pyogenes* (GPC) (10%), *M catarrhalis* (GNDC) (55% of adults), *M tuberculosis*, fungus (cryptococcosis, histoplasmosis). Immunocompromised: *Candida* sp., CMV, HSV.
Specimen	Throat swab for culture. Place in sterile tube or transport medium. If *N gonorrhoeae* suspected, use chocolate agar or Thayer-Martin media. If *C diphtheriae* suspected, use Tinsdale or blood agar. Throat swabs are routinely cultured for group A streptococcus only. If other organisms are suspected, this must be stated. Throat culture is about 70% sensitive for group A streptococcus. "Rapid" tests for group A streptococcus can speed diagnosis and aid in the treatment of family members. However, false-negative results may lead to underdiagnosis and failure to treat.	Diagnosis is made by clinical picture of upper respiratory infection with hoarseness.
Comments	Controversy exists over how to evaluate patients with sore throat. Some authors suggest culturing all patients and then treating only those with positive cultures. In patients with compatible histories, be sure to consider pharyngeal abscess or epiglottitis, both of which may be life-threatening. Complications include pharyngeal abscess and Lemierre syndrome (infection with fusobacterium sp.), which can progress to sepsis and multi-organ failure. Clin Infect Dis 1997;25:574. Int J Pediatr Otorhinolaryngol 1998;45:51. J Clin Microbiol 1998;36:3468. Ann Intern Med 2001;134:506.	Laryngitis usually occurs with common cold or influenzal syndromes. Fungal laryngeal infections occur most commonly in immunocompromised patients (AIDS, cancer, organ transplants, corticosteroid therapy, diabetes mellitus). Consider acid reflux for chronic cases. Ann Otol Rhinol Laryngol 1993;102:209. Head Neck 1996;18:455. J Infect Dis 1996;174:636. J Voice 1998;12:91.

	UPPER AIRWAY
	Laryngotracheobronchitis

Organism	Specimen/Diagnostic Tests	Comments
Laryngotracheobronchitis Infant/child: RSV (50–75%) (bronchiolitis), adenovirus, parainfluenza virus (croup), B pertussis (GNCB) (whooping cough), other viruses, including rhinovirus, coronavirus, influenza. Adolescent/adult: Usually viruses, M pneumoniae, C pneumoniae, B pertussis. Chronic adult: S pneumoniae (GPDC), H influenzae (GNCB), M catarrhalis (GNDC), klebsiella (GNR), other Enterobacteriaceae (GNR), viruses (eg, influenza), aspergillus (allergic bronchopulmonary aspergillosis). Chronic obstructive airway disease: Viral (25–50%), S pneumoniae (GPC), H influenzae (GNCB), S aureus (GPC), Enterobacteriaceae (GNR), anaerobes (<10%).	Nasopharyngeal aspirate for respiratory virus DFA, for viral culture (rarely indicated), and for PCR for B pertussis. PCR for pertussis is test of choice; culture and DFA are less sensitive. Cellular examination of early morning sputum will show many PMNs in chronic bronchitis. Sputum Gram stain and culture for ill adults. In chronic bronchitis, mixed flora are usually seen with oral flora or colonized H influenzae or S pneumoniae on culture. Paired sera for viral, mycoplasmal, and chlamydial titers can help make a diagnosis retrospectively in infants and children but are not clinically useful except for seriously ill patients.	Chronic bronchitis is diagnosed when sputum is coughed up on most days for at least 3 consecutive months for more than 2 successive years. Bacterial infections are usually secondary infections of initial viral or mycoplasma-induced inflammation. Airway endoscopy can aid in the diagnosis of bacterial tracheitis in children. Infect Dis Clin North Am 1998;12:671. Mayo Clin Proc 1998;73:1102. Pediatr Infect Dis J 1998;17:827. Monaldi Arch Chest Dis 1999;54:43. Can Respir J 1999;6:40A.

UPPER AIRWAY		
Epiglottitis		
Epiglottitis Child: *H influenzae* type B (GNCB). Adult: *S pyogenes* (GPC), *H influenzae*. HIV: Candida	Blood for bacterial culture: positive in 50–100% of children with *H influenzae*. Lateral neck x-ray may show an enlarged epiglottis but has a low sensitivity (31%).	Acute epiglottitis is a rapidly moving cellulitis of the epiglottis and represents an airway emergency. Epiglottitis can be confused with croup, a viral infection of gradual onset that affects infants and causes inspiratory and expiratory stridor. Airway management is the primary concern, and an endo-tracheal tube should be placed or tracheostomy performed as soon as the diagnosis of epiglottitis is made in children. A tracheostomy set should be at the bedside for adults. Mayo Clin Proc 1998;73:1102. Pediatr Infect Dis J 1999;18:490. Am J Otolaryngol 2001;22:268. Postgrad Med 2002;112:81.

	LUNG
	Community-acquired pneumonia

Organism	Specimen/Diagnostic Tests	Comments
Community-acquired pneumonia Neonate: *E coli* (GNR), group A or B streptococcus (GPC), *S aureus* (GPC), pseudomonas sp (GNR), *C trachomatis*. Infant/child (<5 years): Virus, *S pneumoniae* (GPC), *H influenzae* (GNCB), *S aureus*. Age 5–40 years: Virus, *M pneumoniae*, *C pneumoniae* (formerly known as TWAR strain), *C psittaci*, *S pneumoniae*, legionella sp. Age >40 without other disease: *S pneumoniae* (GPDC), *M catarrhalis* (GNDC), *S aureus* (GPC), *M catarrhalis* (GNDC), *C pneumoniae*, legionella sp. (GNR), *C pseudodiphtheriticum* (GPR), *S pyogenes* (GPC), *K pneumoniae* (GNR), Enterobacteriaceae (GNR), *N meningitidis* (GNDC), viruses (eg, influenza). Cystic fibrosis: *P aeruginosa* (GNR), *Burkholderia cepacia*. Elderly: *S pneumoniae* (GPDC), *H influenzae* (GNCB), *S aureus* (GPC), Enterobacteriaceae (GNR), *M catarrhalis* (GNDC), group B streptococcus (GPC), legionella (GNR), nocardia (GPR), influenza. Aspiration: *S pneumoniae* (GPDC), *K pneumoniae* (GNR), Enterobacteriaceae (GNR), bacteroides sp. and other oral anaerobes. Fungal: *H capsulatum*, *C immitis*, *B dermatitidis* Exposure to birthing animals, sheep: *C burnetii* (Q fever), rabbits: *F tularensis* (tularemia), deer mice: hantavirus, birds: *C psittaci*.	Sputum for Gram stain desirable; culture, if empiric therapy fails or patient is seriously ill. An adequate specimen should have <10 epithelial cells and >25 PMNs per low-power field. Special sputum cultures for legionella are available. DFA for legionella has a sensitivity of 25–70% and a specificity of 95%. (Positive predictive value is low in areas of low disease prevalence.) Blood for bacterial cultures (2 sets), especially in ill patients. Pleural fluid for bacterial culture if significant effusion is present. Bronchoalveolar lavage or brushings for bacterial, fungal, and viral antigen tests and AFB culture in immunocompromised patients and atypical cases. Paired sera for *M pneumoniae* complement fixation testing can diagnose infection retrospectively. Serologic tests for *C pneumoniae*, *C psittaci* strains, and Q fever are available. Serologic tests and PCR for hantavirus (IgM and IgG) are available. Other special techniques (bronchoscopy with telescoping plugged catheter on protected brush, transthoracic fine-needle aspiration, or, rarely, open lung biopsy) can be used to obtain specimens for culture in severe cases, in immunocompromised patients, or in cases with negative conventional cultures and progression despite empiric antibiotic therapy. PCR for *M pneumoniae*, legionella sp., and *C pneumoniae* are available.	About 60% of cases of community-acquired pneumonia have an identifiable microbial cause. Pneumatoceles suggest *S aureus* but are also reported with pneumococcus, group A streptococcus, *H influenzae*, and Enterobacteriaceae (in neonates). An "atypical pneumonia" presentation (diffuse pattern on chest x-ray with lack of organisms on Gram stain of sputum) should raise suspicion of mycoplasma, legionella, or chlamydial infection. Consider hantavirus pulmonary syndrome if pulmonary symptoms follow afebrile illness. Clin Infect Dis 1998;27:566. Clin Infect Dis 1998;26:811. Infect Dis Clin North Am 1998;12:689. Aspirations are most commonly associated with stroke, alcoholism, drug abuse, sedation, and periodontal disease. Lancet 1998;352:1295. Can Respir J 1999;6(Suppl A):15. Clin Infect Dis 2000;31:37. Am J Respir Crit Care Med 2001;163:1703.

LUNG	
Anaerobic pneumonia	**Hospital-acquired pneumonia**
Sputum Gram stain and culture for anaerobes are of little value because of contaminating oral flora. Bronchoalveolar sampling (brush or aspirate) for Gram stain will usually make an accurate diagnosis. As contamination is likely with a bronchoscope alone, a Bartlett tube should be used. Percutaneous transthoracic needle aspiration may be useful for culture and for cytology to demonstrate coexistence of an underlying carcinoma. Blood cultures are usually negative (80%).	Aspiration is the most important background feature of lung abscess. Without clear-cut risk factors such as alcoholism, coma, or seizures, bronchoscopy is often performed to rule out neoplasm. Infect Dis Clin North Am 1998;12:781. Respiration 1999;66:95.
Sputum Gram stain and culture for bacteria (aerobic and anaerobic) and fungus (if suspected). Blood cultures for bacteria are often negative (80%). Endotracheal aspirate or bronchoalveolar sample for bacterial and fungal culture in selected patients.	Most cases are related to aspiration. Hospital-acquired aspiration pneumonia is associated with intubation and the use of broad-spectrum antibiotics. A strong association between aspiration pneumonia and swallowing dysfunction is demonstrable by videofluoroscopy. Mendelson syndrome is due to acute aspiration of gastric contents (eg, during anesthesia or drowning). Am J Med 1998;105:319. Infect Dis Clin North Am 1998;12:761. Chest 1999;115:28S. Arch Intern Med 2000;160:192.

Anaerobic pneumonia/lung abscess

Usually polymicrobial: bacteroides sp. (15% *B fragilis*), peptostreptococcus prevotella sp., porphyromonas sp., fusobacterium sp., microaerophilic streptococcus, veillonella, *S aureus*, *P aeruginosa*, type 3 *S pneumoniae* (rare), klebsiella (rare).

Hospital-acquired pneumonia

P aeruginosa (GNR), klebsiella (GNR), *S aureus* (GPC), acinetobacter (GNR), Enterobacteriaceae (GNR), *S pneumoniae* (GPDC), *H influenzae* (GNCB), influenza virus, RSV, legionella (GNR), oral anaerobes. Mendelson syndrome (see comments): No organisms initially, then pseudomonas, Enterobacteriaceae, *S aureus*, *S pneumoniae*.

	LUNG	
	Pneumonia in immunocompromised host	
Organism	**Specimen/Diagnostic Tests**	**Comments**
Pneumonia in the immuno-compromised host Child with HIV infection: Lymphoid interstitial pneumonia (LIP). AIDS: *M avium* (31%), *P carinii* (13%), CMV (11%), *H capsulatum* (7%), *S pneumoniae* (GPDC), *H influenzae* (GNCB), *P aeruginosa* (GNR), Enterobacteriaceae (GNR), *C neoformans*, *C pseudodiphtheriticum* (GPR), *M tuberculosis* (AFB), *C immitis*, *P marneffei*, *Rhodococcus equi* (GPR). Neutropenic: *S aureus* (GPC), Pseudomonas sp. (GNR), klebsiella, enterobacter (GNR), bacteroides sp. and other oral anaerobes, legionella, candida, aspergillus, mucor. Transplant recipients: CMV (60–70%), *P aeruginosa* (GNR), *S aureus* (GPC), *S pneumoniae* (GPDC), legionella (GNR), RSV, influenza virus, *P carinii*, aspergillus, *P boydii*, nocardia sp., strongyloides.	Expectorated sputum for Gram stain and bacterial culture, if purulent. Sputum induction or bronchiolar lavage for Giemsa or methenamine silver staining or DFA for *P carinii* trophozoites or cysts; for mycobacterial, fungal staining and culture, for legionella culture, and for CMV culture. Blood for CMV antigenemia or PCR from transplant patients. Blood or bone marrow fungal culture for histoplasmosis (positive in 50%), coccidioidomycosis (positive in 30%). Blood culture for bacteria. Blood cultures are more frequently positive in HIV-infected patients with bacterial pneumonia and often are the only source where a specific organism is identified; bacteremic patients have higher mortality rates. Histoplasma polysaccharide antigen positive in 90% of AIDS patients with disseminated histoplasmosis; antigen increases ≥ 2 RIA units with relapse. Immunodiffusion or CIE is useful for screening for, and CF for confirmation of, suspected histoplasmosis or coccidioidomycosis. Serum cryptococcal antigen when pulmonary cryptococcosis is suspected. Serum lactate dehydrogenase (LDH) levels are elevated in 63% and hypoxemia with exercise (PaO₂ < 75 mm Hg) occurs in 57% of PCP cases.	In PCP, the sensitivities of the various diagnostic tests are: sputum induction 80% (in experienced labs), bronchoscopy with lavage 90–97%, transbronchial biopsy 94–97%. In PCP, chest x-ray may show interstitial (36%) or alveolar (25%) infiltrates or may be normal (39%), particularly if leukopenia is present. Recurrent episodes of bacterial pneumonia are common. Kaposi sarcoma of the lung is a common neoplastic process that can imitate infection in homosexual and African HIV-infected patients. Infect Dis Clin North Am 1998;12:781. J Thorac Imaging 1998;13:247. Clin Infect Dis 1999;28:341. Haematologica 1999;84:71. Respiration 1999;66:95.

LUNG
Mycobacterial pneumonia

Mycobacterial pneumonia *M tuberculosis* (MTb), *M kansasii*, *M avium-intracellulare* complex (MAC) (AFB, acid-fast beaded rods).	Sputum for AFB stain and culture. First morning samples are best, and at least three samples are required. Culture systems detect mycobacterial growth in as little as several days to 6 weeks. Bronchoalveolar lavage for AFB stain and culture or gastric washings for AFB culture can be used if sputum tests are negative. Sputum or bronchoalveolar lavage for PCR to MTb available for confirmation of smear positive (99%), less sensitive for smear negative (75%). CT- or ultrasound-guided transthoracic fine-needle aspiration cytology can be used if clinical or radiographic features are nonspecific or if malignancy is suspected. Blood culture for MTb (15%).	AFB found on sputum stain do not necessarily make the diagnosis of tuberculosis, because *M kansasii* and MAC look identical. Tuberculosis is very common in HIV-infected patients, in whom the chest x-ray appearance may be atypical and occasionally (4%) may mimic PCP (especially in patients with CD4 cell counts <200/μL). In one study, only 2% of patients sent for sputum induction for PCP had tuberculosis. Consider HIV testing if MTb is diagnosed. Delayed diagnosis of pulmonary tuberculosis is common (up to 20% of cases), especially among patients who are older or who do not have respiratory symptoms. In any patient with suspected tuberculosis, respiratory isolation is required. Chest 1998;114:317. Respiration 1998;65:163. CMAJ 1999;160:1725. Chest Surg Clin North Am 1999;9:227. Am J Respir Crit Care Med 2000;161(4 part 1):1376. Clin Infect Dis 2000;31:633.

	LUNG	
	Empyema	
Organism	**Specimen/Diagnostic Tests**	**Comments**
Empyema Neonate: *E coli* (GNR), group A or B streptococcus (GPC), *S aureus* (GPC), pseudomonas sp (GNR). Infant/child (<5 years): *S aureus* (GPC), *S pneumoniae* (GPC), *H influenzae* (GNCB), anaerobes. Child (>5 years)/adult, acute: *S pneumoniae* (GPC), group A streptococcus (GPC), *S aureus* (GPC), *H influenzae* (GNCB), legionella. Child (>5 years)/adult, chronic: Anaerobic streptococci, bacteroides sp., prevotella sp., porphyromonas sp., fusobacterium sp. (anaerobes 36–76%), Enterobacteriaceae, *E coli*, *Klebsiella pneumoniae*, *M tuberculosis*.	Pleural fluid for cell count (WBCs 25,000–100,000/μL, mostly PMNs), protein (>50% of serum), glucose (< serum, often very low), pH (<7.20), LDH (>60% of serum). (See Pleural fluid profiles, p 384.) Blood cultures for bacteria. Sputum for Gram stain and bacterial culture. Special culture can also be performed for legionella when suspected. Pleural fluid for Gram stain and bacterial culture (aerobic and anaerobic).	Chest tube drainage is paramount. The clinical presentation of empyema is nonspecific. Chest CT with contrast is helpful in demonstrating pleural fluid accumulations due to mediastinal or subdiaphragmatic processes and can identify loculated effusions, bronchopleural fistulae, and lung abscesses. About 25% of cases result from trauma or surgery. Bronchoscopy is indicated when the infection is unexplained. Occasionally, multiple thoracenteses may be needed to diagnose empyema. Clin Chest Med 1998;19:363. Curr Opin Pulm Med 1998;4:185. Semin Respir Infect 1999;14:18. Semin Respir Infect 1999;14:82. Chest 2000;118:1158.

HEART AND VESSELS	
Pericarditis	**Tuberculous Pericarditis**
Viral pericarditis is usually diagnosed clinically (precordial pain, muffled heart sounds, pericardial friction rub, cardiomegaly). The diagnosis is rarely aided by microbiologic tests. CT and MRI may demonstrate pericardial thickening. Bacterial pericarditis is usually secondary to surgery, immunosuppression (including HIV), esophageal rupture, endocarditis with ruptured ring abscess, extension from lung abscess, aspiration pneumonia or empyema, or sepsis with pericarditis. Emerg Med Clin North Am 1998;16:665. Am Heart J 1999;137:516. Clin Cardiol 1999;22:334. Cleve Clin J Med 2000;67:903. Heart 2000;84:449	Spread from nearby caseous mediastinal lymph nodes or pleurisy is the most common route of infection. Acutely, serofibrinous pericardial effusion develops with substernal pain, fever, and friction rub. Tamponade may occur. Tuberculosis accounts for 4% of cases of acute pericarditis, 7% of cases of cardiac tamponade, and 6% of cases of constrictive pericarditis. One-third to one-half of patients develop constrictive pericarditis despite drug therapy. Constrictive pericarditis occurs 2–4 years after acute infection. J Infect 1997;35:215. Clin Infect Dis 2001;33:954.
In acute pericarditis, specific bacterial diagnosis is made in only 19%. Pericardial fluid aspirate for Gram stain and bacterial culture (aerobic and anaerobic). In acute pericarditis, only 54% have pericardial effusions. Blood for buffy coat, stool or throat for enteroviral culture. PCR available in reference laboratories. Surgical pericardial drainage with biopsy of pericardium for culture (22%) and histologic examination. Paired sera for enterovirus (coxsackie) and mycoplasma.	PPD skin testing should be performed (negative in a sizable minority). Pericardial fluid obtained by needle aspiration can show AFB by smear (rare) or culture (low yield). The yield is improved by obtaining three or four repeated specimens for smear and culture. Pericardial biopsy for culture and histologic examination has highest diagnostic yield. Other sources of culture for MTb besides pericardium are available in 50% of patients. Pericardial fluid may show markedly elevated levels of adenosine deaminase.
Pericarditis Viruses: Enteroviruses (coxsackie, echo), influenza, Epstein-Barr, HZV, mumps, HIV, CMV. Bacteria: *S aureus* (GPC), *S pneumoniae* (GPC), mycoplasma, *S pyogenes* (GPC), Enterobacteriaceae (GNR), *N meningitidis* (GNDC), haemophilus sp. Fungi: Candida sp., aspergillus, coccidioides (immunocompromised).	**Tuberculous pericarditis** *Mycobacterium tuberculosis* (MTb, AFB, acid-fast beaded rods).

	HEART AND VESSELS
	Infectious myocarditis

Organism	Specimen / Diagnostic Tests	Comments
Infectious myocarditis Enteroviruses (especially coxsackie B), adenovirus, influenza virus, HIV, *Borrelia burgdorferi* (Lyme disease), scrub typhus, *Rickettsia rickettsii* (Rocky Mountain spotted fever), *Coxiella burnetii* (Q fever), *Mycoplasma pneumoniae*, *Chlamydia pneumoniae*, *C diphtheriae* (GPR), *Trichinella spiralis* (trichinosis), *Trypanosoma cruzi* (Chagas disease), toxoplasma.	Endomyocardial biopsy for pathologic examination, PCR, and culture in selected cases. Indium-111 antimyosin antibody imaging is more sensitive than endomyocardial biopsy. Stool or throat swab for enterovirus culture. Blood for enterovirus PCR (reference labs) and culture of white cells. Paired sera for coxsackie B, *M pneumoniae*, *C pneumoniae*, scrub typhus, *R rickettsii*, *C burnetii*, trichinella, toxoplasma. Single serum for HIV, *B burgdorferi*, *T cruzi*. Gallium scanning is sensitive but not specific for myocardial inflammation. Antimyosin antibody scintigraphy has a high specificity but a lower sensitivity for the detection of myocarditis.	Acute infectious myocarditis should be suspected in a patient with dynamically evolving changes in ECG, echocardiography, and serum CK levels and symptoms of an infection. The value of endomyocardial biopsy in such cases has not been established. In contrast, an endomyocardial biopsy is needed to diagnose lymphocytic or giant cell myocarditis. The incidence of myocarditis in AIDS may be as high as 46%. Many patients with acute myocarditis progress to dilated cardiomyopathy. Am J Med 1997;102:459. Emerg Med Clin North Am 1998;16:665. J Am Coll Cardiol 1998;32:1371. J Infect 1998;37:99. Adv Intern Med 1999;44:293. Circulation 1999;99:2011. New Engl J Med 2000;343:1388.

HEART AND VESSELS		
Infective endocarditis		
Infective endocarditis Viridans group streptococci (GPC), enterococcus (GPC), nutritionally deficient streptococcus (GPC), *S aureus* (GPC), coagulase-negative staphylococci (GPC), *Erysipelothrix rhusiopathiae* (GPR), brucella (GNR), *Coxiella burnetii, C pneumoniae.* Slow-growing fastidious GNRs: *H parainfluenzae, H aphrophilus,* actinobacillus, cardiobacterium, capnocytophaga, eikenella, kingella (HACEK).	Blood cultures for bacteria. Three blood cultures are sufficient in 97% of cases. Blood cultures are frequently positive with gram-positive organisms but can be negative with gram-negative or anaerobic organisms. If the patient is not acutely ill, therapy can begin after cultures identify an organism. Transesophageal echocardiography (TEE) can help in diagnosis by demonstrating the presence of valvular vegetations (sensitivity >90%), prosthetic valve dysfunction, valvular regurgitation, secondary "jet" or "kissing" lesions, and paravalvular abscess. SPECT immunoscintigraphy with antigranulocyte antibody can be used in cases of suspected infective endocarditis if echocardiography is non-diagnostic.	Patients with congenital or valvular heart disease should receive prophylaxis before dental procedures or surgery of the upper respiratory, genitourinary, or gastrointestinal tract. In left-sided endocarditis, patients should be watched carefully for development of valvular regurgitation or ring abscess. The size and mobility of valvular vegetations on TEE can help to predict the risk of arterial embolization. Am J Med 1999;107:198. Clin Infect Dis 1999;28:106. Clin Infect Dis 1999;29:1. Clin Infect Dis 1999;46:275. Infect Dis Clin North Am 1999;13:833. J Infection 1999;39:27. J Infection 1999;38:87. Postgrad Med J 1999;75:540. N Engl J Med 2001;345:1318. Clin Infect Dis 2002;34:1576. Pediatr Infect Dis J 2002;21:265. WMJ 2002;101:24.

	HEART AND VESSELS	
	Prosthetic valve infective endocarditis	
Organism	**Specimen/Diagnostic Tests**	**Comments**
Prosthetic valve infective endocarditis (PVE) Early (<2 months): coagulase-negative staphylococci (usually *S epidermidis* with 80%–87% methicillin-resistant) (GPC) (27%), *S aureus* (GPC) (20%), Enterobacteriaceae (GNR), enterococcus (GPC), diphtheroids (GPR), candida (yeast). Late (>2 months): viridans group streptococci (GPC) (42%), coagulase-negative staphylococci (22–30%), *S aureus* (11%), enterococcus (GPC), Enterobacteriaceae.	Blood cultures for bacteria and yeast. Three sets of blood cultures are sufficient in 97% of cases. Draw before temperature spike. Although more invasive, TEE is superior in predicting which patients with infective endocarditis have perivalvular abscess or prosthetic valve dysfunction and which are most susceptible to systemic embolism.	In a large series using perioperative prophylaxis, the incidences of early and late-onset PVE were 0.78% and 1.1%, respectively. The portals of entry of early-onset PVE are intra-operative contamination and postoperative wound infections. The portals of entry of late-onset PVE appear to be the same as those of native valve endocarditis, and the microbiologic profiles are also similar. Clinically, patients with late-onset PVE resemble those with native valve disease. However, those with early-onset infection are often critically ill, more often have other complicating problems, are more likely to go into shock, and are more likely to have conduction abnormalities due to ring abscess. Clin Infect Dis 1997;24:884. Circulation 1998;98:2936. J Infect 1999;39:27.

HEART AND VESSELS		
Infectious thrombophlebitis		
Infectious thrombophlebitis Associated with venous catheters: *S aureus* (GPC) (65–78%), coagulase-negative staphylococci (GPC), candida sp. (yeast), pseudomonas sp. (GNR), Enterobacteriaceae (GNR). Hyperalimentation with catheter: Candida sp., *Malassezia furfur* (yeast). Indwelling venous catheter (eg, Broviac, Hickman, Gershom): *S aureus*, coagulase-negative staphylococci, diphtheroids (GPR), pseudomonas sp., Enterobacteriaceae, candida sp. Postpartum or postabortion pelvic thrombophlebitis: Bacteroides (GNR), Enterobacteriaceae, clostridium (GPR), streptococcus (GPC).	Blood cultures for bacteria (positive in 80–90%). Catheter tip for bacterial culture to document etiology. More than 15 colonies (CFUs) suggests colonization or infection. CT and MRI are the studies of choice in the evaluation of puerperal septic pelvic thrombophlebitis.	Thrombophlebitis is an inflammation of the vein wall. Infectious thrombophlebitis is associated with microbial invasion of the vessel and is associated with bacteremia and thrombosis. Risk of infection from an indwelling peripheral venous catheter goes up significantly after 4 days. AJR Am J Roentgenol 1997;169:1039. Pediatr Infect Dis J 1997;16:63. Infection 1999;27(Suppl 1):S11. Support Care Cancer 1999;7:386. World J Surg 1999;23:589.

	ABDOMEN	
	Gastritis	Infectious esophagitis

Organism	Specimen/Diagnostic Tests	Comments
Gastritis *Helicobacter pylori*	Serum for antibody test (76–90% sensitivity but low specificity) (see p 98). Stool for antigen detection test (90%) and [^{13}C] and [^{14}C] urea breath test (99%) are specific noninvasive tests. Gastric mucosal biopsy for rapid urea test (89%), culture (89%), histology (92%), and PCR (99%) (reference laboratories).	Also associated with duodenal ulcer, gastric carcinoma, and gastroesophageal reflux disease. Proton pump inhibitors may cause false-negative urea breath tests and fecal antigen tests, and should be withheld for at least 7 days before testing. Aliment Pharmacol Ther 1998;12 (Suppl 1):61. J Clin Microbiol 1999;37:3328. J Gastroenterol 1999;34(Suppl 11):67. J Clin Microbiol 2000;38:13. Am J Gastroenterol 2000;95:72. Arch Intern Med 2000;160:1285. Gastrointest Endosc 2002;52:20.
Infectious esophagitis Candida sp. (yeast), HSV, CMV, VZV, *Helicobacter pylori* (GNR), cryptosporidium. (Rare causes: *M tuberculosis* [AFB], aspergillus, histoplasma, blastomyces, HIV).	Barium esophagram reveals abnormalities in the majority of cases of candidal esophagitis. Endoscopy with biopsy and brushings for culture and cytology has the highest diagnostic yield (57%) and should be performed if clinically indicated or if empiric antifungal therapy is unsuccessful.	Thrush and odynophagia in an immunocompromised patient warrants empiric therapy for candida. Factors predisposing to infectious esophagitis include HIV infection, exposure to radiation, cytotoxic chemotherapy, recent antibiotic therapy, corticosteroid therapy, and neutropenia. Am J Gastroenterol 1998;93:394, 2239. Am J Gastroenterol 1999;94:339. Am J Gastroenterol 2000;95(9):2171. Compr Ther 2000 26(3):163.

ABDOMEN		
Infectious colitis/dysentery		
Infectious colitis/dysentery Infant: *E coli* (enteropathogenic). Child/adult without travel, afebrile, no gross blood or WBCs in stool: Rotavirus, caliciviruses (eg, Norwalk agent), *E coli* (GNR). Child/adult with fever, bloody stool or history of travel to subtropics/tropics (varies with epidemiology): *Campylobacter jejuni* (GNR), *E coli* (GNR) (enterotoxigenic, enteroinvasive, enteropathogenic, enteroaggregative, diarrhea-associated hemolytic and cytolethal distending toxin-producing, enterohemorrhagic O157:H7), shigella (GNR), salmonella (GNR), *Yersinia enterocolitica* (GNR), *Clostridium difficile* (GPR), aeromonas (GNR), plesiomonas (GNR), vibrio (GNR), cryptosporidium, *Entamoeba histolytica, Giardia lamblia,* cyclospora, strongyloides, edwardsiella (GNR). Child/adult with vomiting and no fever: *S aureus* (GPC), *Bacillus cereus* (GPR).	Stool for occult blood helpful in diagnosis of *E coli* O157:H7, salmonella, shigella, campylobacter, and *E histolytica.* Stool for culture and ova and parasites (3 specimens); the sensitivity of culture is 72%, but its specificity is 100%. Special stool culture techniques are needed for yersinia, *E coli* O157:H7, vibrio, aeromonas, plesiomonas, and *C difficile.* Stool cultures for salmonella, shigella, and campylobacter are not helpful from patients who have been hospitalized for >3 days. Specific examination for *C difficile* or its toxin is appropriate for patients who have been hospitalized for >3 days. *C difficile* tissue culture assay has a high sensitivity (94–100%) and specificity (99%). Immunodiagnosis of *G lamblia, E histolytica, Cryptosporidium parvum* cysts in stools is highly sensitive and specific. Proctosigmoidoscopy is indicated in patients with chronic or recurrent diarrhea or in diarrhea of unknown cause for smears of aspirates and biopsy. Culture of a biopsy specimen has a slightly higher sensitivity than routine stool culture. Obtain rectal and jejunal biopsies on HIV-infected patients, culture for bacterial pathogens and Mycobacteria (eg, MAC), and perform modified acid-fast stains for cryptosporidium, isospora, and cyclospora.	Acute dysentery is diarrhea with bloody, mucoid stools, tenesmus, and pain on defecation and implies an inflammatory invasion of the colonic mucosa. BUN and serum electrolytes may be indicated for supportive care. Severe dehydration is a medical emergency. Necrotizing enterocolitis is a fulminant disease of premature newborns; cause is unknown, but human breast milk is protective. Air in the intestinal wall (pneumatosis intestinalis), in the portal venous system, or in the peritoneal cavity seen on plain x-ray can confirm diagnosis. 30–50% of these infants will have bacteremia or peritonitis. Risk factors for infectious colitis include poor hygiene and immune compromise (infancy, advanced age, corticosteroid or immunosuppressive therapy, HIV infection). Am Fam Physician 1998;58:1769. J Diarrhoeal Dis Res 1998;16:248. Adv Pediatr 1999;46:353. Annu Rev Med 1999;50:355. Clin Lab Med 1999;19:553, 691. Emerg Infect Dis 1999;5:607. Clin Infect Dis 2001;32:331. Diagn Microbiol Infect Dis 2001;41:93. Gastroenterol Clin North Am 2001;30:693. Gastroenterol Clin North Am 2001;30:779. J Gastroenterol Hepatol 2002;17:467.

	ABDOMEN
	Antibiotic-associated colitis

Organism	Specimen/Diagnostic Tests	Comments
Antibiotic-associated pseudomembranous colitis *Clostridium difficile* (GPR) toxin, *Clostridium perfringens* (GPR), *Staphylococcus aureus* (GPC), *Klebsiella oxytoca* (GNR), *Candida albicans* (yeast).	Send stool for *C difficile* cytotoxin B by tissue culture (sensitivity 100%, specificity 97%) or toxin A or A and B by less sensitive immunoassay, EIA (sensitivity 70–90%, specificity 99%). Testing two stools on different days will increase sensitivity; toxin testing for test-of-cure is not recommended. Fecal WBCs are present in 30–50% of cases. The toxin is very labile and can be present in infants with no disease. Stool culture is not recommended because nontoxigenic strains occur. Colonoscopy and visualization of characteristic 1–5 mm raised yellow plaques provides the most rapid diagnosis. However, an ultrasound appearance of grossly thickened bowel wall with luminal narrowing or CT findings of thickened bowel wall, presence of an "accordion" sign, heterogeneous contrast enhancement pattern ("target sign"), pericolonic stranding, ascites, pleural effusion, and subcutaneous edema can suggest the diagnosis of pseudomembranous colitis.	Antibiotics cause changes in normal intestinal flora, allowing overgrowth of *C difficile* and elaboration of toxin. Other risk factors for *C difficile*-induced colitis are GI manipulations, advanced age, female sex, inflammatory bowel disease, HIV, chemotherapy, and renal disease. *C difficile* nosocomial infection can be controlled by handwashing. Antibiotic-associated diarrhea may include uncomplicated diarrhea, colitis, or pseudomembranous colitis. Only 10–20% of cases are caused by infection with *C difficile*. Most clinically mild cases are due to functional disturbances of intestinal carbohydrate or bile acid metabolism, to allergic and toxic effects of antibiotics on intestinal mucosa, or to their pharmacologic effects on motility. Clin Infect Dis 1998;27:702. Dig Dis 1998;16:292. Dis Colon Rectum 1998;41:1435. J Antimicrob Chemother 1998;41 (Suppl C):29, 59. Digestion 1999;60:91. Hepatogastroenterology 1999;46:343. Int J Antimicrob Agents 2000;16:521. Arch Intern Med 2002;162:2177. Curr Gastroenterol Rep 2002;4:279. N Engl J Med 2002;346:334.

ABDOMEN		
Diarrhea in HIV		

Diarrhea in the HIV-infected host		
Same as child-adult infectious colitis with addition of CMV, cryptosporidium, *Isospora belli*, microsporidia (*Enterocytozoon bieneusi*), *C difficile*, *Giardia intestinalis*, MAC (AFB), HSV, *Entamoeba histolytica*, ?HIV.	Stool for stain for fecal leukocytes, culture (especially for salmonella, shigella, yersinia, and campylobacter), *C difficile* toxin, ova and parasite examination, and AFB smear. Multiple samples are often needed. Proctosigmoidoscopy with fluid aspiration and biopsy is indicated in patients with chronic or recurrent diarrhea or in diarrhea of unknown cause for smears of aspirates (may show organisms) and histologic examination and culture of tissue. Rectal and jejunal biopsies may be necessary, especially in patients with tenesmus or bloody stools. Need modified acid-fast stain for cryptosporidium, isospora, and cyclospora. Intranuclear inclusion bodies on histologic exam suggest CMV. Immunodiagnosis of giardia, cryptosporidium, and *E histolytica* cysts in stool is highly sensitive and specific.	Most patients with HIV infection will develop diarrhea at some point in their illness. Cryptosporidium causes a chronic debilitating diarrheal infection that rarely remits spontaneously and is still without effective treatment. Diarrhea seems to be the result of malabsorption and produces a cholera-like syndrome. Between 15% and 50% of HIV-infected patients with diarrhea have no identifiable pathogen. Gastrointest Endosc Clin North Am 1998;8:857. Am J Gastroenterol 1999;94:596. Arch Intern Med 1999;159:1473. J Infect Dis 1999;179(Suppl 3):S454. Arch Intern Med 2001;161:525. Diagn Microbiol Infect Dis 2001;41:93. Gastroenterol Clin North Am 2001;30:637. Gastroenterol Clin North Am 2001;30:693. Gastroenterol Clin North Am 2001;30:779.

	ABDOMEN	
	Peritonitis	
Organism	**Specimen/Diagnostic Tests**	**Comments**
Peritonitis Spontaneous or primary (associated with nephrosis or cirrhosis) peritonitis (SBP): Enterobacteriaceae (GNR) (69%), *S pneumoniae* (GPC), group A streptococcus (GPC), *S aureus* (GPC), anaerobes (5%). Secondary (bowel perforation, hospital acquired, or antecedent antibiotic therapy): Enterobacteriaceae, enterococcus (GPC), *Bacteroides fragilis* group (GNR), *Pseudomonas aeruginosa* (GNR) (3–15%). Chronic ambulatory peritoneal dialysis (CAPD): Coagulase-negative staphylococci (GPC) (43%), *S aureus* (14%), streptococcus sp (12%), Enterobacteriaceae (14%), *Pseudomonas aeruginosa*, corynebacterium sp. (GPR), candida (2%), aspergillus (rare), cryptococcus (rare).	Peritoneal fluid sent for WBC (>1000/μL in SPB, >100/μL in CAPD) with PMN (>250/μL in SBP and secondary peritonitis, 50% PMN in CAPD); total protein (>1 g/dL); glucose (<50 mg/dL), and LDH (>225 units/mL) in secondary; pH (<7.35 in 57% of SBP). Gram stain (sensitivity 22–77% for SBP), and culture of large volumes often in blood culture bottles. (See Ascitic fluid profiles, p 364.) Blood cultures for bacteria positive in 85% of SBP cases. Catheter-related infection is associated with a WBC >500/μL.	In nephrotic patients, Enterobacteriaceae and *S aureus* are most frequent. In cirrhotics, 69% of cases are due to Enterobacteriaceae. Cirrhotic patients with low ascitic fluid protein levels (≤1 g/dL) and high bilirubin level or low platelet count are at high risk of developing spontaneous bacterial peritonitis. "Bacterascites," a positive ascitic fluid culture without an elevated PMN count, is seen in 8% of cases of SBP and probably represents early infection. In secondary peritonitis, factors influencing the incidence of postoperative complications and death include age, presence of certain concomitant diseases, site of origin of peritonitis, type of admission, and the ability of the surgeon to eliminate the source of infection. Clin Infect Dis 1998;27:669. Eur J Clin Microbiol Infect Dis 1998;17:542. J Am Soc Nephrol 1998;9:1956. Gastroenterology 1999;117:414. Langenbecks Arch Surg 1999;384:24. J Hepatol 2000;32:142. Aliment Pharmacol Ther 2001;15:1851.

ABDOMEN		
Tuberculous peritonitis/enterocolitis		
Tuberculous peritonitis/ enterocolitis *Mycobacterium tuberculosis* (MTb, AFB, acid-fast beaded rods).	Ascitic fluid for appearance (clear, hemorrhagic or chylous), RBCs (can be high), WBCs (>1000/µL, >70% lymphs), protein (>3.5 g/dL), serum/ascites albumin gradient (<1.1), LDH (>90 units/L), AFB culture (<50% positive). (See Ascitic fluid profiles, p 364.) With coexistent chronic liver disease, protein level and SAAG are usually not helpful, but LDH >90 units/L is a useful predictor. Culture or AFB smear from other sources (especially from respiratory tract) can help confirm diagnosis. Abdominal ultrasound may demonstrate free or loculated intra-abdominal fluid, intra-abdominal abscess, ileocecal mass, and retroperitoneal lymphadenopathy. Ascites with fine, mobile septations shown by ultrasound and peritoneal and omental thickening detected by CT strongly suggest tuberculous peritonitis. Marked elevations of serum CA 125 have been noted; levels decline to normal with anti-tuberculous therapy. Diagnosis of enterocolitis rests on biopsy of colonic lesions via endoscopy if pulmonary or other extra-pulmonary infection cannot be documented. Diagnosis is best confirmed by laparoscopy with peritoneal biopsy and culture. Operative procedure may be needed to relieve obstruction or for diagnosis.	Infection of the intestines can occur anywhere along the GI tract but occurs most commonly in the ileo-cecal area or mesenteric lymph nodes. It often complicates pulmonary infection. Peritoneal infection usually is an extension of intestinal disease. Symptoms may be minimal even with extensive disease. In the United States, 29% of patients with abdominal tuberculosis have a normal chest x-ray. Presence of AFB in the feces does not correlate with intestinal involvement. Rays 1998;23:115. Eur J Surg 1999;165:158. South Med J 1999;92:406. Clin Infect Dis 2000;31:70. Scand J Gastroenterol 2001;36:528.

	ABDOMEN	
	Diverticulitis	**Liver abscess**

	Organism	Specimen/Diagnostic Tests	Comments
Diverticulitis	Enterobacteriaceae (GNR), bacteroides sp. (GNR), enterococcus (GPC in chains).	Identification of organism is not usually sought. Ultrasonography or flat and upright x-rays of abdomen are crucial to rule out perforation (free air under diaphragm) and to localize abscess (air-fluid collections). Barium enema can (82%) show presence of diverticula. Avoid enemas in acute disease because increased intraluminal pressure may cause perforation. Ultrasound (85%) and CT (79–98%) have greater accuracy in the evaluation of patients with diverticulitis. Specificities of barium enema, ultrasound, and CT are 81–84%. Thin-section helical CT is also able to reveal inflamed diverticula in acute diverticulitis by demonstrating an enhancing pattern of the colonic wall. Urinalysis will reveal urinary tract involvement, if present.	Pain usually is localized to the left lower quadrant because the sigmoid and descending colon are the most common sites for diverticula. It is important to rule out other abdominal disease (eg, colon carcinoma, Crohn's disease, ischemic colitis), appendicitis, and gynecologic disorders. Dis Colon Rect 1998;41:1023. N Engl J Med 1998;338:1521. Radiology 1998;208:611. AJR Am J Roengenol 1999;172:601. Am J Gastroenterol 1999;94:1310. Surg Endosc 1999;13:430. Int Surg 2001;86:1991.
Liver abscess	Usually polymicrobial: Enterobacteriaceae, especially klebsiella (GNR), enterococcus (GPC in chains), bacteroides sp. (GNR), actinomyces (GPR), S aureus (GPC in clusters), candida sp., *Entamoeba histolytica.*	CT scan with contrast and ultrasonography are the most accurate tests for the diagnosis of liver abscess. Antibodies against *E histolytica* should be obtained on all patients. (See Amebic serology, p 46.) Complete removal of abscess material obtained via surgery or percutaneous aspiration is recommended for culture and direct examination for *E histolytica*. *E histolytica* has been described with modern techniques as a complex of two species, the commensal parasite *E dispar* and the pathogenic parasite. Stool for antigen detection is sensitive and can distinguish the two species. Chest x-ray is often useful with raised hemidiaphragm, right pleural effusion, or right basilar atelectasis in 41% of patients. Elevation of serum alkaline phosphatase level in 78%.	Travel to and origin in an endemic area are important risk factors for amebic liver abscess. 60% of patients have a single lesion; 40% have multiple lesions. Biliary tract disease is the most common underlying disease, followed by malignancy (biliary tract or pancreatic), colonic disease (diverticulitis), diabetes mellitus, liver disease, and alcoholism. Ann Emerg Med 1999;34:351. West J Med 1999;170:104. World J Surg 1999;23:102. BMJ 2001;322:537. Trends Parasitol 2001;17:280. Clin Liver Dis 2002;6:203.

ABDOMEN		
Cholangitis/cholecystitis		
Cholangitis/cholecystitis Enterobacteriaceae (GNR) (68%), enterococcus (GPC in chains) (14%), *Pseudomonas aeruginosa* (GNR), bacteroides (GNR) (10%), clostridium sp. (GPR) (7%), microsporidia (*Enterocytozoon bienusi*) cryptosporidia, *Ascaris lumbricoides*, *Opisthorchis viverrini*, *O felineus, Clonorchis sinensis, Fasciola hepatica, Echinococcus granulosus, E multilocularis*, hepatitis C virus, hepatitis B virus, CMV.	Ultrasonography is the best test to quickly demonstrate gallstones or phlegmon around the gallbladder or dilation of the biliary tree. (See Abdominal Ultrasound, p 269.) CT scanning is useful in cholangitis in detecting the site and cause of obstruction but may fail to detect stones in the common bile duct. In acute cholecystitis, ultrasonography is superior to MR cholangiography in evaluating gallbladder wall thickening. However, MR cholangiography is superior to ultrasound in depicting cystic duct and gallbladder neck stones and in evaluating cystic duct obstruction. Radionuclide scans can demonstrate cystic duct obstruction. (See p 269.) Blood cultures for bacteria.	90% of cases of acute cholecystitis are calculous, 10% are acalculous. Risk factors for acalculous disease include prolonged illness, fasting, hyperalimentation, HIV infection, and carcinoma of the gallbladder or bile ducts. Biliary obstruction and cholangitis can develop before biliary dilation is detected. Common bile duct obstruction secondary to tumor or pancreatitis seldom results in infection (0–15%). There is a high incidence of acalculous cholecystitis in AIDS patients with CD4 counts <200/μL, due to cryptosporidium, CMV, yeast, tuberculosis, and *M avium-intracellulare*. Observation of gallbladder contraction on hepatobiliary scintigraphy after intravenous cholecystokinin excludes acalculous cholecystitis. Hepatology 1999;30:325. Radiology 1999;211:373. Clin Radiol 2000;55:25. BMJ 2002;325:639.

	GENITOURINARY
	Urinary tract infection

Organism	Specimen/Diagnostic Tests	Comments
Urinary tract infection (UTI)/cystitis/pyuria-dysuria syndrome Enterobacteriaceae (GNR, especially *E coli*), *Chlamydia trachomatis*, *Staphylococcus saprophyticus* (GPC) (in young women), enterococcus (GPC), group B streptococci (GPC), candida sp. (yeast), *N gonorrhoeae* (GNCB), HSV, adenovirus, *Corynebacterium glucuronolyticum* (GPR), *Ureaplasma urealyticum* (GPR).	Urinalysis and culture reveal the two most important signs: bacteriuria and pyuria (>10 WBCs/μL). 30% of patients have hematuria. Cystitis (95%) is diagnosed by ≥10² CFU/mL of bacteria; other urinary infections (90%) by ≥10⁵ CFU/mL. Culture is generally not necessary for uncomplicated cystitis in women. Combination of current symptoms (eg, dysuria, frequency, and hematuria) and prior history yields a ≥90% probability of UTI. However, pregnant women should be screened for asymptomatic bacteriuria and promptly treated. Both Gram stain for bacteria and dipstick analysis for nitrite and leukocyte esterase perform similarly in detecting UTI in children and are superior to microscopic analysis for pyuria. Nitrite or leukocyte esterase maybe negative in 19% of patients with bacteremia. Intravenous pyelogram and cystoscopy should be performed in women with recurrent or childhood infections, all young boys with UTI, men with recurrent or complicated infection, and patients with symptoms suggestive of obstruction or renal stones. (See Intravenous pyelogram, p 277.) DNA amplification tests for chlamydia and gonorrhea are available.	Most men with UTIs have a functional or anatomic genitourinary abnormality. In catheter-related UTI, cure is unlikely unless the catheter is removed. In asymptomatic catheter-related UTI, antibiotics should be given only if patients are at risk for sepsis (old age, underlying disease, diabetes mellitus, pregnancy). Up to one-third of cases of acute cystitis have "silent" upper tract involvement. Am J Med 1999;106:636. BMJ 1999;318:770. Nephrol Dial Transplant 1999;14:2746. J Clin Microbiol 1999;37:3051. Pediatrics 1999;103(4 Part 1):843. Postgrad Med 1999;105:181. Urol Clin North Am 1999;26:821. Am J Med 2002;113(Suppl A):145. JAMA 2002;287:2701.

GENITOURINARY
Prostatitis

Prostatitis

Acute and chronic: Enterobacteriaceae (GNR, *E coli* [80%]), pseudomonas sp. (GNR), enterococcus (GPC in chains), CMV.

Urinalysis shows pyuria.
Urine culture usually identifies causative organism. Prostatic massage is useful in chronic prostatitis to retrieve organisms but is contraindicated in acute prostatitis (it may cause bacteremia). Bacteriuria is first cleared by antibiotic treatment. Then urine cultures are obtained from first-void, bladder, and postprostatic massage urine specimens. A higher organism count in the postprostatic massage specimen localizes infection to the prostate (91%).

Acute prostatitis is a severe illness characterized by fever, dysuria, and a boggy or tender prostate.
Chronic prostatitis often has no symptoms of dysuria or perineal discomfort and a normal prostate examination.
Nonbacterial prostatitis (prostatodynia) represents 90% of prostatitis cases. Its etiology is unknown, although chlamydia antigen can be found in up to 25% of patients.

Clin Microbiol Rev 1998;11:604.
Int J Clin Pract 1998;52:540.
Am J Med 1999;106:327.
Sex Transm Infect 1999;75(Suppl 1):S46.
Urol Clin North Am 1999;26:737.
Curr Opin Urol 2001;11:87.
J Eur Acad Dermatol Venereol 2002;16:253.

	GENITOURINARY	
	Pyelonephritis	**Perinephric abscess**

Organism	Specimen/Diagnostic Tests	Comments
Pyelonephritis Acute, uncomplicated (usually young women): Enterobacteriaceae (especially *E coli*) (GNR), enterococci (GPC in chains), *S aureus* (GPC). Complicated (older women, men; postcatheterization, obstruction, post-renal transplant): Enterobacteriaceae (especially *E coli*), *Pseudomonas aeruginosa* (GNR), enterococcus (GPC), *Staphylococcus saprophyticus* (GPC), *S aureus* (GPC).	Urine culture is indicated when pyelonephritis is suspected. Urinalysis will usually show pyuria ($\geq$5 WBC/hpf) and may show WBC casts. Blood cultures for bacteria if sepsis is suspected. In uncomplicated pyelonephritis, ultrasonography is not necessary. In severe cases, however, ultrasound is the optimal procedure for ruling out urinary tract obstruction, pyonephrosis, and calculi. Doppler ultrasonography (88%) has a specificity of 100% for acute pyelonephritis. Intravenous pyelogram in patients with recurrent infection will show irregularly outlined renal pelvis with caliectasis and cortical scars. (See Intravenous pyelogram, p 277.)	Patients usually present with fever, chills, nausea, vomiting, and costovertebral angle tenderness. 20–30% of pregnant women with untreated bacteriuria develop pyelonephritis. Clin Obstet Gynecol 1998;41:515. Int J Antimicrob Ag 1999;11:257. Urol Clin North Am 1999;26:753. Am J Med 2002;113(Suppl 1A):14S.
Perinephric abscess Associated with staphylococcal bacteremia: *S aureus* (GPC). Associated with pyelonephritis: Enterobacteriaceae (GNR), candida sp. (yeast), coagulase-negative staphylococci (GPC).	CT scan with contrast is more sensitive than ultrasound in imaging abscess and confirming diagnosis. (See Abdominal CT, p 276.) Urinalysis may be normal or may show pyuria. Urine culture (positive in 60–72%). Blood cultures for bacteria (positive in 20–40%). Bacterial culture of abscess fluid via needle aspiration or drainage (percutaneous or surgical).	Most perinephric abscesses are the result of extension of an ascending urinary tract infection. Often they are very difficult to diagnose. They should be considered in patients who fail to respond to antibiotic therapy, in patients with anatomic abnormalities of the urinary tract, and in patients with diabetes mellitus. Hosp Pract (Off Ed) 1997;32(6):40. Infect Dis Clin North Am 1997;11:663. J Urol 2002;168(4 Pt 1):1337.

GENITOURINARY		
Urethritis		**Epididymitis/orchitis**
Urethritis (gonococcal and nongonococcal) Gonococcal (GC): *Neisseria gonorrhoeae* (GNDC). Nongonococcal (NGU): *Chlamydia trachomatis* (50%), *Ureaplasma urealyticum, Trichomonas vaginalis,* HSV, *Mycoplasma genitalium,* unknown (35%).	Urethral discharge collected with urethral swab usually shows ≥4 WBCs per oil-immersion field, Gram stain (identify gonococcal organisms as gram-negative intracellular diplococci). PMNs (in GC, >95% of WBCs are PMNs, in NGU usually <80% are PMNs). Urethral discharge for GC culture (80%) or ligase chain reaction (LCR) (>95%) (usually not needed for diagnosis); urine (90–95%) or urethral discharge (97%) for detection of *C trachomatis* by LCR amplification or wet mount for *T vaginalis*. Culture or nonamplified assays are considerably less sensitive for diagnosis of *C trachomatis*. VDRL should be checked in all patients because of high incidence of associated syphilis.	About 50% of patients with GC will have concomitant NGU infection. Always treat sexual partners. Recurrence may be secondary to failure to treat partners. Half of the cases of NGU are not due to *C trachomatis;* frequently, no pathogen can be isolated. Persistent or recurrent episodes with adequate treatment of patient and partners may warrant further evaluation for other causes (eg, prostatitis). Dermatol Clinic 1998;16:723. MMWR Morb Mortal Wkly Rep 1998;47(RR-1):1. Aust Fam Physician 1999;28:333. Clin Infect Dis 1999;28(Suppl 1):S66. FEMS Immunol Med Microbiol 1999;24:437. Sex Transm Infect 1999;75(Suppl 1):S9
Epididymitis/orchitis Age <35 years, homosexual men: *Chlamydia trachomatis,* GNDC *U urealyticum, E coli* (GNR), *Enterococcus faecalis* (GPC), *P aeruginosa* (GNR). Age >35 years, or children: Enterobacteriaceae (especially *E coli*) (GNR), pseudomonas sp. (GNR), salmonella (GNR), *Haemophilus influenzae* (GNCB), VZV, mumps. Immunosuppression: *H influenzae, Mycobacterium tuberculosis* (AFB), candida sp. (yeast), CMV.	Urinalysis may reveal pyuria. Patients aged >35 years will often have midstream pyuria and scrotal edema. Culture urine and expressible urethral discharge when present. Prostatic secretions for Gram stain and bacterial culture are helpful in older patients. When testicular torsion is considered, Doppler ultrasound or radionuclide scan can be useful in diagnosis. Ultrasonography in tuberculous epididymitis shows enlargement of the epididymis (predominantly in the tail) and marked heterogeneity in texture. Other sonographic findings include a hypoechoic lesion of the testis with associated sinus tract or extratesticular calcifications.	Testicular torsion is a surgical emergency that is often confused with orchitis or epididymitis. Sexual partners should be examined for signs of sexually transmitted diseases. In non-sexually transmitted disease, evaluation for underlying urinary tract infection or structural defect is recommended. Clin Infect Dis 1998;26:942. Sex Transm Infect 1999;75(Suppl 1):S51. BJU Int 1999;84:827. Drugs 1999;57:743. J Androl 2002;23:453.

	GENITOURINARY
	Vaginitis/vaginosis

Organism	Specimen/Diagnostic Tests	Comments
Vaginitis/vaginosis Candida sp. (yeast), *Trichomonas vaginalis*, *Gardnerella vaginalis* (GPR), bacteroides (non-*fragilis*) (GNR), mobiluncus (GPR), peptostreptococcus (GPC), *Mycoplasma hominis*, groups A and B streptococci (GPC), HSV.	Vaginal discharge for appearance (in candidiasis, area is pruritic with thick "cheesy" discharge: in trichomoniasis, copious foamy, yellow-green or discolored discharge), pH (about 4.5 for candida; 5.0–7.0 in trichomonas; 5.0–6.0 with bacterial), saline ("wet") preparation (motile organisms seen in trichomonas; cells covered with organisms—clue cells—in gardnerella; yeast and hyphae in candida, "fishy" odor on addition of KOH with gardnerella infection). Vaginal fluid pH as a screening test for bacterial vaginosis showed a sensitivity of 74.3%, but combined with clinical symptoms and signs its sensitivity increased to 81.3%. (See Vaginitis table, p 402.) Atrophic vaginitis is seen in postmenopausal patients, often with bleeding, scant discharge, and pH 6.0–7.0 Cultures for gardnerella are not useful and are not recommended. Culture for *T vaginalis* has greater sensitivity than wet mount. Culture for groups A and B streptococci and rare causes of bacterial vaginosis may be indicated. Gram stain of discharge is more reliable than wet mount for diagnosis of bacterial vaginosis (93% vs. 70%, respectively).	Bacterial vaginosis results from massive overgrowth of anaerobic vaginal bacterial flora (especially gardnerella). Serious infectious sequelae associated with bacterial vaginosis include abscesses, endometritis and pelvic inflammatory disease. There is also a danger of miscarriage, premature rupture of the membranes, and premature labor. Int J Gynaecol Obstet 1999;66:143. Pediatr Clin North Am 1999;46:733. Sex Transm Infect 1999;75(Suppl 1):S16, S21. Am Fam Physician 2000;62:1095. Clin Infect Dis 2000;31:1225. AIDS Patient Care STDS 2002;16:367.

	GENITOURINARY	
	Cervicitis	
Cervicitis, mucopurulent *Chlamydia trachomatis* (50%), *N gonorrhoeae* (GNDC) (8%), HSV.	Cervical swab specimen for appearance (yellow or green purulent material), cell count (>10 WBCs per high-power oil immersion field and culture (58–80%) or nucleic acid assay (93%) for GC; urine for nucleic acid assay (93%) for GC; urine (80–92%) or cervical swab (97%) for detection of *C trachomatis* by nucleic acid amplification. Culture (52%) or nonamplified assays (50–80%) are considerably less sensitive for diagnosis of *C trachomatis*.	Because of the danger of false-positive amplified nucleic acid assays, culture is the preferred method in cases of suspected child abuse. In one study of pregnant women, a wet mount preparation of endocervical secretions with <10 PMNs per high-power field had a negative predictive value of 99% for gonococcus-induced cervicitis and of 96% for *C trachomatis*-induced cervicitis. In family planning clinics, however, a mucopurulent discharge with >10 PMNs/hpf had a low positive predictive value of 29.2% for *C trachomatis*-related cervicitis. Mucopurulent discharge may persist for 3 months or more even after appropriate therapy. Curr Probl Dermatol 1996;24:110. CMAJ 1998;158:41. J Clin Microbiol 1998;36:1630. Am J Obstet Gynecol 1999;181:283. Eur J Clin Microbiol Infect Dis 1999;18:142. Clin Infect Dis 2000;31:1225.

	GENITOURINARY	
	Salpingitis	**Chorioamnionitis/endometritis**

Organism

Salpingitis/pelvic inflammatory disease (PID)

Usually polymicrobial: *N gonorrhoeae* (GNDC), *Chlamydia trachomatis*, bacteroides, peptostreptococcus, *G vaginalis*, and other anaerobes, Enterobacteriaceae (GNR), streptococci (GPC in chains), *Mycoplasma hominis* (debatable).

Chorioamnionitis/endometritis

Group B streptococcus (GPC), *E coli* (GNR), *Listeria monocytogenes* (GPR), *Mycoplasma hominis*, *Ureaplasma urealyticum*, *Gardnerella vaginalis*, enterococci (GPC), viridans streptococci (GPC), bacteroides (GNR), prevotella (GNR), and other anaerobic flora, *Chlamydia trachomatis*, group A streptococcus (GPC).

Specimen/Diagnostic Tests

Gram stain and culture or amplified nucleic acid assays of urethral or endocervical exudate.
Ultrasonographic findings include thickened fluid-filled tubes, polycystic-like ovaries, and free pelvic fluid. MRI imaging findings for PID (95%) include fluid-filled tube, pyosalpinx, tubo-ovarian abscess, or polycystic-like ovaries and free fluid.
Laparoscopy supplemented by microbiologic tests and fimbrial biopsy is the diagnostic standard for PID. Transvaginal ultrasonography (81%) has a lower specificity than MRI.
Laparoscopy is the most specific test to confirm the diagnosis of PID.
VDRL should be checked in all patients because of the high incidence of associated syphilis.

Amniotic fluid for Gram stain, leukocyte esterase, glucose levels <10–20 mg/dL, and aerobic and anaerobic culture; blood for culture. Sonographic evaluation of fetus can be helpful, but findings are nonspecific.

Comments

PID typically progresses from cervicitis to endometritis to salpingitis. PID is a sexually transmitted disease in some cases, not in others.
All sexual partners should be examined.
All IUDs should be removed.
Some recommend that all patients with PID be hospitalized.
A strategy of identifying, testing, and treating women at increased risk for cervical chlamydial infection can lead to a reduced incidence of PID.
Dermatol Clin 1998;16:747.
Lippincott Primary Care 1998;2:307.
Clin Infect Dis 1999;28 (Suppl 1):S29.
Radiology 1999;210:209.
Eur J Obstet Gynecol Reprod Biol 2000;92:189.
Sex Transm Infect 2002;78:18.

Risk factors include bacterial vaginosis, preterm labor, duration of labor, parity, internal fetal monitoring.
Semin Perinatol 1998;22:242.
Pediatrics 1999;103:78.

BONE	
Osteomyelitis	
Osteomyelitis *Staphylococcus aureus* (GPC) (about 60% of all cases). Infant: *S aureus*, Enterobacteriaceae (GNR), groups A and B streptococci (GPC). Child (<3 years): *H influenzae* (GNCB), *S aureus*, streptococci. Child (>3 years) to adult: *S aureus*, *Pseudomonas aeruginosa.* Postoperative: *S aureus*, Enterobacteriaceae, pseudomonas sp (GNR), *Bartonella henselae* (GNR). Joint prosthesis: Coagulase-negative staphylococci, peptostreptococcus (GPC), *Propionibacterium acnes* (GPR), viridans streptococci (GPC in chains). Immunocompromised patients (eg, elderly, HIV-infected): *M tuberculosis.*	Blood cultures for bacteria are positive in about 60%. Cultures of percutaneous needle biopsy or open bone biopsy are needed if blood cultures are negative and osteomyelitis is suspected. Imaging with bone scan or gallium/indium scan (sensitivity 95%, specificity 60–70%) can localize areas of suspicion. Technetium methylene diphosphonate bone scan can suggest osteomyelitis days or weeks before plain bone films. Plain bone films are abnormal in acute cases after about 2 weeks of illness (33%). Indium-labeled WBC scan is useful in detecting abscesses. Ultrasound to detect subperiosteal abscesses and ultrasound-guided aspiration can assist in diagnosis and management of osteomyelitis. Ultrasound can differentiate acute osteomyelitis from vaso-occlusive crisis in patients with sickle cell disease. CT scan aids in detecting sequestra. When bone x-rays and scintigraphy are negative, MRI (98%) is useful for detecting early osteomyelitis (specificity 89%), in defining extent, and in distinguishing osteomyelitis from cellulitis. Myelography, CT, or MRI is indicated to rule out epidural abscess in vertebral osteomyelitis.	Hematogenous or contiguous infection (eg, infected prosthetic joint, chronic cutaneous ulcer) may lead to osteomyelitis in children (metaphyses of long bones) or adults (vertebrae, metaphyses of long bones). Hematogenous osteomyelitis in drug addicts occurs in unusual locations (vertebrae, clavicle, ribs). In infants, osteomyelitis is often associated with contiguous joint involvement. Acta Radiologica 1998;39:523. J Pediatr Orthop 1998;18:552. J Comput Assist Tomogr 1998;22:437. Clin Radiol 1999;54:636. Pediatr Surg Int 1999;15:363. J Trauma 2002:52:1210. Pediatr Infect Dis J 2002;21:432.

JOINT		
Bacterial/septic arthritis		
Organism	Specimen/Diagnostic Tests	Comments
Bacterial/septic arthritis Infant (<3 months): *S aureus* (GPC), Enterobacteriaceae (GNR), *Kingella kingae* (GNCB), *Haemophilus influenzae* (GNCB). Child (3 months to 6 years): *S aureus* (35%), *H influenzae*, group A streptococcus (GPC), (10%), Enterobacteriaceae (6%), *Borrelia burgdorferi* (Lyme). Adult, STD not likely: *S aureus* (40%), group A streptococcus (27%), Enterobacteriaceae (23%), *Streptobacillus moniliformis* (GNR), brucella (GNR), *Mycobacterium marinum* (AFB). Adult, STD likely: *N gonorrhoeae* (GNDC) (disseminated gonococcal infection [DGI]). Prosthetic joint, postoperative or following intraarticular injection: Coagulase-negative staphylococci (40%), *S aureus* (20%), viridans streptococci (GPC in chains), enterococci (GPC), peptostreptococcus (GPC), *Propionibacterium acnes* (GPR), Enterobacteriaceae, pseudomonas sp.	Joint aspiration (synovial) fluid for WBCs (in nongonococcal infection, mean WBC is 100,000/μL). Gram stain (best on centrifuged concentrated specimen; positive in one-third of cases), culture (non gonococcal infection in adults [85–95%], DGI [25%]). (See Synovial fluid profiles, p 391.) Yield of culture is greatest if 10 mL of synovial fluid is inoculated into a large volume of culture media, such as a blood culture bottle, within 1 hour after collection. Blood cultures for bacteria may be useful, especially in infants; nongonococcal infection in adults (50%); DGI (13%). *B burgdorferi* serology for Lyme disease. Genitourinary, throat, or rectal culture: DGI may be diagnosed by positive culture from a nonarticular source and by a compatible clinical picture. In difficult cases, MRI can help differentiate septic arthritis from transient synovitis.	It is important to obtain synovial fluid and blood for culture before starting antimicrobial treatment. Septic arthritis is usually hematogenously acquired. Prosthetic joint and diminished host defenses secondary to cancer, HIV, liver disease, or hypogammaglobulinemia are common predisposing factors. Nongonococcal bacterial arthritis is usually monarticular (and typically affects one knee joint). DGI is the most common cause of septic arthritis in urban centers and is usually polyarticular with associated tenosynovitis. Lancet 1998;351:197. Am J Orthop 1999;28:168. Pediatr Emerg Care 1999;15:40. Radiology 1999;211:459. Joint Bone Spine 2000;67:11.

	MUSCLE	SKIN
	Gas gangrene	**Impetigo**

	Gas gangrene	Impetigo
Gas gangrene	Diagnosis should be suspected in areas of devital-ized tissue when gas is discovered by palpation (subcutaneous crepitation) or x-ray. Gram stain of foul-smelling, brown, or blood-tinged watery exudate can be diagnostic with gram-positive rods and a remarkable absence of neutrophils. Anaerobic culture of discharge is confirmatory.	Gas gangrene occurs in the setting of a contaminated wound. *C perfringens* produces potent exotoxins, including alpha toxin and theta toxin, which depresses myocardial contractility, induces shock, and causes direct vascular injury at the site of infection. Infections with enterobacter or *E coli* and mixed anaerobic and anaerobic infections can also cause gas formation. These agents cause cellulitis rather than myonecrosis. Clin Infect Dis 1999;28:159. Trends Microbiol 1999;7:104. Obstet Gynecol Surv 2002;57:53.
Clostridium perfringens (GPR). (80–95%), other clostridium sp.		
Impetigo	Gram stain, culture, and smear for HSV and VZV antigen detection by DFA of scrapings from lesions may be useful in differentiating impetigo from other vesicular or pustular lesions (HSV, VZV, contact dermatitis). DFA smear can be performed by scraping the contents, base, and roof of vesicle and applying to glass slide. After fixing, the slide is stained with DFA for identification of HSV or VZV.	Impetigo neonatorum requires prompt treatment and protection of other infants (isolation). Polymicrobial aerobic-anaerobic infections are pre-sent in some patients. Patients with recurrent impetigo should have cul-tures of the anterior nares to exclude carriage of *S aureus*. Aust Fam Physician 1998;27:735. Practitioner 1998;242:405. Clin Microbiol Rev 2000;13:470. Pediatr Ann 2000;29:26.
Infant (impetigo neonatorum): Staphylococcus (GPC). Nonbullous or "vesicular": *S pyogenes* (GPC), *S aureus* (GPC), anaerobes. Bullous: *S aureus*.		

SKIN

Cellulitis

Organism	Specimen/Diagnostic Tests	Comments
Cellulitis	Skin culture: In spontaneous cellulitis, isolation of the causative organism is difficult. In traumatic and postoperative wounds, Gram stain may allow rapid diagnosis of staphylococcal or clostridial infection. Culture of wound or abscess material after disinfection of the skin site will almost always yield the diagnosis. MRI can aid in diagnosis of secondary abscess formation, necrotizing fasciitis, or pyomyositis. Frozen section of biopsy specimen may be useful.	Cellulitis has long been considered to be the result of an antecedent bacterial invasion with subsequent bacterial proliferation. However, the difficulty in isolating putative pathogens from cellulitic skin has cast doubt on this theory. Predisposing factors for cellulitis include diabetes mellitus, edema, peripheral vascular disease, venous insufficiency, leg ulcer or wound, tinea pedis, dry skin, obesity, and prior history of cellulitis.
Spontaneous, traumatic wound: Polymicrobial: *S aureus* (GPC), groups A, C, and G streptococci (GPC), enterococci (GPC), Enterobacteriaceae (GNR), *Clostridium perfringens* (GPR), *Clostridium tetani*, pseudomonas sp. (GNR) (if water exposure).		Consider updating antitetanus prophylaxis for all wounds.
Postoperative wound (not GI or GU): *S aureus*, group A streptococcus, Enterobacteriaceae, pseudomonas sp.		In the diabetic, and in postoperative and traumatic wounds, consider prompt surgical debridement for necrotizing fasciitis. With abscess formation, surgical drainage is the mainstay of therapy and may be sufficient.
Postoperative wound (GI or GU): Must add bacteroides sp., anaerobes, enterococcus (GPC), groups B or C streptococci.		Hemolytic streptococcal gangrene may follow minor trauma and involves specific strains of streptococcus.
Diabetes mellitus: Polymicrobial: *S pyogenes*, enterococcus, *S aureus*, Enterobacteriaceae, anaerobes.		AJR Am J Roentgenol 1998;170:615.
Bullous lesions, sea water contaminated abrasion, after raw water seafood consumption: *Vibrio vulnificus* (GNR).		BMJ 1999;318:1591.
Vein graft donor site: Streptococcus.		Diagn Microbiol Infect Dis 1999;34:325.
Decubitus ulcers: Polymicrobial: *S aureus*, anaerobic streptococci, Enterobacteriaceae, pseudomonas sp., bacteroides sp.		Lippincott Primary Care Pract 1999;3:59.
Necrotizing fasciitis, type 1: Streptococcus, anaerobes, Enterobacteriaceae; type 2: Group A streptococcus (hemolytic streptococcal gangrene).		Am Fam Physician 2002;66:119.

BLOOD		
Bacteremia of unknown source		
Bacteremia of unknown source Neonate (<4 days): Group B streptococcus (GPC), *E coli* (GNR), klebsiella (GNR), enterobacter (GNR), *S aureus* (GPC), coagulase-negative staphylococci (GPC). Neonate (>5 days): Add *H influenzae* (GNCB). Child (nonimmunocompromised): *H influenzae, S pneumoniae* (GPDC), *N meningitidis* (GNDC), *S aureus*. Adult (IV drug use): *S aureus* or viridans group streptococci (GPC). Adult (catheter-related, "line" sepsis): *S aureus*, coagulase-negative staphylococci, *Corynebacterium jeikeium* (GPR), pseudomonas sp., candida sp., *Malassezia furfur* (yeast). Adult (splenectomized): *S pneumoniae, H influenzae, N meningitidis*. Neutropenia (<500 PMN): Enterobacteriaceae, pseudomonas sp., *S aureus*, coagulase-negative staphylococcus, viridans group streptococcus. Parasites: Babesia, ehrlichia, plasmodium sp., filarial worms. Immunocompromised: Bartonella sp. (GNR), herpesvirus 8 (HHV8), *Mycobacterium avium-intracellulare* (AFB).	Blood cultures are mandatory for all patients with fever and no obvious source of infection. Often they are negative, especially in neonates. Cultures (2 sets) should be drawn at onset of febrile episode. Culture should never be drawn from an IV line or from a femoral site. Culture and Gram stain of urine, wounds, and other potentially infected sites provide a more rapid diagnosis than blood cultures.	Occult bacteremia affects approximately 5% of febrile children ages 2–36 months. In infants, the findings of an elevated total WBC count (>15,000) and absolute neutrophil count (ANC >10,000) were equally sensitive in predicting bacteremia, but the ANC was more specific. Predisposing factors in adults include IV drug use, neutropenia, cancer, diabetes mellitus, venous catheterization, hemodialysis, and plasmapheresis. Catheter-related infection in patients with long-term venous access (Broviac, Hickman, etc) may be treated successfully without removal of the line, but recurrence of bacteremia is frequent. Switching needles during blood cultures does not decrease contamination rates and increases the risk of needle-stick injuries. Am J Clin Pathol 1998;109:221. Ann Emerg Med 1998;31:679. Pediatrics 1998;102(1 Part 1):67. Infect Dis Clin North Am 1999;13:397. Infect Dis Clin North Am 1999;13:483. Infect Dis Clin North Am 2001;15:1009. J Intraven Nurs 2001;24:180.

6

Diagnostic Imaging: Test Selection and Interpretation

Benjamin M. Yeh, MD, and Susan D. Wall, MD

HOW TO USE THIS SECTION

Information in this chapter is arranged anatomically from superior to inferior. It would not be feasible to include all available imaging tests in one chapter in a book this size, but we have attempted to summarize the essential features of those examinations that are most frequently ordered in modern clinical practice or those that may be associated with difficulty or risk. Indications, advantages and disadvantages, contraindications, and patient preparation are presented. Costs of the studies are approximate and represent averages reported from several large medical centers.

$$\$ = <\$250$$
$$\$\$ = \$250–\$750$$
$$\$\$\$ = \$750–\$1000$$
$$\$\$\$\$ = >\$1000$$

RISKS OF CT AND ANGIOGRAPHIC INTRAVENOUS CONTRAST AGENTS

While intravenous contrast is an important tool in radiology, it is not without substantial risks. Minor reactions (nausea, vomiting, hives) occur with an overall incidence between 1% and 12%. Major reactions (laryngeal edema, bronchospasm, cardiac arrest) occur in 0.16–2 cases per 1000 patients. Deaths have been reported in 1 : 170,000 to 1 : 40,000 cases. Patients with an allergic history (asthma, hay fever, allergy to foods or drugs) are at increased risk. A history of reaction to contrast material is associated with an increased risk of a subsequent severe reaction. Prophylactic measures that may be required in such cases include H$_1$ and H$_2$ blockers and corticosteroids.

In addition, there is a risk of contrast-induced renal failure, which is usually mild and reversible. Persons at increased risk for potentially *irreversible* renal damage include patients with preexisting renal disease (particularly diabetics with high serum creatinine concentrations), multiple myeloma, and severe hyperuricemia.

MRI INTRAVENOUS CONTRAST AGENTS

Contrast agents used in MRI are different from those used in most other radiology studies. Contrast-induced renal failure is not associated with MRI intravenous contrast. Minor reactions occur with an overall incidence of approximately 0.066%. Major reactions occur in 0.001%. Most MRI contrast agents are teratogenic and contraindicated in pregnancy.

In summary, intravenous contrast should be viewed in the same manner as other medications—ie, risks and benefits must be balanced before an examination using this pharmaceutical is ordered.

Test	Indications	Advantages	Disadvantages/Contraindications	Preparation
HEAD				
HEAD **Computed tomography (CT)** $$$	Evaluation of acute craniofacial trauma, acute neurologic dysfunction (<72 hours) from suspected intracranial or subarachnoid hemorrhage. Further characterization of intracranial masses identified by MRI (presence or absence of calcium or involvement of the bony calvarium). Evaluation of sinus disease and temporal bone disease.	Rapid acquisition makes it the modality of choice for trauma. Superb spatial resolution. Superior to MRI in detection of hemorrhage within the first 24–48 hours.	Artifacts from bone may interfere with detection of disease at the skull base and in the posterior fossa. Generally limited to transaxial views. Direct coronal images of paranasal sinuses and temporal bones are routinely obtained if patient can lie prone. **Contraindications and risks:** Caution in pregnancy because of the potential harm of ionizing radiation to the fetus. See Risks of CT and Angiographic Intravenous Contrast Agents, p 245.	Normal hydration. Sedation of agitated patients. Recent serum creatinine determination if intravenous contrast is to be used.
HEAD **Magnetic resonance imaging (MRI)** $$$$	Evaluation of essentially all intracranial disease except those listed above for CT.	Provides excellent tissue contrast resolution, multiplanar capability. Can detect flowing blood and cryptic vascular malformations. Can detect demyelinating and dysmyelinating disease. No beam-hardening artifacts such as can be seen with CT. No ionizing radiation.	Subject to motion artifacts. Inferior to CT in the setting of acute trauma because it is insensitive to acute hemorrhage, incompatible with traction devices, inferior in detection of bony injury and foreign bodies, and requires longer image acquisition time. Special instrumentation required for patients on life support. **Contraindications and risks:** Contraindicated in patients with cardiac pacemakers, intracranial metallic foreign bodies, intracranial aneurysm clips, cochlear implants, and some artificial heart valves.	Sedation of agitated patients. Screening CT or plain radiograph images of orbits if history suggests possible metallic foreign body in the eye.

Test	Indications	Advantages	Disadvantages/Contraindications	Preparation
BRAIN			**BRAIN**	
			MRA/MRV	**Brain scan**
BRAIN **Magnetic resonance angiography/venography (MRA/MRV)** $$$$	Evaluation of cerebral arteriovenous malformations, intracranial aneurysm, and blood supply of vascular tumors as aid to operative planning (MRA). Evaluation of dural sinus thrombosis (MRV).	No ionizing radiation. No iodinated contrast needed.	Subject to motion artifacts. Special instrumentation required for patients on life support. **Contraindications and risks:** Contraindicated in patients with cardiac pacemakers, intraocular metallic foreign bodies, intracranial aneurysm clips, cochlear implants, and some artificial heart valves.	Sedation of agitated patients. Screening CT or plain radiograph images of orbits if history suggests possible metallic foreign body in the eye.
BRAIN **Brain scan (radionuclide)** $$	Confirmation of brain death.	Confirmation of brain death not impeded by hypothermia or barbiturate coma. Can be portable.	Limited resolution. Delayed imaging required with some agents. Cannot be used alone to establish diagnosis of brain death. Must be used in combination with clinical examination or cerebral angiography to establish diagnosis. **Contraindications and risks:** Caution in pregnancy because of the potential harm of ionizing radiation to the fetus.	Premedicate with potassium perchlorate when using TcO4 in order to block choroid plexus uptake.

BRAIN				
Brain PET/SPECT				**Cisternography**
BRAIN **Positron emission tomography** (PET)/single photon emission (SPECT) brain scan $$$	Evaluation of suspected dementia. Evaluation of medically refractory seizures.	Provide functional information. Can localize seizure focus prior to surgical excision. Up to 82% positive predictive value for Alzheimer's dementia in appropriate clinical settings. Provide cross-sectional images and therefore improved lesion localization compared with planar imaging techniques.	Limited resolution compared with MRI and CT. Limited application in work-up of dementia due to low specificity of images and fact that test results do not alter clinical management. **Contraindications and risks:** Caution in pregnancy because of potential harm of ionizing radiation to the fetus.	Requires lumbar puncture to deliver radiopharmaceutical.
BRAIN **Cisternography** (radionuclide) $$	Evaluation of hydrocephalus (particularly normal pressure), CSF rhinorrhea or otorrhea, and ventricular shunt patency.	Provides functional information. Can help distinguish normal pressure hydrocephalus from senile atrophy. Can detect CSF leaks.	Requires multiple delayed imaging sessions up to 48–72 hours after injection. **Contraindications and risks:** Caution in pregnancy because of the potential harm of ionizing radiation to the fetus.	Sedation of agitated patients. For suspected CSF leak, pack the patient's nose or ears with cotton pledgets prior to administration of dose. Must follow strict sterile precautions for intrathecal injection.

Test	Indications	Advantages	Disadvantages/Contraindications	Preparation
			NECK	
			MRI	**MRA**
NECK **Magnetic resonance imaging** (MRI) $$$$	Evaluation of the upper aero-digestive tract. Staging of neck masses. Differentiation of lymphadenopathy from blood vessels. Evaluation of head and neck malignancy, thyroid nodules, parathyroid adenoma, lymphadenopathy, retropharyngeal abscess, brachial plexopathy.	Provides excellent tissue contrast resolution. Tissue differentiation of malignancy or abscess from benign tumor often possible. Sagittal and coronal planar imaging possible. Multiplanar capability especially advantageous regarding brachial plexus. No iodinated contrast needed to distinguish lymphadenopathy from blood vessels.	Subject to motion artifacts, particularly those of carotid pulsation and swallowing. Special instrumentation required for patients on life support. **Contraindications and risks:** Contraindicated in patients with cardiac pacemakers, intraocular metallic foreign bodies, intracranial aneurysm clips, cochlear implants, and some artificial heart valves.	Sedation of agitated patients. Screening CT or plain radiograph images of orbits if history suggests possible metallic foreign body in the eye.
NECK **Magnetic resonance angiography** (MRA) $$$$	Evaluation of carotid bifurcation atherosclerosis, cervicocranial arterial dissection.	No ionizing radiation. No iodinated contrast needed. MRA of the carotid arteries can be a sufficient preoperative evaluation regarding critical stenosis when local expertise exists.	Subject to motion artifacts, particularly from carotid pulsation and swallowing. Special instrumentation required for patients on life support. **Contraindications and risks:** Contraindicated in patients with cardiac pacemakers, intraocular metallic foreign bodies, intracranial aneurysm clips, cochlear implants, and some artificial heart valves.	Sedation of agitated patients. Screening CT or plain radiograph images of orbits if history suggests possible metallic foreign body in the eye.

	NECK		THYROID
	CT	**Ultrasound**	**Ultrasound**

Examination	Indications / Uses	Advantages	Comments / Contraindications	Patient Preparation
NECK Computed tomography (CT) $$$$	Evaluation of the upper aerodigestive tract. Staging of neck masses for patients who are not candidates for MRI. Evaluation of suspected abscess.	Rapid. Superb spatial resolution. Can guide percutaneous fine-needle aspiration of possible tumor or abscess.	Adequate intravenous contrast enhancement of vascular structures is mandatory for accurate interpretation. **Contraindications and risks:** Contraindicated in pregnancy because of the potential harm of ionizing radiation to the fetus. See Risks of CT and Angiographic Intravenous Contrast Agents, p 245.	Normal hydration. Sedation of agitated patients. Recent serum creatinine determination.
NECK Ultrasound (US) $$	Patency and morphology of arteries and veins. Evaluation of thyroid and parathyroid. Guidance for percutaneous fine-needle aspiration biopsy of neck lesions.	Can detect and monitor atherosclerotic stenosis of carotid arteries noninvasively and without iodinated contrast.	Technically demanding, operator-dependent. Patient must lie supine and still for 1 hour.	None.
THYROID Ultrasound (US) $$	Determination as to whether a palpable nodule is a cyst or solid mass and whether single or multiple nodules are present. Assessment of response to suppressive therapy. Screening patients with a history of prior radiation to the head and neck. Guidance for biopsy.	Noninvasive. No ionizing radiation. Can be portable. Can image in all planes.	Cannot distinguish between benign and malignant lesions unless local invasion is demonstrated. Technique very operator-dependent. **Contraindications and risks:** None.	None.

	THYROID
	Thyroid uptake and scan

Test	Indications	Advantages	Disadvantages/Contraindications	Preparation
THYROID **Thyroid uptake and scan** (radionuclide) $$	Uptake indicated for evaluation of clinical hypothyroidism, hyperthyroidism, thyroiditis, effects of thyroid-stimulating and -suppressing medications, and for calculation of therapeutic radiation dosage. Scanning indicated for above as well as evaluation of palpable nodules, mediastinal mass, and screening of patients with history of head and neck irradiation. Total body scanning used for postoperative evaluation of thyroid metastases.	Demonstrates both morphology and function. Can identify ectopic thyroid tissue and "cold" nodules that have a greater risk of malignancy. Imaging of total body with one dose (^{131}I).	Substances interfering with test include iodides in vitamins and medicines, antithyroid drugs, steroids, and intravascular contrast agents. Delayed imaging is required with iodides (^{123}I, 6 hours and 24 hours; ^{131}I total body, 72 hours). Test may not visualize thyroid gland in subacute thyroiditis. **Contraindications and risks:** Not advised in pregnancy because of the risk of ionizing radiation to the fetus (iodides cross placenta and concentrate in fetal thyroid). Significant radiation exposure occurs in total body scanning with ^{131}I; patients should be instructed about precautionary measures by nuclear medicine personnel.	Administration of dose after a 4- to 6-hour fast aids absorption. Discontinue all interfering substances prior to test, especially thyroid-suppressing medications: T_3 (1 week), T_4 (4–6 weeks), propylthiouracil (2 weeks).

| | THYROID | | | PARATHYROID |
	Radionuclide therapy			Radionuclide scan
THYROID **Thyroid therapy** (radionuclide) $$$	Hyperthyroidism and some thyroid carcinomas (papillary and follicular types are amenable to treatment, whereas medullary and anaplastic types are not).	Noninvasive alternative to surgery.	Rarely, radiation thyroiditis may occur 1–3 days after therapy. Hypothyroidism occurs commonly as a long-term complication. Higher doses that are required to treat thyroid carcinoma may result in pulmonary fibrosis. **Contraindications and risks:** Contraindicated in pregnancy and lactation. Contraindicated in patients with metastatic disease to the brain, because treatment may result in brain edema and subsequent herniation, and in those <20 years of age because of possible increased risk of thyroid cancer later in life. After treatment, a patient's activities are restricted to limit total exposure of any member of the general public until radiation level is ≤0.5 rem. High doses for treatment of thyroid carcinoma may necessitate hospitalization.	After treatment, patients must isolate all bodily secretions from household members.
PARATHYROID **Parathyroid scan** (radionuclide) $$	Evaluation of suspected parathyroid adenoma.	Identifies hyperfunctioning tissue, which is useful when planning surgery.	Small adenomas (<500 mg) may not be detected. **Contraindications and risks:** Caution in pregnancy is advised because of the risk of ionizing radiation to the fetus.	Requires strict patient immobility during scanning.

Test	Indications	Advantages	Disadvantages/Contraindications	Preparation
CHEST				
CHEST **Chest radiograph** $	Evaluation of pleural and parenchymal pulmonary disease, mediastinal disease, cardiogenic and noncardiogenic pulmonary edema, congenital and acquired cardiac disease. Screening for traumatic aortic rupture (though angiogram is the standard and spiral CT is playing an increasing role). Evaluation of possible pneumothorax (expiratory upright film) or free flowing fluid (decubitus views).	Inexpensive. Widely available.	Difficult to distinguish between causes of hilar enlargement (ie, vasculature versus adenopathy). **Contraindications and risks:** Caution in pregnancy because of the potential harm of ionizing radiation to the fetus.	None.
CHEST **Computed tomography** (CT) $$$	Evaluation of trauma to the thorax. Differentiation of mediastinal and hilar lymphadenopathy from vascular structures. Evaluation and staging of primary and metastatic lung neoplasm. Characterization of pulmonary nodules. Differentiation of parenchymal versus pleural process (ie, lung abscess versus empyema). Evaluation of interstitial lung disease (1-mm thin sections), aortic dissection, and aneurysm.	Rapid. Superb spatial resolution. Can guide percutaneous fine-needle aspiration of possible tumor or abscess.	Patient cooperation required for appropriate breath-holding. Generally limited to transaxial views. **Contraindications and risks:** Contraindicated in pregnancy because of the potential harm of ionizing radiation to the fetus. See Risks of CT and Angiographic Intravenous Contrast Agents, p 245.	Preferably NPO for 2 hours prior to study. Normal hydration. Sedation of agitated patients. Recent serum creatinine determination.

	CHEST	LUNG
	MRI	**Ventilation-perfusion scan**
	Sedation of agitated patients. Screening CT of the orbits if history suggests possible metallic foreign body in the eye.	Current chest radiograph is mandatory for interpretation.

CHEST **Magnetic resonance imaging (MRI)** $$$$	Evaluation of mediastinal masses. Discrimination between hilar vessels and enlarged lymph nodes. Tumor staging (especially when invasion of vessels or pericardium is suspected). Evaluation of aortic dissection, aortic aneurysm, congenital and acquired cardiac disease.	Provides excellent tissue contrast resolution and multiplanar capability. No beam-hardening artifacts such as can be seen with CT. No ionizing radiation.	Subject to motion artifacts. **Contraindications and risks:** Contraindicated in patients with cardiac pacemakers, intracranial metallic foreign bodies, intraocular aneurysm clips, cochlear implants, and some artificial heart valves.
LUNG **Ventilation-perfusion scan** (radionuclide) $\dot{V}$ = $$ $\dot{Q}$ = $$ $\dot{V}$ + $\dot{Q}$ = $$$-$$$$	Evaluation of pulmonary embolism or burn inhalation injury. Preoperative evaluation of patients with chronic obstructive pulmonary disease and of those who are candidates for pneumonectomy.	Noninvasive. Provides functional information in preoperative assessment. Permits determination of differential and regional lung function in preoperative assessment. Documented pulmonary embolism is extremely rare with normal perfusion scan.	Patients must be able to cooperate for ventilation portion of the examination. There is a high proportion of intermediate probability studies in patients with underlying lung disease. The likelihood of pulmonary embolism ranges from 20%–80% in these cases. A patient who has a low probability scan still has a chance ranging from nil to 19% of having a pulmonary embolus. **Contraindications and risks:** Patients with severe pulmonary artery hypertension or significant right-to-left shunts should have fewer particles injected. Caution advised in pregnancy because of risk of ionizing radiation to the fetus.

	LUNG
	CT

Test	Indications	Advantages	Disadvantages/Contraindications	Preparation
LUNG **Computed tomography** (CT) $$$	Evaluation of clinically suspected pulmonary embolism.	Rapid. Sensitivity and specificity values likely about 90% for the CT diagnosis of pulmonary emboli involving main to segmental artery branches in unselected patients. Overall, CT sensitivity may be higher than ventilation-perfusion scintigraphy. Allows determination of causes other than pulmonary embolism for dyspnea.	Accuracy of CT in diagnosing pulmonary embolism depends on the size of the pulmonary artery involved and the size of the thrombus. Sensitivity and accuracy of CT decreases for small, subsegmental emboli (sensitivity rates of 53–63% have been reported). Respiratory motion artifacts can be a problem in dyspneic patients. High-quality study requires breath-holding of approximately 20 seconds. Specific imaging protocol utilized which limits diagnostic information for other abnormalities. **Contraindications and risks:** Contraindicated in pregnancy because of potential harm of ionizing radiation to fetus. See Risks of CT and Angiographic Intravenous Contrast Agents, p 245.	Large gauge intravenous access (minimum 20-gauge) required. Prebreathing oxygen may help dyspneic patients perform adequate breath hold. Normal hydration. Preferably NPO for 2 hours prior to study. Recent serum creatinine determination.

LUNG				
Pulmonary angiography				
LUNG **Pulmonary angiography** $$$$	Suspected pulmonary embolism with equivocal results on ventilation-perfusion scan or when definitive diagnosis especially important because of contraindication to anticoagulation. Arteriovenous malformation, pulmonary sequestration, vasculitides, vascular occlusion by tumor or inflammatory disease.	Remains the standard for diagnosis of acute and chronic pulmonary embolism.	Invasive. Requires catheterization of the right heart and pulmonary artery. **Contraindications:** Elevated pulmonary artery pressure (>70 mm Hg) or elevated right ventricular end-diastolic pressure (>20 mm Hg).	Ventilation-perfusion scan for localization of right versus left lung. Electrocardiogram, especially to exclude left bundle branch block (in such cases, temporary cardiac pacemaker should be placed before the catheter is introduced into the pulmonary artery).

	BREAST			
	Mammogram			
Test	Indications	Advantages	Disadvantages/Contraindications	Preparation
BREAST Mammo-gram $	Screening for breast cancer in asymptomatic women: (1) every 1–2 years between ages 40 and 49; (2) every year after age 50. If prior history of breast cancer, mammogram should be performed yearly at any age. Indicated at any age for symptoms (palpable mass, bloody discharge) or before breast surgery.	Newer film screen techniques generate lower radiation doses (0.1–0.2 rad per film, mean glandular dose). A 23% lower mortality has been demonstrated in patients screened with combined mammogram and physical exam compared to physical exam alone. In a screening population, more than 40% of cancers are detected by mammography alone and cannot be palpated on physical exam.	Detection of breast masses is more difficult in patients with radiographically dense breasts. Breast compression may cause patient discomfort. In a screening population, 9% of cancers are detected by physical examination alone and are not detectable by mammography. **Contraindications and risks:** Radiation from repeated mammograms can theoretically cause breast cancer; however, the benefits of screening mammograms greatly outweigh the risks.	None.

HEART				Ventriculography
	Myocardial perfusion scan			
HEART **Myocardial perfusion scan** (thallium scan, technetium-99m methoxyisobutyl isonitrile (sestamibi) scan, others) $-$$-$$$ (broad range)	Evaluation of atypical chest pain. Detection of presence, location, and extent of myocardial ischemia.	Highly sensitive for detecting physiologically significant coronary stenosis. Noninvasive. Able to stratify patients according to risk for myocardial infarction. Normal examination associated with average risk of cardiac death or nonfatal myocardial infarction of <1% per year.	The patient must be carefully monitored during treadmill or pharmacologic stress—optimally, under the supervision of a cardiologist. False-positive results may be caused by exercise-induced spasm, aortic stenosis, or left bundle branch block; false-negative results may be caused by inadequate exercise, mild or distal disease, or balanced diffuse ischemia. **Contraindications and risks:** Aminophylline (inhibitor of dipyridamole) is a contraindication to the use of dipyridamole. Treadmill or pharmacologic stress carries a risk of arrhythmia, ischemia, infarct, and, rarely, death. Caution in pregnancy because of the risk of ionizing radiation to the fetus.	In case of severe peripheral vascular disease, severe pulmonary disease, or musculoskeletal disorder, pharmacologic stress with dipyridamole or other agents may be used. Tests should be performed in the fasting state. Patient should not exercise between stress and redistribution scans.
HEART **Radionuclide ventriculography** (multigated acquisition [MUGA]) $$-$$$-$$$$	Evaluation of patients with ischemic heart disease and other cardiomyopathies. Evaluation of response to pharmacologic therapy and effects of cardiotoxic drugs.	Noninvasive. Ejection fraction is a reproducible index that can be used to follow course of disease and response to therapy.	Gated data acquisition may be difficult in patients with severe arrhythmias. **Contraindications and risks:** Recent infarct is a contraindication to exercise ventriculography (arrhythmia, ischemia, infarct, and rarely death may occur with exercise). Caution is advised in pregnancy because of the risk of ionizing radiation to the fetus.	Requires harvesting, labeling, and re-injecting the patient's red blood cells. Sterile technique required in handling of red cells.

Test	Indications	Advantages	Disadvantages/Contraindications	Preparation
		ABDOMEN		
	KUB		**Ultrasound**	
ABDOMEN Abdominal plain radiograph (KUB [kidneys, ureters, bladder] x-ray) $	Assessment of bowel gas patterns (eg, to distinguish ileus from obstruction). To rule out pneumoperitoneum, order an upright abdomen and chest radiograph (acute abdominal series).	Inexpensive. Widely available.	Supine film alone is inadequate to rule out pneumoperitoneum (see indications). Obstipation may obscure lesions. **Contraindications and risks:** Contraindicated in pregnancy because of the risk of ionizing radiation to the fetus.	None.
ABDOMEN Ultrasound (US) $$	Differentiation of cystic versus solid lesions of the liver and kidneys, intra- and extrahepatic biliary ductal dilation, cholelithiasis, gallbladder wall thickness, pericholecystic fluid, peripancreatic fluid and pseudocyst, primary and metastatic liver carcinoma, hydronephrosis, abdominal aortic aneurysm, appendicitis, ascites.	Noninvasive. No ionizing radiation. Can be portable. Imaging in all planes. Can guide percutaneous fine-needle aspiration of tumor or abscess.	Technique very operator-dependent. Organs (particularly pancreas and distal aorta) may be obscured by bowel gas. Presence of barium obscures sound waves. **Contraindications and risks:** None.	NPO for 6 hours.

ABDOMEN				
CT				
Computed tomography (CT) $$$–$$$$	Morphologic evaluation of all abdominal and pelvic organs. Differentiation of intraperitoneal versus retroperitoneal disorders. Evaluation of abscess, trauma, mesenteric and retroperitoneal lymphadenopathy, bowel obstruction, obstructive biliary disease, pancreatitis, appendicitis, peritonitis, and carcinomatosis, splenic infarction, retroperitoneal hemorrhage. Staging of malignancy in the liver, pancreas, kidneys, and other abdominopelvic organs and spaces. Sensitive in predicting that pancreatic carcinoma is unresectable. Excellent screening tool for evaluation of suspected renal and ureteral calculi. CT angiography valuable in the evaluation of the aorta and its branches. Can provide preoperative assessment of abdominal aortic aneurysm size, proximal and distal extent, relationship to renal arteries, and presence of anatomic anomalies. CT colonography useful in patients with failed colonography or patients unable to undergo colonoscopy.	Rapid. Superb spatial resolution. Not limited by overlying bowel gas, as with ultrasound. Can guide fine-needle aspiration and percutaneous drainage procedures. Noncontrast spiral CT is superior to plain abdominal radiography, ultrasound, and intravenous urography in determination of size and location of renal and ureteral calculi.	Barium or Hypaque, surgical clips, and metallic prostheses can cause artifacts and degrade image quality. **Contraindications and risks:** Contraindicated in pregnancy because of the potential harm of ionizing radiation to the fetus. See Risks of CT and Angiographic Intravenous Contrast Studies, p 245.	Preferably NPO for 4–6 hours. Normal hydration. Opacification of gastrointestinal tract with water-soluble oral contrast (Gastrografin). Sedation of agitated patients. Recent serum creatinine determination.

		ABDOMEN	
		MRI	Mesenteric angiography

Test	Indications	Advantages	Disadvantages/Contraindications	Preparation
ABDOMEN **Magnetic resonance imaging (MRI)** $$$$	Preoperative staging of renal cell carcinoma. Differentiation of benign nonhyperfunctioning adrenal adenoma from malignant adrenal mass. Complementary to CT in evaluation of liver lesions (especially metastatic disease and possible tumor invasion of hepatic or portal veins). Differentiation of benign cavernous hemangioma (>2 cm in diameter) from malignancy. Differentiation of retroperitoneal lymphadenopathy from blood vessels or the diaphragmatic crus.	Provides excellent tissue contrast resolution, multiplanar capability. No beam-hardening artifacts such as can be seen with CT. No ionizing radiation.	Subject to motion artifacts. Gastrointestinal opacification not yet readily available. Special instrumentation required for patients on life support. **Contraindications and risks:** Contraindicated in patients with cardiac pacemakers, intraocular metallic foreign bodies, intracranial aneurysm clips, cochlear implants, and some artificial heart valves.	NPO for 4–6 hours. Intramuscular glucagon to inhibit peristalsis. Sedation of agitated patients. Screening CT or plain radiograph images of orbits if history suggests possible metallic foreign body in the eye.
ABDOMEN **Mesenteric angiography** $$$$	Gastrointestinal hemorrhage that does not resolve with conservative therapy and cannot be treated endoscopically. Localization of gastrointestinal bleeding site. Acute mesenteric ischemia, intestinal angina, splenic or other splanchnic artery aneurysm. Evaluation of possible vasculitis, such as polyarteritis nodosa. Detection of islet cell tumors not identified by other studies. Abdominal trauma.	Therapeutic embolization of gastrointestinal hemorrhage is often possible.	Invasive. Patient may need to remain supine with leg extended for 6 hours following the procedure to protect the common femoral artery at the catheter entry site. **Contraindications and risks:** Allergy to iodinated contrast material may require corticosteroid and H₁ blocker or H₂ blocker premedication. Contraindicated in pregnancy because of the potential harm of ionizing radiation to the fetus. Contrast nephrotoxicity, especially with preexisting impaired renal function due to diabetes mellitus or multiple myeloma; however, any creatinine elevation following the procedure is usually reversible (see p 245).	NPO for 4–6 hours. Good hydration to limit possible renal insult due to iodinated contrast material. Recent serum creatinine determination, assessment of clotting parameters, reversal of anticoagulation. Performed with conscious sedation. Requires cardiac, respiratory, blood pressure, and pulse oximetry monitoring.

GASTROINTESTINAL		
	UGI	**Enteroclysis**
Study	GI — Upper GI study (UGI) — $$	GI — Enteroclysis — $$
Indications	Double-contrast barium technique demonstrates esophageal, gastric, and duodenal mucosa for evaluation of inflammatory disease and other subtle mucosal abnormalities. Single-contrast technique is suitable for evaluation of possible outlet obstruction, peristalsis, gastroesophageal reflux and hiatal hernia, esophageal cancer and varices. Water-soluble contrast (Gastrografin) is suitable for evaluation of anastomotic leak or gastrointestinal perforation. Evaluates esophageal motility.	Barium fluoroscopic study for location of site of intermittent partial small bowel obstruction. Evaluation of extent of Crohn disease or small bowel disease in patient with persistent gastrointestinal bleeding and normal UGI and colonic evaluations. Evaluation of metastatic disease to the small bowel.
Advantages	Good evaluation of mucosa with double-contrast examination. No sedation required. Less expensive than endoscopy.	Clarifies lesions noted on more traditional barium examination of the small bowel. Best means of establishing small bowel as normal.
Limitations / Contraindications and risks	Aspiration of water-soluble contrast material may occur, resulting in severe pulmonary edema. Leakage of barium from a perforation may cause granulomatous inflammatory reaction. Identification of a lesion does not prove it to be the site of blood loss in patients with gastrointestinal bleeding. Barium precludes endoscopy and body CT examination. Retained gastric secretions prevent mucosal coating with barium. **Contraindications and risks:** Contraindicated in pregnancy because of the potential harm of ionizing radiation to the fetus.	Requires nasogastric or orogastric tube placement and manipulation to beyond the ligament of Treitz. **Contraindications and risks:** Radiation exposure is substantial, because lengthy fluoroscopic examination is required. Therefore, the test is contraindicated in pregnant women and should be used sparingly in children and women of childbearing age.
Preparation	NPO for 8 hours.	Clear liquid diet for 24 hours. Colonic cleansing.

| | | GASTROINTESTINAL | |
		Small bowel follow-through	Peroral pneumocolon
Test		GI **Small bowel follow-through** $$	GI **Peroral pneumocolon** $
Indications		Barium fluoroscopic study for location of site of intermittent partial small bowel obstruction. Evaluation of extent of Crohn disease or small bowel disease in patient with persistent gastrointestinal bleeding and normal UGI and colonic evaluations. Evaluation of metastatic disease to the small bowel.	Fluoroscopic evaluation of the terminal ileum by insufflating air per rectum after orally ingested barium has reached the cecum.
Advantages		Less invasive and better tolerated than enteroclysis. May be combined with UGI.	Best evaluation of the terminal ileum. Can be performed concurrently with UGI.
Disadvantages/Contraindications		Less diagnostic power than enteroclysis for mucosal detail. Requires nasogastric or orogastric tube placement and manipulation to beyond the ligament of Treitz. **Contraindications and risks:** Radiation exposure is substantial, because lengthy fluoroscopic examination is required. Therefore, the test is contraindicated in pregnant women and should be used sparingly in children and women of childbearing age.	Undigested food in the small bowel interferes with the evaluation. **Contraindications and risk:** Contraindicated in pregnancy because of the potential harm of ionizing radiation to the fetus.
Preparation		Clear liquid diet for 24 hours. Colonic cleansing.	Clear liquid diet for 24 hours.

GASTROINTESTINAL				
			Barium enema	CT colonography
GI **Barium enema** (BE) $$	Double-contrast technique for evaluation of colonic mucosa in patients with suspected inflammatory bowel disease or neoplasm. Single-contrast technique for investigation of possible fistulous tracts, bowel obstruction, large palpable masses in the abdomen, diverticulitis, and for examination of debilitated patients.	Good mucosal evaluation. No sedation required.	Retained fecal material limits study. Requires patient cooperation. Marked diverticulosis precludes evaluation of possible neoplasm in that area. Evaluation of right colon occasionally incomplete or limited by reflux of barium across ileocecal valve and overlapping opacified small bowel. Use of barium delays subsequent colonoscopy and body CT. **Contraindications and risks:** Contraindicated in patients with toxic megacolon and immediately after full-thickness colonoscopic biopsy.	Colon cleansing with enemas, cathartic, and clear liquid diet (1 day in young patients, 2 days in older patients). Intravenous glucagon (which inhibits peristalsis) sometimes given to distinguish colonic spasm from a mass lesion.
GI **CT colonography** $$	Thin section CT for evaluation of possible colonic polyps and masses.	Has ability to evaluate extracolonic intra-abdominal disease (AAA, renal cell cancer, kidney stones). No IV contrast. Less invasive than colonoscopy.	Retained fecal material limits study. Requires patient cooperation. If polyps or masses are found, patient will need to undergo colonoscopy or sigmoidoscopy for tissue diagnosis.	Requires colonic preparation that varies from institution to institution.

		GASTROINTESTINAL	
		Hypaque enema	Esophageal reflux study
Preparation		Colonic cleansing is desirable but not always necessary.	NPO for 4–6 hours. During test, patient must be able to consume 300 mL of liquid.
Disadvantages/Contraindications		Demonstrates only colonic morphologic features and not mucosal changes. **Contraindications and risks:** Contraindicated in patients with toxic megacolon. Hypertonic solution may lead to fluid imbalance in debilitated patients and children.	Incomplete emptying of esophagus may mimic reflux. Abdominal binder—used to increase pressure in the lower esophagus—may not be tolerated in patients who have undergone recent abdominal surgery. **Contraindications and risks:** Contraindicated in pregnancy because of the potential harm of ionizing radiation to the fetus.
Advantages		Water-soluble contrast medium is evacuated much faster than barium because it does not adhere to the mucosa. Therefore, Hypaque enema can be followed immediately by oral ingestion of barium for evaluation of possible distal small bowel obstruction.	Noninvasive and well tolerated. More sensitive for reflux than fluoroscopy, endoscopy, and manometry; sensitivity similar to that of acid reflux test. Permits quantitation of reflux. Can also identify aspiration into the lung fields.
Indications		Water-soluble contrast for fluoroscopic evaluation of sigmoid or cecal volvulus, anastomotic leak, or other perforation. Differentiation of colonic versus small bowel obstruction. Therapy for obstipation.	Evaluation of heartburn, regurgitation, recurrent aspiration pneumonia.
Test		GI **Hypaque enema** $$	GI **Esophageal reflux study** (radionuclide) $$

GASTROINTESTINAL	
Gastric emptying study	**GI bleeding scan**
GI **Gastric emptying study** (radionuclide) $$	GI **GI bleeding scan** (labeled red cell scan, radionuclide) $$–$$$
Evaluation of dumping syndrome, vagotomy, gastric outlet obstruction due to inflammatory or neoplastic disease, effects of drugs, and other causes of gastroparesis (eg, diabetes mellitus).	Evaluation of upper or lower gastrointestinal blood loss. Distinguishing hemangioma of the liver from other mass lesions of the liver.
Gives functional information not available by other means.	Noninvasive compared with angiography. Longer period of imaging possible, which aids in detection of intermittent bleeding. Labeled red cells and sulfur colloid can detect bleeding rates as low as 0.05–0.10 mL/min (angiography requires rate of about 0.5 mL/min). 90% sensitivity for blood loss >500 mL/24 h.
Reporting of meaningful data requires adherence to standard protocol and establishment of normal values. **Contraindications and risks:** Contraindicated in pregnancy because of the potential harm of ionizing radiation to the fetus.	Bleeding must be active during time of imaging. Presence of free TcO_4 (poor labeling efficiency) can lead to gastric, kidney, and bladder activity that can be misinterpreted as sites of bleeding. Uptake in hepatic hemangioma, varices, arteriovenous malformation, abdominal aortic aneurysm, and bowel wall inflammation can also lead to false-positive examination. **Contraindications and risks:** Contraindicated in pregnancy because of the potential harm of ionizing radiation to the fetus.
NPO for 4–6 hours. During test, patient must be able to eat a 300-g meal consisting of both liquids and solids.	Sterile technique required during in vitro labeling of red cells.

	BLOOD
	Indium scan

Test	Indications	Advantages	Disadvantages/Contraindications	Preparation
BLOOD **Leukocyte scan** (indium scan, labeled white blood cell [WBC] scan, technetium-99m hexa-methylpro-pyleneamine oxime [Tc99m-HMPAO]-labeled WBC scan, radio-nuclide) $$–$$$	Evaluation of fever of unknown origin, suspected abscess, pyelonephritis, osteomyelitis, inflammatory bowel disease. Examination of choice for evaluation of suspected vascular graft infection.	Highly specific (98%) for infection (in contrast to gallium). Highly sensitive in detecting abdominal source of infection. In patients with fever of unknown origin, total body imaging is advantageous compared with CT scan or ultrasound. Preliminary imaging as early as 4 hours is possible with indium but less sensitive (30–50% of abscesses are detected at 24 hours).	24-hour delayed imaging may limit the utility of indium scan in critically ill patients. False-negative scans occur with antibiotic administration or in chronic infection. Perihepatic or splenic infection can be missed because of normal leukocyte accumulation in these organs; liver and spleen scan is necessary adjunct in this situation. False-positive scans occur with swallowed leukocytes, bleeding, indwelling tubes and catheters, surgical skin wound uptake, and bowel activity due to inflammatory processes. Pulmonary uptake is nonspecific and has low predictive value for infection. Patients must be able to hold still during relatively long acquisition times (5–10 minutes). Tc99m-HMPAO WBC may be suboptimal for detecting infection involving the genitourinary and gastrointestinal tracts because of normal distribution of the agent to these organs. **Contraindications and risks:** Contraindicated in pregnancy because of the hazard of ionizing radiation to the fetus. High radiation dose to spleen.	Leukocytes from the patient are harvested, labeled in vitro, and then reinjected; process requires 12 hours. Scanning takes place 24 hours after injection of indium-labeled WBC and 1–2 hours after injection of Tc99m-HMPAO WBC. Homologous donor leukocytes should be used in neutropenic patients.

GALLBLADDER			
		Ultrasound	HIDA scan
GALLBLADDER **Ultrasound (US)** $	Demonstrates cholelithiasis (95% sensitive), gallbladder wall thickening, pericholecystic fluid, intra- and extrahepatic biliary dilation.	Noninvasive. No ionizing radiation. Can be portable. Imaging in all planes. Can guide fine-needle aspiration, percutaneous transhepatic cholangiography, and biliary drainage procedures.	Technique very operator-dependent. Presence of barium obscures sound waves. Difficult in obese patients. Administration of excessive pain medication prior to exam limits accuracy of diagnosing acute cholecystitis. **Contraindications and risks:** None	Preferably NPO for 6 hours to enhance visualization of gallbladder.
GALLBLADDER **Hepatic iminodiacetic acid scan (HIDA)** $$	Evaluation of suspected acute cholecystitis or common bile duct obstruction. Evaluation of bile leaks, biliary atresia, and biliary enteric bypass patency.	95 percent sensitivity and 99% specificity for diagnosis of acute cholecystitis. Hepatobiliary function assessed. Defines pathophysiology underlying acute cholecystitis. Rapid. Can be performed in patients with elevated serum bilirubin. No intravenous contrast used.	Does not demonstrate the cause of obstruction (eg, tumor or gallstone). Not able to evaluate biliary excretion if hepatocellular function is severely impaired. Sensitivity may be lower in acalculous cholecystitis. False-positive results can occur with hyperalimentation, prolonged fasting, and acute pancreatitis. **Contraindications and risks:** Contraindicated in pregnancy because of the potential harm of ionizing radiation to the fetus.	NPO for at least 4 hours but preferably less than 24 hours. Premedication with cholecystokinin can prevent false-positive examination in patients who are receiving hyperalimentation or who have been fasting longer than 24 hours. Avoid administration of morphine prior to examination if possible.

		PANCREAS/BILIARY TREE			
Test	Indications	Advantages	Disadvantages/Contraindications	Preparation	
				ERCP	MRCP
PANCREAS/ BILIARY TREE **Endoscopic retrograde cholangiopancreatography (ERCP)** $$$$	Primary sclerosing cholangitis, AIDS-associated cholangitis, and cholangiocarcinomas. Demonstrates cause, location, and extent of extrahepatic biliary obstruction (eg, choledocholithiasis). Can diagnose chronic pancreatitis.	Avoids surgery. Less invasive than percutaneous transhepatic cholangiography. If stone is suspected, ERCP offers therapeutic potential (sphincterotomy and extraction of common bile duct stone). Finds gallstones in up to 14% of patients with symptoms but negative ultrasound. Plastic or metallic stent placement may be possible in patients with obstruction.	Requires endoscopy. May cause pancreatitis (1%), cholangitis (<1%), peritonitis, hemorrhage (if sphincterotomy performed), and death (rare). **Contraindications and risks:** Relatively contraindicated in patients with concurrent or recent (<6 weeks) acute pancreatitis or suspected pancreatic pseudocyst. Contraindicated in pregnancy because of the potential harm of ionizing radiation to the fetus.	NPO for 6 hours. Sedation required. Vital signs should be monitored by the nursing staff. Not possible in patient who has undergone Roux-en-Y hepaticojejunostomy.	
PANCREAS/ BILIARY TREE **Magnetic resonance cholangiopancreatography (MRCP)** $$$	Evaluation of intra- and extrahepatic biliary and pancreatic duct dilatation, and the cause of obstruction.	Noninvasive. No ionizing radiation. Imaging in all planes. Can image ducts beyond the point of obstruction.	Special instrumentation required for patients on life support. **Contraindications and risks:** Contraindicated in patients with cardiac pacemakers, intraocular metallic foreign bodies, intracranial aneurysm clips, cochlear implants, and some artificial heart valves.		Preferably NPO for 6 hours.

LIVER				
Ultrasound			**CT**	
LIVER **Ultrasound** (US) $	Differentiation of cystic versus solid intrahepatic lesions. Evaluation of intra- and extra-hepatic biliary dilation, primary and metastatic liver tumors, and ascites. Evaluation of patency of portal vein, hepatic arteries, and hepatic veins.	Noninvasive. No radiation. Can be portable. Imaging in all planes. Can guide fine-needle aspiration, percutaneous transhepatic cholangiography, and biliary drainage procedures.	Technique very operator-dependent. Presence of barium obscures sound waves. More difficult in obese patients. The presence of fatty liver or cirrhosis can limit the sensitivity of ultrasound for focal mass lesions. **Contraindications and risks:** None.	Preferably NPO for 6 hours.
LIVER **Computed tomography** (CT) $$$–$$$$	Suspected metastatic or primary tumor, gallbladder carcinoma, biliary obstruction, abscess.	Excellent spatial resolution. Can direct percutaneous fine-needle aspiration biopsy. Excellent evaluation of hepatic vasculature.	Requires iodinated contrast material administered intravenously. **Contraindications and risks:** Contraindicated in pregnancy because of the potential harm of ionizing radiation to the fetus. See Risks of CT and Angiographic Intravenous Contrast Agents, p 245.	NPO for 4–6 hours. Recent creatinine determination. Administration of oral contrast material for opacification of stomach and small bowel. Specific hepatic protocol with arterial, portal venous, and delayed images used for evaluation of neoplasm.

			LIVER		
Test	Indications	Advantages	Disadvantages/Contraindications	Preparation

Test	Indications	Advantages	Disadvantages/Contraindications	Preparation
LIVER **Computed tomographic arterial portography (CTAP)** $$$$	Assessment of number, location, and resectability of metastatic liver tumors.	Sensitive to number of liver lesions (good for lesion detection). Provides cross-sectional imaging for segmental localization of liver tumors.	Invasive, requiring percutaneous catheter placement in the superior mesenteric artery. Patient must remain supine with leg extended for 6 hours following the procedure to protect the common femoral artery at the catheter entry site. Useful for lesion detection but does not permit characterization of lesions. May not be possible in patients with cirrhosis where portal hypertension limits delivery of contrast material to liver.	NPO for 4–6 hours. Recent creatinine determination. Requires some conscious sedation.
LIVER **Magnetic resonance imaging (MRI)** $$$$	Characterization of hepatic lesions, including suspected cyst, hepatocellular carcinoma, focal nodular hyperplasia, and metastasis. Suspected metastatic or primary tumor. Differentiation of benign cavernous hemangioma from malignant tumor. Evaluation of hemochromatosis, hemosiderosis, fatty liver, and suspected focal fatty infiltration.	Requires no iodinated contrast material. Provides excellent tissue contrast resolution, multiplanar capability.	Subject to motion artifacts, particularly those of respiration. Special instrumentation required for patients on life support. **Contraindications and risks:** Contraindicated in patients with cardiac pacemakers, intraocular metallic foreign bodies, intracranial aneurysm clips, cochlear implants, some artificial heart valves.	Screening CT or plain radiograph images of orbits if history suggests possible metallic foreign body in the eye. Intramuscular glucagon is used to inhibit intestinal peristalsis.

LIVER/BILIARY TREE			
PTC			
LIVER/ BILIARY TREE **Percutaneous transhepatic cholangiogram** (PTC) $$$	Evaluation of biliary obstruction in patients in whom ERCP has failed or patients with Roux-en-Y hepaticojejunostomy.	Best examination to assess site and morphology of obstruction close to the hilum (as opposed to ERCP, which is better for distal obstruction). Can characterize the nature of diffuse intrahepatic biliary disease such as primary sclerosing cholangitis. Provides guidance and access for percutaneous transhepatic biliary drainage and possible stent placement to treat obstruction.	Invasive; requires special training. Performed with conscious sedation. **Contraindications and risks:** Ascites may present a contraindication.	NPO for 4–6 hours. Sterile technique, assessment of clotting parameters, correction of coagulopathy. Performed with conscious sedation.

Test	Indications	Advantages	Disadvantages/Contraindications	Preparation
	LIVER			**LIVER/SPLEEN**
	Hepatic angiography			**Liver, spleen scan**
LIVER **Hepatic angiography** $$$$	Preoperative evaluation for liver transplantation, vascular malformations, trauma, Budd-Chiari syndrome, portal vein patency (when ultrasound equivocal) prior to transjugular intrahepatic portosystemic shunt (TIPS) procedure. In some cases, evaluation of hepatic neoplasm or transcatheter embolotherapy of hepatic malignancy.	Gold standard assessment of hepatic arterial anatomy, which is highly variable. More accurate than ultrasound with respect to portal vein patency when the latter suggests occlusion.	Invasive. Patient must remain supine with leg extended for 6 hours following the procedure to protect the common femoral artery at the catheter entry site. **Contraindications and risks:** Allergy to iodinated contrast material may require corticosteroid and H₁ blocker or H₂ blocker premedication. Contraindicated in pregnancy because of the potential harm of ionizing radiation to the fetus. Contrast nephrotoxicity may occur, especially with preexisting impaired renal function due to diabetes mellitus or multiple myeloma; however, any creatinine elevation following the procedure is usually reversible.	NPO for 4–6 hours. Good hydration to limit possible renal insult due to iodinated contrast material. Recent serum creatinine determination, assessment of clotting parameters, reversal of anticoagulation. Performed with conscious sedation. Requires cardiac, respiratory, blood pressure, and pulse oximetry monitoring.
LIVER-SPLEEN **Liver, spleen scan** (radionuclide) $$	Identification of functioning splenic tissue to localize an accessory spleen or evaluate suspected functional asplenia. Assessment of size, shape, and position of liver and spleen. Characterization of a focal liver mass with regard to inherent functioning reticuloendothelial cell activity (in particular focal nodular hyperplasia). Confirmation of patency and distribution of hepatic arterial perfusion catheters.	May detect isodense lesions missed by CT. Useful to detect location of active GI bleed (see GI bleeding scan, p 267).	Diminished sensitivity for small lesions (less than 1.5–2.0 cm) and deep lesions. SPECT increases sensitivity (can detect lesions of 1.0–1.5 cm). Nonspecific; unable to distinguish solid versus cystic or inflammatory versus neoplastic tissue. Lower sensitivity for diffuse hepatic tumors. **Contraindications and risks:** Caution in pregnancy advised because of the risk of ionizing radiation to the fetus.	None.

	PANCREAS		ADRENAL
	CT	**Ultrasound**	**MIBG scan**

Modality	Indications	Comments	Contraindications and risks	Patient preparation
PANCREAS **Computed tomography (CT)** $$$–$$$$	Evaluation of pancreatic and biliary obstruction and possible adenocarcinoma. Staging of pancreatic carcinoma. Evaluation of complications and causes of acute pancreatitis.	Can guide fine-needle biopsy or placement of a drainage catheter. Can identify early necrosis in pancreatitis.	Optimal imaging requires special protocol, including precontrast plus arterial and venous phase contrast-enhanced images. **Contraindications and risks:** Contraindicated in pregnancy because of the potential harm of ionizing radiation to the fetus. See Risks of CT and Angiographic Intravenous Contrast Agents, p 245.	Preferably NPO for 4–6 hours. Normal hydration. Opacification of gastrointestinal tract with oral Gastrografin. Sedation of agitated patients. Recent serum creatinine determination.
PANCREAS **Ultrasound (US)** $	Identification of peripancreatic fluid collections, pseudocysts, and pancreatic ductal dilation.	Noninvasive. No radiation. Can be portable. Imaging in all planes. Can guide fine-needle aspiration or placement of drainage catheter.	Pancreas may be obscured by overlying bowel gas. Technique very operator dependent. Presence of barium obscures sound waves. Less sensitive than CT. **Contraindications and risks:** None.	Preferably NPO for 6 hours.
ADRENAL **MIBG (meta-iodobenzyl-guanidine)** (radionuclide) $$$$	Suspected pheochromocytoma when CT is negative or equivocal. Also useful in evaluation of neuroblastoma, carcinoid, and medullary carcinoma of thyroid.	Test is useful for localization of pheochromocytomas (particularly extra-adrenal). 80–90% sensitive for detection of pheochromocytoma.	High radiation dose to adrenal gland. High cost and limited availability of MIBG. Delayed imaging (at 1, 2, and 3 days) necessitates return of patient. **Contraindications and risks:** Contraindicated in pregnancy because of the risk of ionizing radiation to the fetus. Because of the relatively high dose of ^{131}I, patients should be instructed about precautionary measures by nuclear medicine personnel.	Administration of Lugol's iodine solution (to block thyroid uptake) prior to and following administration of MIBG.

	GENITOURINARY		
	CT	**Ultrasound**	**MRI**
Test	GENITO-URINARY **Computed tomography (CT)** $$$	GENITO-URINARY **Ultrasound (US)** $$	GENITO-URINARY **Magnetic resonance imaging (MRI)** $$$$
Indications	Evaluation for possible kidney or ureteral stones. Evaluation of staging of renal parenchymal tumors, hydronephrosis, pyelonephritis, and perinephric abscess.	Evaluation of renal morphology, hydronephrosis, size of prostate, and residual urine volume. Differentiation of cystic versus solid renal lesions.	Staging of cancers of the uterus, cervix, and prostate. Can provide information additional to what is obtained by CT in some cases of cancer of the kidney and urinary bladder.
Advantages	Rapid. Can guide percutaneous procedures. Excellent spatial resolution.	Noninvasive. No radiation. Can be portable. Imaging in all planes. Can guide fine-needle aspiration or placement of drainage catheter.	Provides excellent tissue contrast resolution, multiplanar capability. No beam-hardening artifacts such as can be seen with CT. No ionizing radiation.
Disadvantages/Contraindications	Generally limited to transaxial views. **Contraindications and risks:** Caution in pregnancy because of the risk of ionizing radiation to the fetus. See Risks of CT and Angiographic Intravenous Contrast Agents, p 245.	Technique very operator-dependent. More difficult in obese patients. **Contraindications and risks:** None.	Subject to motion artifacts. Gastrointestinal opacification not yet readily available. Special instrumentation required for patients on life support. **Contraindications and risks:** Contraindicated in patients with cardiac pacemakers, intraocular metallic foreign bodies, intracranial aneurysm clips, cochlear implants, and some artificial heart valves.
Preparation	Sedation of agitated patients.	Preferably NPO for 6 hours. Full urinary bladder required for pelvic studies.	Sedation of agitated patients. Screening CT or plain radiograph images of orbits if history suggests possible metallic foreign body in the eye.

GENITOURINARY

Imaging Study	Indications	Comments	Contraindications and risks	Patient preparation
GENITOURINARY Intravenous pyelogram (IVP) $$$	Fluoroscopic evaluation of uroepithelial neoplasm, calculus, papillary necrosis, and medullary sponge kidney. Screening for urinary system injury after trauma.	Permits evaluation of collecting system in less invasive manner than retrograde pyelogram. Can assess both renal morphology and function.	Suboptimal evaluation of the renal parenchyma. Does not adequately evaluate cause of ureteral deviation. **Contraindications and risks:** Caution in pregnancy is advised because of the risk of ionizing radiation to the fetus. See Risks of CT and Angiographic Intravenous Contrast Agents, p 245.	Adequate hydration. Colonic cleansing is preferred but not essential. Recent serum creatinine determination.
GENITOURINARY Renal scan (radionuclide) $$	Determination of relative renal function. Evaluation of suspected renal vascular hypertension. Differentiation of a dilated but non-obstructed system from one that has a urodynamically significant obstruction. Evaluation of renal blood flow and function in acute or chronic renal failure. Evaluation of both medical and surgical complications of renal transplant. Estimation of glomerular filtration rate and effective renal plasma flow.	Provides functional information without risk of iodinated contrast used in IVP. Provides quantitative information not available by other means.	Finding of poor renal blood flow does not pinpoint an etiologic diagnosis. Limited utility when renal function is extremely poor. Estimation of glomerular filtration rate and renal plasma flow often is inaccurate. **Contraindications and risks:** Caution in pregnancy because of the risk of ionizing radiation to the fetus.	Normal hydration needed for evaluation of suspected obstructive uropathy because dehydration may result in false-positive examination. Blood pressure should be monitored and an intravenous line started when an angiotensin-converting enzyme (ACE) inhibitor is used to evaluate renal vascular hypertension. Patient should discontinue ACE inhibitor medication for at least 48 hours prior to examination if possible.

(Table header as printed: GENITOURINARY — IVP | Radionuclide scan)

		PELVIS	
		Ultrasound	**MRI**
Preparation		Distended bladder required (only in transabdominal examination).	Intramuscular glucagon is used to inhibit intestinal peristalsis. Sedation of agitated patients. Screening CT or plain radiograph images of orbits if history suggests possible metallic foreign body in the eye. An endorectal device (radiofrequency coil) is used for prostate MRI.
Disadvantages/Contraindications		Transabdominal scan has limited sensitivity for uterine or ovarian pathology. Vaginal probe has limited field of view and therefore may miss large masses outside the pelvis. **Contraindications and risks:** None.	Subject to motion artifacts. Special instrumentation required for patients on life support. **Contraindications and risks:** Contraindicated in patients with cardiac pacemakers, intraocular metallic foreign bodies, intracranial aneurysm clips, cochlear implants, and some artificial heart valves.
Advantages		Use of a vaginal probe enables very early detection of intrauterine pregnancy and ectopic pregnancy and does not require a full bladder.	Provides excellent tissue contrast resolution, multiplanar capability. No beam-hardening artifacts such as can be seen with CT. No ionizing radiation. Best imaging evaluation of cancer of the uterus, cervix, prostate, and bladder.
Indications		Evaluation of ovarian mass, enlarged uterus, vaginal bleeding, pelvic pain, possible ectopic pregnancy, and infertility. Monitoring of follicular development. Localization of intrauterine device.	Evaluation of gynecologic malignancies, particularly endometrial, cervical, and vaginal carcinoma. Evaluation of prostate, bladder, and rectal carcinoma. Evaluation of congenital anomalies of the genitourinary tract. Useful in distinguishing lymphadenopathy from vasculature.
Test		PELVIS **Ultrasound** (US) $$	PELVIS **Magnetic resonance imaging** (MRI) $$$$

	BONE			
	Bone scan			
BONE **Bone scan, whole body** (radio-nuclide) $$–$$$	Evaluation of primary or metastatic neoplasm, osteomyelitis, arthritis, metabolic disorders, trauma, avascular necrosis, joint prosthesis, and reflex sympathetic dystrophy. Evaluation of clinically suspected but radiographically occult fractures. Identification of stress fractures.	Can examine entire osseous skeleton or specific area of interest. Highly sensitive compared with plain film radiography for detection of bone neoplasm. In osteomyelitis, bone scan may be positive much earlier (24 hours) than plain film (10–14 days).	Nonspecific. Correlation with plain film radiographs often necessary. Limited utility in patients with poor renal function. Poor resolution in distal extremities, head, and spine; in these instances, SPECT is often useful. Sometimes difficult to distinguish osteomyelitis from cellulitis or septic joint; dual imaging with gallium or with indium-labeled leukocytes can be helpful. False-negative results for osteomyelitis can occur following antibiotic therapy and within the first 24 hours after trauma. In avascular necrosis, bone scan may be "hot," "cold," or normal, depending on the stage. **Contraindications and risks:** Caution in pregnancy because of the risk of ionizing radiation to the fetus.	Patient should be well hydrated and void frequently after the procedure.

Test	Indications	Advantages	Disadvantages/Contraindications	Preparation
SPINE				
CT				
SPINE **Computed tomography** (CT) $$$	Evaluation of structures that are not well visualized on MRI, including ossification of the posterior longitudinal ligament, tumoral calcification, osteophytic spurring, retropulsed bone fragments after trauma. Also used for patients in whom MRI is contraindicated.	Rapid. Superb spatial resolution. Can guide percutaneous fine-needle aspiration of possible tumor or abscess.	Generally limited to transaxial views. Coronal and sagittal reformation images can be generated. MRI unequivocally superior in evaluation of the spine nerve roots and cord, except for conditions mentioned in Indications. Artifacts from metal prostheses degrade images. **Contraindications and risks:** Contraindicated in pregnancy because of the potential harm of ionizing radiation to the fetus. See Risks of CT and Angiographic Intravenous Contrast Agents, p 245.	Normal hydration. Sedation of agitated patients.
MRI				
SPINE **Magnetic resonance imaging** (MRI) $$$$	Diseases involving the spine and cord except where CT is superior (ossification of the posterior longitudinal ligament, tumoral calcification, osteophytic spurring, retropulsed bone fragments after trauma).	Provides excellent tissue contrast resolution, multiplanar capability. No beam-hardening artifacts such as can be seen with CT. No ionizing radiation.	Less useful in detection of calcification, small spinal vascular malformations, acute spinal trauma (because of longer acquisition time, incompatibility with life support devices, and inferior detection of bony injury). Subject to motion artifacts. Special instrumentation required for patients on life support. **Contraindications and risks:** Contraindicated in patients with cardiac pacemakers, intraocular metallic foreign bodies, intracranial aneurysm clips, cochlear implants, and some artificial heart valves.	Sedation of agitated patients. Screening CT or plain radiograph images of orbits if history suggests possible metallic foreign body in the eye.

	MUSCULOSKELETAL			VASCULATURE
	MRI			Ultrasound
MUSCULOSKELETAL SYSTEM **Magnetic resonance imaging (MRI)** $$$$	Evaluation of joints except where a prosthesis is in place. Extent of primary or malignant tumor (bone and soft tissue). Evaluation of aseptic necrosis, bone and soft tissue infections, marrow space disease, and traumatic derangements.	Provides excellent tissue contrast resolution, multiplanar capability. No beam-hardening artifacts such as can be seen with CT. No ionizing radiation.	Subject to motion artifacts. Less able than CT to detect calcification, ossification, and periosteal reaction. Special instrumentation required for patients on life support. **Contraindications and risks:** Contraindicated in patients with cardiac pacemakers, intraocular metallic foreign bodies, intracranial aneurysm clips, cochlear implants, and some artificial heart valves.	Sedation of agitated patients. Screening CT or plain radiograph images of orbits if history suggests possible metallic foreign body in the eye.
VASCULATURE **Ultrasound (US)** $$	Evaluation of deep venous thrombosis, extremity grafts, patency of inferior vena cava, portal vein, and hepatic veins. Carotid doppler indicated for symptomatic carotid bruit, atypical transient ischemic attack, monitoring after endarterectomy, and baseline prior to major vascular surgery. Surveillance of TIPS patency and flow.	Noninvasive. No radiation. Can be portable. Imaging in all planes.	Technique operator-dependent. Ultrasound not sensitive to detection of ulcerated plaque. May be difficult to diagnose tight stenosis versus occlusion (catheter angiography may be necessary). May be difficult to distinguish acute from chronic deep venous thrombosis. **Contraindications and risks:** None.	None.

	AORTA			
	Angiography			
Test	Indications	Advantages	Disadvantages/Contraindications	Preparation
AORTA AND ITS BRANCHES Angiography $$$	Peripheral vascular disease, abdominal aortic aneurysm, renal artery stenosis (atherosclerotic and fibromuscular disease), visceral ischemia, thoracic aortic dissection, gastrointestinal hemorrhage, vasculitis, abdominal tumors, arteriovenous malformations, abdominopelvic trauma. Preoperative evaluation for aortofemoral bypass reconstructive surgery. Postoperative assessment of possible graft stenosis, especially femoral to popliteal or femoral to distal (foot or ankle).	Can localize atherosclerotic stenosis and assess the severity by morphology, flow, and pressure gradient. Provides assessment of stenotic lesions and access for percutaneous transluminal balloon dilation as well as stent treatment of iliac stenoses. Provides access for thrombolytic therapy of acute or subacute occlusion of native artery or bypass graft.	Invasive. Patient must remain supine with leg extended for 6 hours following the procedure to protect the common femoral artery at the catheter entry site. **Contraindications and risks:** Allergy to iodinated contrast material may require corticosteroid and H_1 blocker or H_2 blocker premedication. Contraindicated in pregnancy because of the potential harm of ionizing radiation to the fetus. Contrast nephrotoxicity may occur, especially with preexisting impaired renal function due to diabetes mellitus or multiple myeloma; however, any creatinine elevation that occurs after the procedure is usually reversible.	NPO for 4–6 hours. Good hydration to limit possible renal insult due to iodinated contrast material. Recent serum creatinine determination, assessment of clotting parameters, reversal of anticoagulation. Performed with conscious sedation. Requires cardiac, respiratory, blood pressure, and pulse oximetry monitoring as well as noninvasive studies of peripheral vascular disease to verify indication for angiography and to guide the examination.

AORTA AND ITS BRANCHES **Computed tomography angiography** (CTA) $$$	Preoperative assessment of aortic aneurysm. Evaluation of abdominal trauma. Evaluation of possible aortic injury.	Rapid. Excellent spatial resolution. Evaluates calcified vascular plaques.	Limited functional and hemodynamic evaluation. **Contraindications and risks:** Contraindicated in pregnancy because of potential harm of ionizing radiation to the fetus. See Risks of CT and Angiographic Intravenous Contrast Agents, p 245.	Sedation of agitated patients. Hydration.	CTA	AORTA
AORTA AND ITS BRANCHES **Magnetic resonance angiography** (MRA) $$$$	Can provide preoperative assessment of abdominal aortic aneurysm to determine aneurysm size, proximal and distal extent, relationship to renal arteries, and presence of anatomic anomalies. Permits evaluation of the hemodynamic and functional significance of renal artery stenosis.	No ionizing radiation. No iodinated contrast needed.	Subject to motion artifacts. Special instrumentation required for patients on life support. **Contraindications and risks:** Contraindicated in patients with cardiac pacemakers, intraocular metallic foreign bodies, intracranial aneurysm clips, cochlear implants, and some artificial heart valves.	Sedation of agitated patients. Screening CT or plain radiograph images of orbits if history suggests possible metallic foreign body in the eye.	MRA	

7

Basic Electrocardiography*

Fred M. Kusumoto, MD

HOW TO USE THIS SECTION

This chapter includes criteria for the diagnosis of basic electrocardiographic waveforms and cardiac arrhythmias. It is intended for use as a reference and assumes a basic understanding of the electrocardiogram (ECG).

Electrocardiographic interpretation is a "stepwise" procedure, and the first steps are to study and characterize the cardiac rhythm.

Step One (Rhythm)

Categorize what you see in the 12-lead ECG or rhythm strip, using the three major parameters that allow for systematic analysis and subsequent diagnosis of the rhythm:

1. Mean rate of the QRS complexes (slow, normal, or fast).
2. Width of the QRS complexes (wide or narrow).
3. Rhythmicity of the QRS complexes (characterization of spaces between QRS complexes) (regular or irregular).

Step Two (Morphology)

Step 2 consists of examining and characterizing the morphology of the cardiac waveforms.

1. Examine for atrial abnormalities and bundle branch blocks (BBBs) (pp 306–308).
2. Assess the QRS axis and the causes of axis deviations (pp 310–311).
3. Examine for signs of left ventricular hypertrophy (pp 311–312).

---

* Adapted, with permission, from Evans GT Jr.: *ECG Interpretation Cribsheets,* 4th ed. Ring Mountain Press, 1999.

4. Examine for signs of right ventricular hypertrophy (p 313).

5. Examine for signs of myocardial infarction, if present (pp 315–324).

6. Bear in mind conditions that may alter the ability of the ECG to diagnose a myocardial infarction (p 324).

7. Examine for abnormalities of the ST segment or T wave (pp 325–328).

8. Assess the QT interval (pp 329–332).

9. Examine for miscellaneous conditions (pp 332–335).

STEP ONE: DIAGNOSIS OF THE CARDIAC RHYTHM

A. APPROACH TO DIAGNOSIS OF THE CARDIAC RHYTHM

Most electrocardiograph machines display 10 seconds of data in a standard tracing. A rhythm is defined as three or more successive P waves or QRS complexes.

Categorize the patterns seen in the tracing according to a systematic method. This method proceeds in three steps that lead to a diagnosis based upon the most likely rhythm producing a particular pattern:

1. What is the mean rate of the QRS complexes?

   Slow (<60 bpm): The easiest way to determine this is to count the total number of QRS complexes in a 10-second period. If there are no more than 9, the rate is slow.

   Another method for determining the rate is to count the number of large boxes (0.20 s) between QRS complexes and use the following formula:

   Rate = 300 ÷ (number of large boxes between QRS complexes)

   A slow heart rate (<60 bpm) will have more than five large boxes between QRS complexes.

   Normal (60–100 bpm): If there are 10–16 complexes in a 10-second period, the rate is normal.

   In normal heart rates, the QRS complexes will be separated by 3–5 large boxes.

   Fast (>100 bpm): If there are ≥17 complexes in a 10-second period, the rate is fast.

   Fast heart rates will have fewer than 3 large boxes between QRS complexes.

2. Is the duration of the dominant QRS morphology narrow (<0.12 s) or wide (≥0.12 s)? (Refer to the section below on the QRS duration.)

3. What is the "rhythmicity" of the QRS complexes (defined as the spacing between QRS complexes)? Regular or irregular? (Any change in the spacing of the R-R intervals defines an irregular rhythm.)

Using the categorization above, refer to Tables 7–1 and 7–2 to select a specific diagnosis for the cardiac rhythm.

B. NORMAL HEART RATE

Sinus Rhythm

The sinus node is the primary pacemaker for the heart. Because the sinus node is located at the junction of the superior vena cava and the right atrium, in **sinus rhythm** the atria are activated from "right to left" and "high to low." The P wave in sinus rhythm is upright in lead II and inverted in lead aVR. In lead V_I, the P wave is usually biphasic with a small initial positive deflection due to right atrial activation and a terminal negative deflection due to left atrial activation.

The normal sinus rate is usually between 60 and 100 bpm but can vary significantly. During sleep, when parasympathetic tone is high, **sinus bradycardia** (sinus rates <60 bpm) is a normal finding, and during conditions associated with increased sympathetic tone (exercise, stress), **sinus tachycardia** (sinus rate >100 bpm) is common. In children and young adults, **sinus arrhythmia** (sinus rates that vary by more than 10% during 10 seconds) due to respiration is frequently observed.

TABLE 7–1. SUSTAINED REGULAR RHYTHMS.

Rate	Fast	Normal	Slow
Narrow QRS duration	Sinus tachycardia Atrial tachycardia Atrial flutter (2 : 1 AV conduction) Junctional tachycardia Orthodromic AVRT	Sinus rhythm Ectopic atrial rhythm Atrial flutter (4 : 1 conduction) Accelerated junctional rhythm	Sinus bradycardia Ectopic atrial bradycardia Junctional rhythm
Wide QRS duration	All rhythms listed above under narrow QRS duration, but with BBB or IVCD patterns		
	Ventricular tachycardia Antidromic AVRT	Accelerated ventricular rhythm	Ventricular escape rhythm

Abbreviations: AV, atrioventricular; BBB, bundle branch blocks; IVCD, intraventricular conduction delay.

TABLE 7–2. SUSTAINED IRREGULAR RHYTHMS.

Rate	Fast	Normal	Slow
Narrow QRS duration	Atrial fibrillation Atrial flutter (variable AV conduction) Multifocal atrial tachycardia Atrial tachycardia with AV block (rare)	Atrial fibrillation Atrial flutter (variable AV conduction) Multiform atrial rhythm Atrial tachycardia with AV block (rare)	Atrial fibrillation Atrial flutter (variable AV conduction) Multiform atrial rhythm Sinus rhythm with 2° AV block
Wide QRS duration	All rhythms listed above under narrow QRS duration, but with BBB or IVCD patterns		
	Torsade de pointes Rarely, anterograde conduction of atrial fibrillation over an accessory pathway in patients with WPW syndrome		

Abbreviations: AV, atrioventricular; BBB, bundle branch blocks; IVCD, intraventricular conduction delay; WPW, Wolff-Parkinson-White syndrome.

Ectopic Atrial Rhythm

In some situations, the atria are activated by an ectopic atrial focus rather than the sinus node. In this case, the P wave will have an abnormal shape depending on where the ectopic focus is located. For example, if the focus arises from the left atrium, the P wave will be inverted in leads I and aVL. If the depolarization rate of the ectopic focus is between 60 and 100 bpm, the patient has an **ectopic atrial rhythm.** If the rate is <60 bpm, the rhythm is defined as an ectopic atrial bradycardia.

Atrial Flutter With 4:1 Atrioventricular Conduction

In **atrial flutter**, the atria are activated rapidly (usually 300 bpm) due to a stable reentrant circuit. Most commonly, the reentrant circuit rotates counterclockwise around the tricuspid valve. Because the left atrium and interatrial septum are activated low-to-high, "sawtooth" flutter waves that are inverted in the inferior leads (II, III, and aVF) are usually observed. If every fourth atrial beat is conducted to the ventricles (due to slow conduction in the atrioventricular [AV] node), a relatively normal ventricular rate of 75 bpm will be observed.

Accelerated Junctional Rhythm (page 304)

Premature QRS Activity

It is common to have isolated premature QRS activity that leads to mild irregularity of the heart rhythm. A premature narrow QRS complex is most often due to a normally conducted **premature atrial complex (PAC)** or more rarely a **premature junctional complex (PJC)**. A premature wide QRS complex is usually due to a **premature ventricular complex (PVC)** or to a premature supraventricular complex (PAC or PJC) that conducts to the ventricle with aberrant conduction due to block in one of the bundle branches (pp 306–307). Premature supraventricular complexes (with or without aberrant conduction) are commonly observed phenomena that are not associated with cardiac disease. Although PVCs are observed in normal individuals, they are usually associated with higher risk in patients with cardiac disease.

C. TACHYCARDIA

Tachycardias are normally classified by whether the QRS complex is narrow or wide, and whether the rhythm is regular or irregular. A narrow QRS tachycardia indicates normal activation of the ventricular tissue regardless of the tachycardia mechanism. Narrow QRS tachycardias are frequently grouped together as supraventricular tachycardia (SVT) and can be due to a number of mechanisms described below. This grouping also has clinical utility because SVTs are not usually life-threatening. In addition to QRS width, it is useful to consider the anatomic site from which the tachycardia arises: atrium, atrioventricular junction, ventricle, or utilization of an accessory pathway (Figure 7–1).

Narrow QRS Tachycardia with a Regular Rhythm: Regular SVT (Figure 7–2)

A. Sinus Tachycardia: Under many physiologic conditions, the sinus node will discharge at a rate >100 bpm. In **sinus tachycardia,** an upright P wave will be observed in II and aVF and an inverted P wave will be observed in aVR. The PR interval is usually relatively normal, because conditions associated with sinus tachycardia (most commonly sympathetic activation) also cause more rapid AV conduction.

B. Atrial Tachycardia: Rarely, a single atrial site other than the sinus node fires rapidly. This leads to an abnormally shaped P wave. The specific shape of the P wave will depend on the specific site of **atrial tachycardia.** The PR interval depends on how quickly atrio-

Atrial tachycardias

Atrial flutter

Atrial fibrillation

Atrial tachycardia

Atrial tachycardia (MAT)

Junctional tachycardias

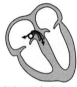

Atrioventricular node reentrant tachycardia

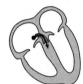

Atrioventricular node automatic tachycardia

Ventricular tachycardias

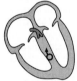

Ventricular tachycardia

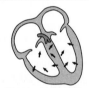

Ventricular fibrillation

Accessory pathway-mediated tachycardias

Orthodromic atrioventricular reentrant tachycardia

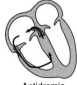

Antidromic atrioventricular reentrant tachycardia

Atrial fibrillation with activation of the ventricles via an accessory pathway and the AV node

Figure 7–1. Anatomic classification of tachycardias. (Adopted from Kusumoto FM: Arrhythmias. In: *Cardiovascular Pathophysiology*, FM Kusumoto (editor), Fence Creek Publishing, 1999.)

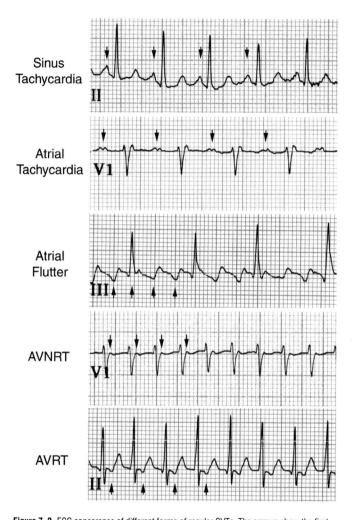

Figure 7–2. ECG appearance of different forms of regular SVTs. The arrows show the first four atrial deflections in each SVT. In *sinus tachycardia*, the P wave has a normal morphology and the PR interval is normal. In *atrial tachycardia*, the P wave is abnormal (positive in V_I) and the PR interval is prolonged because of decremental conduction in the AV node. In *atrial flutter*, inverted "saw-tooth" waves are observed in lead III. In *AVNRT*, a pseudo-R wave due to retrograde atrial activation is observed in lead VI. In *AVRT*, a retrograde P wave is observed in the ST segment because the atria and ventricles are activated sequentially. The P wave is usually located relatively close to the preceding QRS complex because the accessory pathway conducts rapidly.

ventricular conduction occurs. As the atrial tachycardia rate increases, the AV node conduction will slow (decremental conduction) and the PR interval will increase; decremental conduction properties of the AV node prevent rapid ventricular rates in the presence of rapid atrial rates.

C. **Atrial Flutter:** The mechanism for **atrial flutter** is described above. Most commonly atrioventricular conduction occurs with every other flutter wave (2:1 conduction), leading to a heart rate of approximately 150 bpm. In some situations, very rapid ventricular rates can be observed due to 1:1 conduction, or slower rates observed due to 3:1 conduction.

D. **Junctional Tachycardia:** The most common type of tachycardia to arise from tissue near the atrioventricular junction is **AV nodal reentrant tachycardia (AVNRT)**. In AVNRT, two separate parallel pathways of conduction are present within junctional and perijunctional tissue. Usually one of the pathways has relatively rapid conduction properties but a long refractory period ("fast pathway") and the other has slow conduction and a short refractory period ("slow pathway"). In some cases, a premature atrial contraction can block in one of the pathways (usually the fast pathway), conduct down the slow pathway, and activate the fast pathway retrogradely, initiating a reentrant circuit. In rare circumstances, a site within the AV node will fire rapidly due to increased automaticity.

Regardless of mechanism, because the tachycardia originates within the AV junction, the atria and ventricles are activated simultaneously. Most commonly (in approximately 50% of cases), the P wave is buried in the QRS complex and is not seen. In approximately 40% of cases, the retrograde P wave is observed in the terminal portion of the QRS complex. The easiest place to see the retrograde P wave is in lead V_1, where a low-amplitude terminal positive deflection (pseudo-R′ wave) is seen (Figure 7–2). In addition, a terminal negative deflection (pseudo-S wave) is seen in the inferior leads (II, III, and aVF). Finally, in about 10% of cases, the P wave is observed in the initial portion of the QRS complex. The location of the P wave depends on the relative speeds of retrograde activation of the atria and anterograde activation of the ventricles via the His-Purkinje system.

E. **Accessory Pathway–Mediated Tachycardia:** Usually, the AV node and His bundle provide the only path for AV conduction. In approximately 1 in 1000 individuals, an additional AV connection called an accessory pathway is present. The presence of two parallel pathways (the **accessory pathway** and the AV node-His bundle) for AV conduction increases the likelihood that reentrant tachycardias will occur. The most common tachycardia is a reentrant narrow QRS tachycardia in which the ventricles are activivated via the His-Purkinje system and the atria are activated via retrograde activation from the accessory pathway (Figure 7–3). This type of tachycardia is frequently called **orthodromic atrioventricular reentrant tachycardia (AVRT)** because conduction through the AV node and His-Purkinje fibers occurs normally (*ortho* is Greek for straight or normal). Orthodromic AVRT is one cause of SVT; the QRS complexes are narrow and normal-appearing because the ventricles are activated via the AV node and His-Purkinje system, ventricular tissue, an accessory pathway, and atrial tissue. Because the ventricles and atria are activated sequentially, the P wave is most often observed within the ST segment (Figure 7–2). As discussed later, accessory pathways can also be associated with regular and irregular wide complex tachycardias.

Narrow QRS Tachycardias with an Irregular Rhythm: Irregular SVT (Figure 7–4)

A. Atrial Fibrillation: Atrial fibrillation is the most common abnormal fast heat rhythm observed. Atrial fibrillation is most commonly due to multiple chaotic wandering wavelets of reentry that cause irregular activation of the atria. Because the AV node is also activated irregularly, AV conduction is variable and an irregular ventricular rhythm is observed. In atrial fibrillation, the rhythm is often called "irregu-

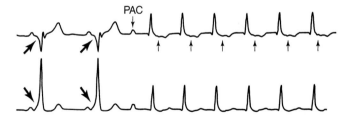

Figure 7–3. Initiation of SVT in a patient with an accessory pathway. During sinus rhythm, the ventricles are activated via the accessory pathway and the AV node-His bundle. Because the accessory pathway conducts rapidly and inserts into regular ventricular myocardium, the PR interval is short and a delta wave is observed (*large arrows*). A PAC blocks in the accessory pathway and travels only down the AV node-His bundle, leading to a narrow QRS complex. The atria are activated retrogradely by the accessory pathway (small arrows) and orthodromic AVRT is initiated. (From Kusumoto FM: Cardiovascular disorders: Heart disease: In: *Pathophysiology of Disease: An Introduction to Clinical Medicine*, 4th ed. SJ McPhee, VR Lingappa, WF Ganong (editors), McGraw-Hill, 2003.)

Atrial fibrillation

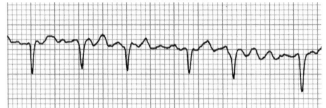

Multifocal atrial tachycardia

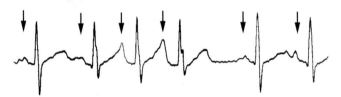

Figure 7–4. ECG appearance of atrial fibrillation and MAT. In atrial fibrillation, continuous chaotic activation of the atria results in continuous low-amplitude fibrillatory waves. In MAT, discrete P waves (*arrows*) and an isoelectric T–P segment are observed.

larly irregular" because there is no organized atrial activity. On the ECG, continuous fibrillatory low-amplitude waves with varying morphology are observed with no easily identifiable isoelectric period. The fibrillatory waves are usually best seen in leads V_1, V_2, II, III, and aVF.

B. **Multifocal Atrial Tachycardia:** In **multifocal atrial tachycardia** (often called **MAT**), several atrial sites beat due to abnormal automaticity. This leads to P waves of three or more different morphologies. The rhythm is usually irregular; the different sites fire at different rates. MAT can be distinguished from atrial fibrillation by discrete P waves and isoelectric periods between the T wave and the P wave. The most common cause of MAT is chronic obstructive pulmonary disease (approximately 60% of cases).

C. **Atrial Flutter With Variable Block:** Atrial flutter can sometimes present as an irregular rhythm because of variable AV block. In this case, although the ventricular rhythm is irregular, there are often relatively constant intervals between the QRS complexes. For example, if the atrial flutter rate is 300 bpm, the possible ventricular rates will be 300 bpm, 150 bpm, 100 bpm, or 75 bpm for 1:1, 2:1, 3:1, and 4:1 AV conduction, respectively.

Wide QRS Complex Tachycardia With a Regular Rhythm

The most common cause of **wide QRS complex tachycardia with a regular rhythm (WCT-RR)** is sinus tachycardia with either right bundle branch block (RBBB) or left bundle branch block (LBBB). However, if a patient with structural heart disease presents with WCT-RR, one assumes a worst-case scenario and the presumptive diagnosis becomes **ventricular tachycardia (VT).** Most commonly, VT originates from a rapid reentrant circuit located at the border of infarcted and normal myocardium. Because the ventricles are not activated via the bundle branches or the Purkinje system, an abnormally wide QRS complex is observed. Any atrial or junctional tachycardias associated with aberrant conduction can also cause a WCT-RR. Finally, in very rare circumstances, patients with accessory pathways will present with **antidromic AVRT** in which the ventricles are activated via the accessory pathway (leading to a wide and bizarre QRS complex) and the atria are activated retrogradely via the His bundle-AV node (*anti* is Greek for against).

The ECG differentiation between regular SVTs with aberrant conduction (sinus tachycardia, atrial tachycardia, atrial flutter, junctional tachycardia, orthodromic AVRT) and VT can sometimes be difficult. Accurate diagnosis of VT is critical because this rhythm is frequently life-threatening. The two principal techniques for identifying VT are the presence of AV dissociation and abnormal QRS morphology.

A. **Atrioventricular Dissociation:** In **AV dissociation,** the atria and ventricles are not related in one-to-one fashion. AV dissociation can be due to several conditions:
   1. Atrioventricular conduction block (p 304).
   2. Slowing of the primary pacemaker, most commonly due to sinus bradycardia or sinus pauses with junctional escape rhythm (p 304).
   3. Acceleration of a subsidiary pacemaker, most commonly due to VT or much less commonly due to junctional tachycardia.

   The most important reason to identify AV dissociation is in wide complex tachycardia for the differentiation of SVT with aberrancy from VT. In VT, the rapid ventricular rate is often associated with

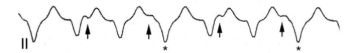

Figure 7–5. Lead II from a wide complex tachycardia. The arrows mark P waves that are not associated with every QRS complex (AV dissociation). The QRS complexes marked with an * are slightly narrower due to partial activation from the preceding P wave (fusion complex).

retrograde block within the His-Purkinje system (ventriculoatrial block). This leads to P waves (from sinus node depolarization) that are not associated in 1 : 1 fashion with the QRS complexes (Figure 7–5). The presence of AV dissociation makes VT the most likely diagnosis in a patient with a regular wide complex tachycardia. In some circumstances, AV dissociation can be identified by the presence of **capture beats** or **fusion beats**. Occasionally, a properly timed P wave will conduct to the ventricles and a portion (fusion beat) or all (capture beat) of ventricular tissue will be activated by the His-Purkinje tissue for one QRS complex. It is always easier to identify AV dissociation rather than AV association; T waves can often be confused for P waves. Always examine the entire ECG for unexpected deflections in the QRS complex, ST segment, and T waves that are dissociated P waves. The P waves will usually be most obvious in the inferior leads (II, III, and aVF) or V_1.

MORPHOLOGY ALGORITHMS FOR IDENTIFYING VT

1. METHOD 1: QUICK METHOD FOR DIAGNOSIS OF VT (REQUIRES LEADS I, V_1, AND V_2)

This method derives from an analysis of typical waveforms of RBBB or LBBB as seen in leads I, V_1, and V_2. If the waveforms do not conform to either the common or uncommon typical morphologic patterns, the diagnosis defaults to VT.

Step One

Determine the morphologic classification of the wide QRS complexes (RB type or LB type), using the criteria below.

A. **Determination of the Morphologic Type of Wide QRS Complexes:** Use lead V_1 only to determine the type of bundle branch block morphology of abnormally wide QRS complexes.

1. **RBBB and RBB type QRS complexes as seen in lead V_1:** A wide QRS complex with a net positive area under the QRS curve is called the right bundle branch "type" of QRS. This does not mean that the QRS conforms exactly to the morphologic criteria for RBBB. Typical morphologies seen in RBBB are shown in the box at left below. Atypical morphologies at the right are most commonly seen in PVCs or during VT.

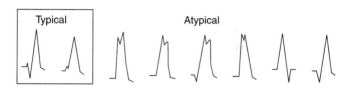

2. **LBBB and LBB-type QRS complexes as seen in lead V_1:** A wide QRS complex with a net negative area under the QRS curve is called a left bundle branch "type" of QRS. This does not mean that the QRS conforms exactly to the morphologic criteria for LBBB. Typical morphologies of LBBB are shown in the box at left below. Atypical morphologies at the right are most commonly seen in PVCs or during VT.

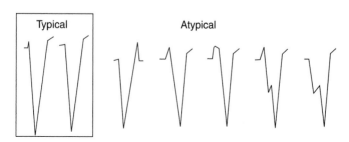

Step Two

Apply criteria for common and uncommon normal forms of either RBBB or LBBB, as described below. The waveforms may not be identical, but the morphologic descriptions must match. If the QRS complexes do not match, the rhythm is probably VT.

A. RBBB: Lead I must have a terminal broad S wave, but the R/S ratio may be <1.

In lead V_1, the QRS complex is usually triphasic but sometimes is notched and monophasic. The latter must have notching on the ascending limb of the R wave, usually at the lower left.

B. LBBB: Lead I must have a monophasic, usually notched R wave and may not have Q waves or S waves.

Both lead V_1 and lead V_2 must have a dominant S wave, usually with a small, narrow R wave. S descent must be rapid and smooth, without notching.

2. Method Two: The Brugada Algorithm for Diagnosis of VT

(Requires all six precordial leads)

Brugada and coworkers reported on a total of 554 patients with WCT-RR whose mechanism was diagnosed in the electrophysiology laboratory. Patients included 384 (69%) with VT and 170 (31%) with SVT with aberrant ventricular conduction.

1. **Is there absence of an RS complex in ALL precordial leads?**

    If Yes ($n = 83$), VT is established diagnosis (sensitivity 21%, specificity 100%). *Note:* Only QR, Qr, qR, QS, QRS, monophasic R, or rSR′ are present. qRs complexes were not mentioned in the Brugada study.

    If No ($n = 471$), proceed to next step.

2. **Is the RS interval >100 ms in ANY ONE precordial lead?**

    If Yes ($n = 175$), VT is established diagnosis (sensitivity 66%, specificity 98%). *Note:* The onset of R to the nadir of S is >100 ms (>2.5 small boxes) in a lead with an RS complex.

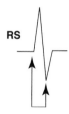

    If No ($n = 296$), proceed to next step.

3. **Is there AV dissociation?**

    If Yes ($n = 59$), VT is established diagnosis (sensitivity 82%, specificity 98%). *Note:* VA block also implies the same diagnosis.

    If No ($n = 237$), proceed to next step. *Note:* Antiarrhythmic drugs were withheld from patients in this study. Clinically, drugs that prolong the QRS duration may give a false-positive sign of VT using this criterion.

4. **Are morphologic criteria for VT present?**

    If Yes ($n = 59$), VT is established diagnosis (sensitivity 99%, specificity 97%). *Note:* RBBB type QRS in V_1 versus LBBB type QRS in V_1 should be assessed as shown in the boxes below.

    If No ($n = 169$)—and if there are no matches for VT in the boxes below—the diagnosis is SVT with aberration (sensitivity 97%, specificity 99%.)

In the presence of **LBBB** type QRS complexes, Brugada used the criteria derived from the study of Kindwall and coworkers (Am J Cardiol 1988;61:1279). ANY of the criteria shown below were highly specific for VT.

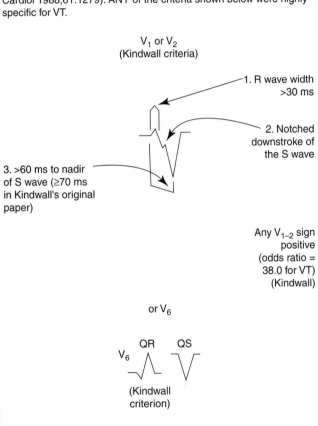

V_1 or V_2
(Kindwall criteria)

1. R wave width >30 ms

2. Notched downstroke of the S wave

3. >60 ms to nadir of S wave (≥70 ms in Kindwall's original paper)

Any V_{1-2} sign positive (odds ratio = 38.0 for VT) (Kindwall)

or V_6

V_6

QR   QS

(Kindwall criterion)

In the presence of **RBBB** type QRS complexes (dominant positive in V_1), a diagnosis of VT can be made by examination of both V_1 and V_6.

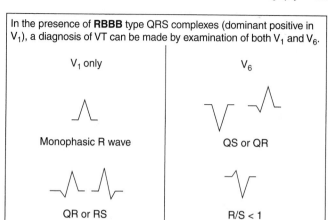

V_1 only	V_6
Monophasic R wave	QS or QR
QR or RS	R/S < 1 (seen with LAD)

3. METHOD THREE: THE GRIFFITH METHOD FOR DIAGNOSIS OF VT (REQUIRES LEADS V_1 AND V_6)

This method derives from an analysis of typical waveforms of RBBB or LBBB as seen in both leads V_1 and V_6. If the waveforms do not conform to the typical morphologic patterns, the diagnosis defaults to VT.

Step One

Determine the morphologic classification of the wide QRS complexes (RB type or LB type), using the criteria above.

Step Two

Apply criteria for normal forms of either RBBB or LBBB, as described below. A negative answer to any of the three questions is inconsistent with either RBBB or LBBB, and the diagnosis defaults to VT.

A. For QRS Complexes With RBBB Categorization:
1. Is there an rSR´ morphology in lead V_1?

2. Is there an RS complex in V$_6$ (may have a small septal Q wave)?

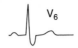

3. Is the R/S ratio in lead V$_6$ > 1?

B. For QRS Complexes With LBBB Categorization:
   1. Is there an rS or QS complex in leads V$_1$ and V$_2$?

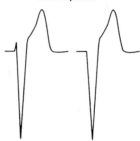

2. Is the onset of the QRS to the nadir of the S wave in lead V$_1$ <70 ms?
3. Is there an R wave in lead V$_6$, without a Q wave?

Wide QRS Tachycardia with an Irregular Rhythm

A. Polymorphic Ventricular Tachycardia and Ventricular Fibrillation
   In **polymorphic ventricular tachycardia** and **ventricular fibrillation,** the ventricles are often activated continuously in chaotic fashion by disorganized wavelets of activation that produce irregular

QRS complexes with no isoelectric periods. Both ventricular fibrillation and polymorphic ventricular tachycardia are life-threatening conditions that require prompt defibrillation. The distinction between ventricular fibrillation and polymorphic ventricular tachycardia is simply based on the amplitude of the QRS complexes and has very little clinical utility. The most common cause of polymorphic ventricular tachycardia and ventricular fibrillation is myocardial ischemia due to coronary artery occlusion.

B. Torsade de Pointes

Torsade de pointes ("twisting of the points") is a specific form of polymorphic VT that is often pause dependent, has a characteristic shifting morphology of the QRS complex, and occurs in the setting of a prolonged QT interval. Torsade de pointes is associated with drug-induced states, congenital long QT syndrome, and hypokalemia (p 329).

C. Atrial Fibrillation with Anterograde Accessory Pathway Activation

If a patient with an accessory pathway develops atrial fibrillation, the ventricles are activated by both the normal AV node-His bundle axis and the accessory pathway. Because the accessory pathway does not have decremental conduction properties, it will allow very rapid activation of the ventricles. The combination of an irregular wide complex rhythm with very rapid rates (250–300 bpm) should arouse suspicion of this scenario, particularly in a young, otherwise healthy patient.

D. Bradycardia

Slow heart rates can be due to failure of impulse formation (sinus node dysfunction) or blocked AV conduction.

Sinus Node Dysfunction

Sinus node dysfunction is manifested in a number of ECG findings. Most commonly, there is a sinus pause with a junctional escape beat. Alternatively, sinus bradycardia can be associated with sinus node dysfunction.

A. Sinus Bradycardia: The normal range of sinus rates changes with age. In infants less than 12 months old, the mean heart rate is 140 bpm with a range of 100–190 bpm. In contrast, the normal range for adults is probably 50–90 bpm. Sinus rates less than 60 bpm are classified as **sinus bradycardia,** but it must be remembered that sinus rates of less than 60 bpm are commonly observed (sleep, athletes). Treatment of sinus bradycardia (usually with a pacemaker) is indicated only when it is associated with symptoms, not because of a specific heart rate.

B. Sinus Pauses: In some individuals, the sinus node abruptly stops firing, leading to **sinus pauses.** Usually an escape rhythm from an ectopic atrial focus or the junction will prevent asystole. Sinus pauses of up to 2 seconds are seen in normal adults. Patients with sinus pauses >3 seconds should be evaluated for the presence of sinus node dysfunction.

C. **Junctional Rhythm:** If the sinus node rate is very low, **sustained junctional rhythm** can sometimes be observed. In junctional rhythm, the QRS is not preceded by a P wave. A retrograde P wave can sometimes be seen in the initial portion or terminal portion of the QRS complex, but most commonly will be "buried" in the QRS complex. Normally junctional rhythms are <60 bpm. Transient junctional rhythm during sleep can be observed in normal individuals, but sinus node dysfunction should be suspected if junctional rhythm is observed when a patient is awake.

In rare circumstances, accelerated junctional rhythms between 60 and 100 bpm are observed due to more rapid depolarization of AV nodal cells. If the junctional rate is faster than the sinus rate, the sinus node will be suppressed by retrograde atrial activation due to repetitive depolarization from the junction. Accelerated junctional rhythms can be present in digitalis toxicity, rheumatic fever, and after cardiac surgery.

AV Block

Because AV conduction normally occurs along a single axis, the AV node and His bundle, **atrioventricular (AV) block** most commonly is due to block at one of these two sites. Block within the His bundle is associated with a worse prognosis, and should be suspected in any form of AV block associated with a wide QRS complex. Electrocardiographically, AV block is usually described as first-degree, second-degree, or third-degree AV block. In **first-degree (1°) AV block,** every P wave is conducted to the ventricles, but there is an abnormal delay between atrial activation and ventricular activation (PR interval >0.2 seconds. In 1° AV block, the ventricular rate is not slow unless sinus bradycardia is also present.

In **second-degree (2°) AV block,** some but not all P waves are conducted to the ventricles. This leads to an irregular ventricular rhythm. Second-degree AV block is usually subclassified as **Mobitz type I** block, **Wenckebach block** or **Mobitz type II block.** In type I 2° AV block, progressive prolongation of the PR interval is observed; in type II 2° AV block, the PR interval remains relatively constant before the blocked P wave. The importance of this distinction is this: type I 2° AV block usually indicates that conduction is blocked within the AV node whereas type II AV block suggests that conduction is blocked within the His bundle (regardless of the width of the QRS complex). The simplest way to differentiate between type I and type II 2° AV block is to compare the PR intervals before and after the block P wave. In type I 2° AV block, the PR interval after the blocked P wave is shorter than the PR interval before the blocked P wave; in type II 2° AV block, the PR intervals are the same.

In **third-degree (3°) or complete AV block,** no P waves are conducted to the ventricles. The P-to-P and QRS-to-QRS intervals are constant and unrelated (AV dissociation). The QRS rate and morphology depend on the site of the subsidiary intrinsic pacemaker. If the block is within the AV node, a lower AV nodal pacemaker often takes over and the rate is 40–50 bpm with a normal-appearing QRS complex (junctional rhythm). If the block is within the His bundle, a ventricular pacemaker with a rate of 20–40 bpm and a wide QRS will be noted **(ventricular escape rhythm).**

STEP TWO: MORPHOLOGIC DIAGNOSIS OF THE CARDIAC WAVEFORMS

A. THE NORMAL ECG: TWO BASIC QRST PATTERNS

The most common pattern is illustrated below and is usually seen in leads I or II and V_{5-6}. There is a small "septal" Q wave <30 ms in duration. The T wave is upright. The normal ST segment, which is never normally iso-electric except sometimes at slow rates (<60 bpm), slopes upward into an upright T wave, whose proximal angle is more obtuse than the distal angle. The normal T wave is never symmetric.

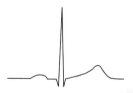

The pattern seen in the right precordial leads, usually V_{1-3}, is shown below. There is a dominant S wave. The J point—the junction between the end of the QRS complex and the ST segment—is usually slightly elevated, and the T wave is upright. The T wave in V_1 may occasionally be inverted as a normal finding in up to 50% of young women and 25% of young men, but this finding is usually abnormal in adult males. V_2 usually has the largest absolute QRS and T wave magnitude of any of the 12 electrocardiographic leads.

B. ATRIAL ABNORMALITIES

Right Atrial Enlargement (RAE)

Diagnostic criteria include a positive component of the P wave in lead V_1 or $V_2 \geq 1.5$ mm. Another criterion is a P wave amplitude in lead II > 2.5 mm. *Note:* A tall, peaked P in lead II may represent RAE but is more commonly due to either chronic obstructive pulmonary disease (COPD) or increased sympathetic tone.

Clinical correlation: RAE is seen with right ventricular hypertrophy (RVH).

Left Atrial Enlargement (LAE)

The most sensitive lead for the diagnosis of LAE is lead V_1, but the criteria for lead II are more specific. Criteria include a terminal negative wave ≥ 1 mm deep and ≥ 40 ms wide (one small box by one small box in area) for lead V_1 and > 40 ms between the first (right) and second (left) atrial components of the P wave in lead II, or a P wave duration > 110 ms in lead II.

Clinical correlations: left ventricular hypertrophy (LVH), coronary artery disease, mitral valve disease, or cardiomyopathy.

C. BUNDLE BRANCH BLOCK

The normal QRS duration in adults ranges from 67–114 ms (Glasgow cohort). If the QRS duration is ≥ 120 ms (three small boxes or more on the electrocardiographic paper), there is usually an abnormality of conduction of the ventricular impulse. The most common causes are either RBBB or LBBB (see p 297). However, other conditions may also prolong the QRS duration.

RBBB is defined by delayed terminal QRS forces that are directed to the right and anteriorly, producing broad terminal positive waves in leads V_1 and aVR and a broad terminal negative wave in lead I.

LBBB is defined by delayed terminal QRS forces that are directed to the left and posteriorly, producing wide R waves in leads that face the left ventricular free wall and wide S waves in the right precordial leads.

RIGHT BUNDLE BRANCH BLOCK

Diagnostic Criteria

The diagnosis of uncomplicated complete RBBB is made when the following criteria are met:

1. Prolongation of the QRS duration to 120 ms or more.

2. An rsr', rsR', or rSR' pattern in lead V_1 or V_2. The R' is usually greater than the initial R wave. In a minority of cases, a wide and notched R pattern may be seen.
3. Leads V_6 and I show a QRS complex with a wide S wave (S duration is longer than the R duration or >40 ms in adults).

(See common and uncommon waveforms for RBBB under Step Two, p 298).

ST–T changes in RBBB

In uncomplicated RBBB, the ST–T segment is depressed and the T wave inverted in the right precordial leads with an R' (usually only in lead V_1 but occasionally in V_2). The T wave is upright in leads I, V_5, and V_6.

LEFT BUNDLE BRANCH BLOCK

Diagnostic Criteria

The diagnosis of uncomplicated complete LBBB is made when the following criteria are met:

1. Prolongation of the QRS duration to 120 ms or more.
2. There are broad and notched or slurred R waves in left-sided precordial leads V5 and V6, as well as in leads I and aVL. Occasionally, an RS pattern may occur in leads V5 and V6 in uncomplicated LBBB associated with posterior displacement of the left ventricle.
3. With the possible exception of lead aVL, Q waves are absent in the left-sided leads, specifically in leads V_5, V_6, and I.
4. The R peak time is prolonged to >60 ms in lead V_5 or V_6 but is normal in leads V_1 and V_2 when it can be determined.
5. In the right precordial leads V_1 and V_3, there are small initial r waves in the majority of cases, followed by wide and deep S waves. The transition zone in the precordial leads is displaced to the left. Wide QS complexes may be present in leads V_1 and V_2 and rarely in lead V_3.

(See common and uncommon waveforms for LBBB under Step Two, p 298).

ST–T Changes in LBBB

In uncomplicated LBBB, the ST segments are usually depressed and the T waves inverted in left precordial leads V_5 and V_6 as well as in leads I and aVL. Conversely, ST segment elevations and positive T waves are recorded in leads V_1 and V_2. Only rarely is the T wave upright in the left precordial leads. As a general rule, ST–T changes in LBBB are usually in the direction opposite the direction of the QRS complex (inverted T waves and ST segment depression if the QRS is upright).

D. INCOMPLETE BUNDLE BRANCH BLOCKS

Incomplete LBBB

The waveforms are similar to those in complete LBBB, but the QRS duration is <120 ms. Septal Q waves are absent in I and V_6. Incomplete LBBB is synonymous with LVH and commonly mimics a delta wave in leads V_5 and V_6.

Incomplete RBBB

The waveforms are similar to those in complete RBBB, but the QRS duration is <120 ms. This diagnosis suggests RVH. Occasionally, in a normal variant pattern, there is an rSr' waveform in lead V_1. In this case, the r' is usually smaller than the initial r wave; this pattern is not indicative of incomplete RBBB.

Intraventricular Conduction Delay or Defect

If the QRS duration is ≥120 ms but typical waveforms of either RBBB or LBBB are not present, there is an intraventricular conduction delay or defect (IVCD). This pattern is common in dilated cardiomyopathy. An IVCD with a QRS duration of ≥170 ms is highly predictive of dilated cardiomyopathy.

E. FASCICULAR BLOCKS (HEMIBLOCKS)

1. LEFT ANTERIOR FASCICULAR BLOCK (LAFB)

Diagnostic Criteria

1. Mean QRS axis from –45 degrees to –90 degrees (possibly –31 to –44 degrees).
2. A qR pattern in lead aVL, with the R peak time, ie, the onset of the Q wave to the peak of the R wave ≥45 ms (slightly more than one small box wide), as shown below.

Clinical correlations: hypertensive heart disease, coronary artery disease, or idiopathic conducting system disease.

2. LEFT POSTERIOR FASCICULAR BLOCK (LPFB)

Diagnostic Criteria

1. Mean QRS axis from +90 degrees to +180 degrees.
2. A qR complex in leads III and aVF, an rS complex in leads aVL and I, with a Q wave ≥40 ms in the inferior leads.

Clinical correlations: LPFB is a diagnosis of exclusion. It may be seen in the acute phase of inferior myocardial injury or infarction or may result from idiopathic conducting system disease.

F. DETERMINATION OF THE MEAN QRS AXIS

The mean electrical axis is the average direction of the activation or repolarization process during the cardiac cycle. Instantaneous and mean electrical axes may be determined for any deflection (P, QRS, ST–T) in the three planes (frontal, transverse, and sagittal). The determination of the electrical axis of a QRS complex is useful for the diagnosis of certain pathologic cardiac conditions.

The Mean QRS Axis in the Frontal Plane (Limb Leads)

Arzbaecher developed the **hexaxial reference system** that allowed for the display of the relationships among the six frontal plane (limb) leads. A diagram of this system is shown below.

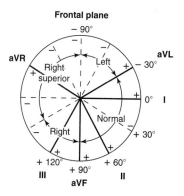

Frontal plane

The normal range of the QRS axis in adults is −30 degrees to +90 degrees.

It is rarely important to precisely determine the degrees of the mean QRS. However, the recognition of abnormal axis deviations is critical because it leads to a presumption of disease. The mean QRS axis is derived from the net area under the QRS curves. The most efficient method of determining the mean QRS axis uses the method of Grant, which requires only leads I and II (see below). If the net area under the QRS curves in these leads is positive, the axis falls between −30 degrees and +90 degrees, which is the normal range of axis in adults. (The only exception to this rule is in RBBB, in which the first 60 ms of the QRS is used. Alternatively, one may use the maximal amplitude of the R and S waves in leads I and II to assess the axis in RBBB.) Abnormal axes are shown below.

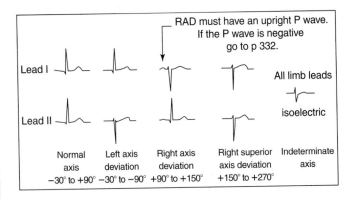

RAD must have an upright P wave. If the P wave is negative go to p 332.

	Lead I	Lead II	
Normal axis	−30° to +90°		
Left axis deviation	−30° to −90°		
Right axis deviation	+90° to +150°		
Right superior axis deviation	+150° to +270°		
Indeterminate axis	All limb leads isoelectric		

Left Axis Deviation (LAD)

The four main causes of left axis deviation are as follows:

A. **Left Anterior Fascicular Block (LAFB):** See criteria above.

B. **Inferior Myocardial Infarction:** There is a pathologic Q wave ≥30 ms either in lead aVF or lead II in the absence of ventricular pre-excitation.

C. **Ventricular Preexcitation (WPW Pattern):** LAD is seen with inferior paraseptal accessory pathway locations. This can mimic inferoposterior myocardial infarction. The classic definition of the Wolff-Parkinson-White (WPW) pattern includes a short PR interval (<120 ms); an initial slurring of the QRS complex, called a delta wave; and prolongation of the QRS complex to >120 ms. However, because this pattern may not always be present despite the presence of ventricular preexcitation, a more practical definition is an absent PR segment and an initial slurring of the QRS complex in any lead. The diagnosis of the WPW pattern usually requires sinus rhythm.

D. COPD: LAD is seen in 10% of patients with COPD.

Right Axis Deviation (RAD)

The four main causes of right axis deviation (RAD) are as follows:

A. Right Ventricular Hypertrophy: This is the most common cause (refer to diagnostic criteria, below). However, one must first exclude acute occlusion of the posterior descending coronary artery, causing LPFB, and exclude also items B and C below.

B. Extensive Lateral and Apical Myocardial Infarction: Criteria include QS or Qr patterns in leads I and aVL and in leads V_{4-6}.

C. Ventricular Preexcitation (WPW Pattern): RAD seen with left lateral accessory pathway locations. This can mimic lateral myocardial infarction.

D. Left Posterior Fascicular Block (LPFB): This is a diagnosis of exclusion (see criteria above).

Right Superior Axis Deviation

This category is rare. Causes include RVH, apical myocardial infarction, VT, and hyperkalemia. Right superior axis deviation may rarely be seen as an atypical form of LAFB.

G. VENTRICULAR HYPERTROPHY

1. LEFT VENTRICULAR HYPERTROPHY

The ECG is very insensitive as a screening tool for LVH, but electrocardiographic criteria are usually specific. Echocardiography is the major resource for this diagnosis.

The best electrocardiographic criterion for the diagnosis of LVH is the Cornell voltage, the sum of the R wave amplitude in lead aVL and the S wave depth in lead V_3, adjusted for sex:

1. RaVL + SV_3 >20 mm (females), >25 mm (males). The R wave height in aVL alone is a good place to start.
2. RaVL >9 mm (females), >11 mm (males).

Alternatively, application of the following criteria will diagnose most cases of LVH.

3. Sokolow-Lyon criteria: $SV_1 + RV_5$ or RV_6 (whichever R wave is taller) >35 mm (in patients age >35).
4. Romhilt-Estes criteria: Points are scored for QRS voltage (1 point), the presence of LAE (1 point), typical repolarization abnormalities in the absence of digitalis (1 point), and a few other findings. The combination of LAE (see above) and typical repolarization abnormalities (see below) (score ≥5 points) will suffice for the diagnosis of LVH even when voltage criteria are not met.
5. $RV_6 > RV_5$ (usually occurs with dilated LV). First exclude anterior myocardial infarction and establish that the R waves in V_5 are >7 mm tall and that in V_6 they are >6 mm tall before using this criterion.

Repolarization Abnormalities

Typical repolarization abnormalities in the presence of LVH are an ominous sign of end-organ damage. In repolarization abnormalities in LVH, the ST segment and T wave are directed opposite to the dominant QRS waveform in all leads. However, this directional rule does not apply either in the transitional lead (defined as a lead having an R wave height equal to the S wave depth) or in the transitional zone (defined as leads adjacent to the transitional lead) or one lead to the left in the precordial leads.

Spectrum of Repolarization Abnormalities

The waveforms below, usually seen in leads I, aVL, V_5, and V_6 but more specifically in leads with dominant R waves, represent hypothetical stages in the progression of LVH.

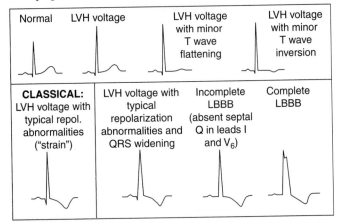

Normal	LVH voltage	LVH voltage with minor T wave flattening	LVH voltage with minor T wave inversion
CLASSICAL: LVH voltage with typical repol. abnormalities ("strain")	LVH voltage with typical repolarization abnormalities and QRS widening	Incomplete LBBB (absent septal Q in leads I and V_6)	Complete LBBB

2. RIGHT VENTRICULAR HYPERTROPHY (RVH)

The ECG is insensitive for the diagnosis of RVH. In 100 cases of RVH from one echocardiography laboratory, only 33% had RAD because of the confounding effects of LV disease. Published electrocardiographic criteria for RVH are listed below, all of which have $\geq 97\%$ specificity.

With rare exceptions, right atrial enlargement is synonymous with RVH.

Diagnostic Criteria

Recommended criteria for the electrocardiographic diagnosis of RVH are as follows:

1. Right axis deviation (> 90 degrees), or
2. An R/S ratio ≥ 1 in lead V_1 (absent posterior MI or RBBB), or
3. An R wave >7 mm tall in V_1 (not the R′ of RBBB), or
4. An rsR′ complex in V_1 (R′ ≥ 10 mm), with a QRS duration of <0.12 s (incomplete RBBB), or
5. An S wave >7 mm deep in leads V_5 or V_6 (in the absence of a QRS axis more negative than +30 degrees), or
6. RBBB with RAD (axis derived from first 60 ms of the QRS). (Consider RVH in RBBB if the R/S ratio in lead I is <0.5.)

A variant of RVH (type C loop) may produce a false-positive sign of an anterior myocardial infarction.

Repolarization Abnormalities

The morphology of repolarization abnormalities in RVH is identical to those in LVH, when a particular lead contains tall R waves reflecting the hypertrophied RV or LV. In RVH, these typically occur in leads V_{1-2} or V_3 and in leads aVF and III. This morphology of repolarization abnormalities due to ventricular hypertrophy is illustrated above. In cases of RVH with massive dilation, all precordial leads may overlie the diseased RV and may exhibit repolarization abnormalities.

H. LOW VOLTAGE OF THE QRS COMPLEX

Low-Voltage Limb Leads Only

Defined as peak-to-peak QRS voltage <5 mm in all limb leads.

Low-Voltage Limb and Precordial Leads

Defined as peak-to-peak QRS voltage <5 mm in all limb leads and <10 mm in all precordial leads. Primary myocardial causes include multiple or massive infarctions; infiltrative diseases such as amyloidosis, sarcoidosis, or hemochromatosis; and myxedema. Extracardiac causes include pericardial effusion, COPD, pleural effusion, obesity, anasarca, and subcutaneous emphysema. When there is COPD, expect to see low voltage in the limb leads as well as in leads V_5 and V_6.

I. PROGRESSION OF THE R WAVE IN THE PRECORDIAL LEADS

The normal R wave height increases from V_1 to V_5. The normal R wave height in V_5 is always taller than that in V_6 because of the attenuating effect of the lungs. The normal R wave height in lead V_3 is usually >2 mm.

"Poor R Wave Progression"

The term "poor R wave progression" (PRWP) is a nonpreferred term because most physicians use this term to imply the presence of an anterior myocardial infarction, although it may not be present. Other causes of small R waves in the right precordial leads include LVH, LAFB, LBBB, cor pulmonale (with the type C loop of RVH), and COPD.

Reversed R Wave Progression (RRWP)

Reversed R wave progression is defined as a loss of R wave height between leads V_1 and V_2 or between leads V_2 and V_3 or between leads V_3 and V_4. In the absence of LVH, this finding suggests anterior myocardial infarction or precordial lead reversal.

J. TALL R WAVES IN THE RIGHT PRECORDIAL LEADS

Etiology

Causes of tall R waves in the right precordial leads include the following:

A. Right Ventricular Hypertrophy: This is the most common cause. There is an R/S ratio ≥ 1 or an R wave height >7 mm in lead V_1.

B. Posterior Myocardial Infarction: There is an R wave ≥ 6 mm in lead V_1 or ≥ 15 mm in lead V_2. One should distinguish the tall R wave of RVH from the tall R wave of posterior myocardial infarction in lead V_1. In RVH, there is a downsloping ST segment and an inverted T wave, usually with right axis deviation. In contrast, in posterior myocardial infarction, there is usually an upright, commonly tall T wave and, because posterior myocardial infarction is usually associated with concomitant inferior myocardial infarction, a left axis deviation.

C. **Right Bundle Branch Block:** The QRS duration is prolonged, and typical waveforms are present (see above).

D. **The WPW Pattern:** Left-sided accessory pathway locations produce prominent R waves with an R/S ratio ≥ 1 in V_1, with an absent PR segment and initial slurring of the QRS complex, usually best seen in lead V_4.

E. **Rare or Uncommon Causes:** The normal variant pattern of early precordial QRS transition (not uncommon); the reciprocal effect of a deep Q wave in leads V_{5-6} (very rare); Duchenne muscular dystrophy dextrocardia (very rare); chronic constrictive pericarditis (very rare); and reversal of the right precordial leads.

K. MYOCARDIAL INJURY, ISCHEMIA, AND INFARCTION

Definitions

A. **Myocardial Infarction:** Pathologic changes in the QRS complex reflect ventricular activation away from the area of infarction.

B. **Myocardial Injury:** Injury always points *outward* from the surface that is injured.

   1. **Epicardial injury:** ST elevation in the distribution of an acutely occluded artery.

   2. **Endocardial injury:** Diffuse ST segment depression, which is really reciprocal to the primary event, reflected as ST elevation in aVR.

C. **Myocardial Ischemia:** Diffuse ST segment depression, usually with associated T wave inversion. It usually reflects subendocardial injury, reciprocal to ST elevation in lead aVR. In ischemia, there may only be inverted T waves with a symmetric, sharp nadir.

D. **Reciprocal Changes:** Passive electrical reflections of a primary event viewed from either the other side of the heart, as in epicardial injury, or the other side of the ventricular wall, as in subendocardial injury.

Steps in the Diagnosis of Myocardial Infarction

The following pages contain a systematic method for the electrocardiographic diagnosis of myocardial injury or infarction, arranged in seven steps. Following the steps will achieve the diagnosis in most cases.

Step 1: Identify the presence of myocardial injury by ST segment deviations.

Step 2: Identify areas of myocardial injury by assessing lead groupings.

Step 3: Define the primary area of involvement and identify the culprit artery producing the injury.

Step 4: Identify the location of the lesion in the artery to risk stratify the patient.

Step 5: Identify any electrocardiographic signs of infarction found in the QRS complexes.

Step 6: Determine the age of the infarction by assessing the location of the ST segment in leads with pathologic QRS abnormalities.

Step 7: Combine all observations into a final diagnosis.

STEPS ONE AND TWO

Identify presence of and areas of myocardial injury.

The GUSTO study of patients with ST segment elevation in two contiguous leads defined four affected areas as set out in Table 7–3.

Two other major areas of possible injury or infarction were not included in the GUSTO categorization because they do not produce ST elevation in two contiguous standard leads. These are:

1. **Posterior Injury:** The most commonly used sign of posterior injury is ST depression in leads V_{1-3}, but posterior injury may best be diagnosed by obtaining posterior leads V_7, V_8, and V_9.

2. **Right Ventricular Injury:** The most sensitive sign of right ventricular injury, ST segment elevation ≥ 1 mm, is found in lead V_4R. A very specific—but insensitive—sign of right ventricular injury or infarction is ST elevation in V_1, with concomitant ST segment depression in V_2 in the setting of ST elevation in the inferior leads.

STEP THREE

Identify the primary area of involvement and the culprit artery.

Primary Anterior Area

ST elevation in two contiguous V_{1-4} leads defines a primary anterior area of involvement. The left anterior descending coronary artery (LAD) is the culprit artery. Lateral (I and aVL) and apical (V_5 and V_6) areas are contiguous

TABLE 7–3. GUSTO STUDY DEFINITIONS.

Area of ST Segment Elevation	Leads Defining This Area
Anterior (Ant)	V_{1-4}
Apical (Ap)	V_{5-6}
Lateral (Lat)	I, aVL
Inferior (Inf)	II, aVF, III

to anterior (V_{1-4}), so ST elevation in these leads signifies more myocardium at risk and more adverse outcomes.

Primary Inferior Area

ST segment elevation in two contiguous leads (II, aVF, or III) defines a primary inferior area of involvement. The right coronary artery (RCA) is usually the culprit artery. Apical (V_5 and V_6), posterior (V_{1-3} or V_{7-9}) and right ventricular (V_4R) areas are contiguous to inferior (II, aVF, and III), so ST elevation in these contiguous leads signifies more myocardium at risk and more adverse outcomes (see below).

The Culprit Artery

In the GUSTO trial, 98% of patients with ST segment elevation in any two contiguous V_{1-4} leads, either alone or with associated changes in leads V_{5-6} or I and aVL, had LAD obstruction. In patients with ST segment elevation only in leads II, aVF, and III, there was RCA obstruction in 86%.

PRIMARY ANTERIOR PROCESS

Acute occlusion of the LAD produces a sequence of changes in the anterior leads (V_{1-4}).

Earliest Findings

A. "Hyperacute" Changes: ST elevation with loss of normal ST segment concavity, commonly with tall, peaked T waves.

B. Acute Injury: ST elevation, with the ST segment commonly appearing as if a thumb has been pushed up into it.

Evolutionary Changes

A patient who presents to the emergency department with chest pain and T wave inversion in leads with pathologic Q waves is most likely to be in the evolutionary or completed phase of infarction. Successful revascularization usually causes prompt resolution of the acute signs of injury or infarction and results in the electrocardiographic signs of a fully evolved infarction. The tracing below shows QS complexes in lead V_2.

A. **Development of Pathologic Q Waves (Infarction):** Pathologic Q waves develop within the first hour after onset of symptoms in at least 30% of patients.

QS complexes
V_2 shown

day 1

B. **ST Segment Elevation Decreases:** T wave inversion usually occurs in the second 24-hour period after infarction.

day 2

C. **Fully Evolved Pattern:** Pathologic Q waves, ST segment rounded upward, T waves inverted.

chronic

PRIMARY INFERIOR PROCESS

A primary inferior process usually develops after acute occlusion of the RCA, producing changes in the inferior leads (II, III, and aVF).

Earliest Findings

The earliest findings are of acute injury (ST segment elevation). The J point may "climb up the back" of the R wave (a), or the ST segment may rise up into the T wave (b).

Evolutionary Changes

ST segment elevation decreases and pathologic Q waves develop. T wave inversion may occur in the first 12 hours of an inferior myocardial infarction—in contrast to that in anterior myocardial infarction.

Right Ventricular Injury or Infarction

With right ventricular injury, there is ST segment elevation, best seen in lead V_4R. With right ventricular infarction, there is a QS complex.

For comparison, the normal morphology of the QRS complex in lead V_4R is shown below. The normal J point averages +0.2 mm.

POSTERIOR INJURY OR INFARCTION

Posterior injury or infarction is commonly due to acute occlusion of the left circumflex coronary artery, producing changes in the posterior leads (V_7, V_8, V_9) or reciprocal ST segment depression in leads V_{1-3}.

Acute Pattern

Acute posterior injury or infarction is shown by ST segment depression in V_{1-3} and perhaps also V_4, usually with upright (often prominent) T waves.

V_2 or V_3 V_2

Chronic Pattern

Chronic posterior injury or infarction is shown by pathologic R waves with prominent tall T waves in leads V_{1-3}.

V_2

STEP FOUR

Identify the location of the lesion within the artery to risk stratify the patient.

Primary Anterior Process

Aside from an acute occlusion of the left main coronary artery, occlusion of the proximal LAD conveys the most adverse outcomes. Four electrocardiographic signs indicate proximal LAD occlusion:

1. ST elevation >1 mm in lead I, in lead aVL, or in both
2. New RBBB
3. New LAFB
4. New first-degree AV block

If the occlusion occurs in a more distal portion of the LAD (after the first diagonal branch and after the first septal perforator), ST segment elevation is observed in the anterior leads but the four criteria described above are not seen. In patients with occlusion of the left main coronary artery, diffuse endocardial injury leads to ST segment elevation in aVR, because this is the only lead that "looks" directly at the ventricular endocardium, and diffuse ST segment depression is observed in the anterior and inferior leads.

Primary Inferior Process

Nearly 50% of patients with inferior myocardial infarction have distinguishing features that may produce complications or adverse outcomes unless successfully managed:

1. Precordial ST segment depression in V_{1-3} (suggests concomitant posterior wall involvement);
2. Right ventricular injury or infarction (identifies a proximal RCA lesion);
3. AV block (implies a greater amount of involved myocardium);
4. The sum of ST segment depressions in leads V_{4-6} exceeds the sum of ST segment depressions in leads V_{1-3} (suggests multivessel disease).

Reciprocal Changes in the Setting of Acute Myocardial Infarction

ST depressions in leads remote from the primary site of injury are felt to be a purely reciprocal change. With successful reperfusion, the ST depressions usually resolve. If they persist, patients more likely have significant three-vessel disease and so-called ischemia at a distance. Mortality rates are higher in such patients.

STEP FIVE

Identify Electrocardiographic Signs of Infarction in the QRS Complexes

The 12-lead ECG shown below contains numbers corresponding to pathologic widths for Q waves and R waves for selected leads (see Table 7–4 for more complete criteria).

One can memorize the above criteria by mastering a simple scheme of numbers that represent the durations of pathological Q waves or R waves. Begin with lead V_1 and repeat the numbers in the box below in the following order. The numbers increase from "any" to 50.

TABLE 7–4. DIAGNOSIS OF MYOCARDIAL INFARCTION.[1]

Infarct Location	ECG Lead	Criterion	Sensitivity	Specificity	Likelihood Ratio (+)	Likelihood Ratio (−)
Inferior	II	Q ≥ 30 ms	45	98	22.5	0.6
	aVF	Q ≥ 30 ms	70	94	11.7	0.3
		Q ≥ 40 ms	40	98	20.0	0.6
		R/Q ≤ 1	50	98	25.0	0.5
Anterior	V₁	Any Q	50	97	16.7	0.5
	V₂	Any Q, or R ≤ 0.1 mV and R ≤ 10 ms, or RV₂ ≤ RV₁	80	94	13.3	0.2
	V₃	Any Q, or R ≤ 0.2 mV, or R ≤ 20 ms	70	93	10.0	0.3
	V₄	Q ≥ 20 ms	40	92	5.0	0.9
		R/Q ≤ 0.5, or R/S ≤ 0.5	40	97	13.3	0.6
Anterolateral (lateral)						
	I	Q ≥ 30 ms R/Q ≤ 1, or R ≤ 2 mm	10 10	98 97	5.0 3.3	0.9 0.9
	aVL	Q ≥ 30 ms	7	97	0.7	1.0
		R/Q ≤ 1	2			
Apical	V₅	Q ≥ 30	5	99	5.0	1.0
		R/Q ≤ 2, or R ≤ 7 mm, or R/S ≤ 2, or notched R	60	91	6.7	0.4
		R/Q ≤ 1, or R/S ≤ 1	25	98	12.5	0.8
	V₆	Q ≤ 30	3	98	1.5	1.0
		R/Q ≤ 3, or R ≤ 6 mm, or R/S ≤ 3, or notched R	40	92	25.0	0.7
		R/Q ≤ 1, or R/S ≤ 1	10	99	10.0	0.9

TABLE 7–4 (CONTINUED).

Infarct Location	ECG Lead	Criterion	Sensitivity	Specificity	Likelihood Ratio (+)	Likelihood Ratio (−)
Posterolateral						
	V_1	R/S ≤ 1	15	97	5.0	0.9
		R ≥ 6 mm, or R ≥ 40 ms	20	93	2.9	0.9
		S ≤ 3 mm	8	97	2.7	0.9
	V_2	R ≥ 15 mm, or R ≥ 50 ms	15	95	3.0	0.9
		R/S ≥ 1.5	10	96	2.5	0.9
		S ≤ 4 mm	2	97	0.7	1.0

[1] Reproduced, with permission, from Haisty WK Jr et al: Performance of the automated complete Selvester QRS scoring system in normal subjects and patients with single and multiple myocardial infarctions. *J Am Coll Cardiol* 1992;19:341.

Key: Notched R = a notch that begins within the first 40 ms of the R wave; Q = Q wave; R/Q = ratio of R wave height to Q wave depth; R = R wave; R/S ratio = ratio of R wave height to S wave depth; $RV_2 ≤ RV_1$ = R wave height in V_2 less than or equal to that in V_1; S = S wave.

Any	Q wave in lead V_1, for anterior MI
Any	Q wave in lead V_2, for anterior MI
Any	Q wave in lead V_3, for anterior MI
20	Q wave ≥ 20 ms in lead V_4, for anterior MI
30	Q wave ≥ 30 ms in lead V_5, for apical MI
30	Q wave ≥ 30 ms in lead V_6, for apical MI

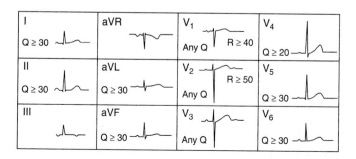

30	Q wave ≥ 30 ms in lead I, for lateral MI
30	Q wave ≥ 30 ms in lead aVL, for lateral MI
30	Q wave ≥ 30 ms in lead II, for inferior MI
30	Q wave ≥ 30 ms in lead aVF, for inferior MI
R40	R wave ≥ 40 ms in lead V_1, for posterior MI
R50	R wave ≥ 50 ms in lead V_2, for posterior MI

Test Performance Characteristics for Electrocardiographic Criteria in the Diagnosis of Myocardial Infarction

Haisty and coworkers studied 1344 patients with normal hearts documented by coronary arteriography and 837 patients with documented myocardial infarction (366 inferior, 277 anterior, 63 posterior, and 131 inferior and anterior) (Table 7–4). (Patients with LVH, LAFB, LPFB, RVH, LBBB, RBBB, COPD, or WPW patterns were excluded from analysis because these conditions can give false-positive results for myocardial infarction.) Shown above are the sensitivity, specificity, and likelihood ratios for the best-performing infarct criteria. Notice that leads III and aVR are not listed: lead III may normally have a Q wave that is both wide and deep, and lead aVR commonly has a wide Q wave.

Mimics of Myocardial Infarction

Conditions that can produce pathologic Q waves, ST segment elevation, or loss of R wave height in the absence of infarction are set out in Table 7–5.

TABLE 7–5. MIMICS OF MYOCARDIAL INFARCTION.

Condition	Pseudoinfarct Location
WPW pattern	Any, most commonly inferoposterior or lateral
Hypertrophic cardiomyopathy	Lateral apical (18%), inferior (11%)
LBBB	Anteroseptal, anterolateral, inferior
RBBB	Inferior, posterior (using criteria from leads V_1 and V_2), anterior
LVH	Anterior, inferior
LAFB	Anterior (may cause a tiny Q in V_2)
COPD	Inferior, posterior, anterior
RVH	Inferior, posterior (using criteria from leads V_1 and V_2), anterior, or apical (using criteria for R/S ratios from leads V_{4-6})
Acute cor pulmonale	Inferior, possibly anterior
Cardiomyopathy (nonischemic)	Any, most commonly inferior (with IVCD pattern), less commonly anterior
Chest deformity	Any
Left pneumothorax	Anterior, anterolateral
Hyperkalemia	Any
Normal hearts	Posterior, anterior

STEP SIX

Determine the Age of the Infarction

An **acute infarction** manifests ST segment elevation in a lead with a pathologic Q wave. The T waves may be either upright or inverted.

An **old** or **age-indeterminate infarction** manifests a pathologic Q wave, with or without slight ST segment elevation or T wave abnormalities.

Persistent ST segment elevation ≥1 mm after a myocardial infarction is a sign of dyskinetic wall motion in the area of infarct. Half of these patients have ventricular aneurysms.

STEP SEVEN

Combine Observations Into a Final Diagnosis

There are two possibilities for the major electrocardiographic diagnosis: myocardial infarction or acute injury. If there are pathologic changes in the QRS complex, one should make a diagnosis of myocardial infarction—beginning with the primary area, followed by any contiguous areas—and state the age of the infarction. If there are no pathologic changes in the QRS complex, one should make a diagnosis of acute injury of the affected segments—beginning with the primary area and followed by any contiguous areas.

L. ST SEGMENTS

Table 7–6 summarizes major causes of ST segment elevations. Table 7–7 summarizes major causes of ST segment depressions or T wave inversions. The various classes and morphologies of ST–T waves as seen in lead V_2 are shown in Table 7–8.

M. U WAVES

Normal U Waves

In many normal hearts, low-amplitude positive U waves <1.5 mm tall that range from 160–200 ms in duration are seen in leads V_2 or V_3. Leads V_2 and V_3 are close to the ventricular mass and small-amplitude signals may be best seen in these leads.

Cause: Bradycardias.

TABLE 7–6. MAJOR CAUSES OF ST SEGMENT ELEVATION.

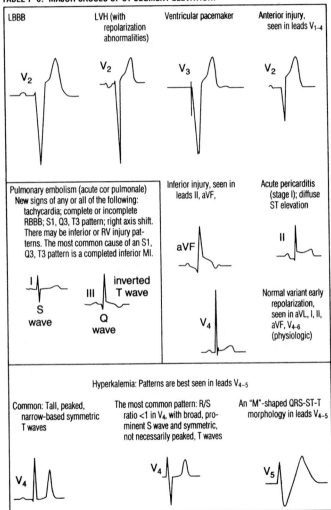

TABLE 7–7. MAJOR CAUSES OF ST SEGMENT DEPRESSION OR T WAVE INVERSION.

Whenever the ST segment or the T wave is directed counter to an expected repolarization abnormality, consider ischemia, healed MI, or drug or electrolyte effect.	In RBBB, there is an obligatory inverted T wave in right precordial leads with an R' (usually only in V_1) or its equivalent (a qR complex in septal MI). An upright T in these leads suggests completed posterior MI.	Altered depolarization RBBB V_1
LBBB V_5	LVH (with repolarization abnormality) V_6	Subarachnoid hemorrhage V_4	RVH **RVH** V_{1-3}
Inferior subendocardial injury II	Posterior subepicardial injury V_2	Anterior subendocardial injury or non-Q wave MI V_5	V_4
Hypokalemia V_4	Digitalis V_4	Antiarrhythmics V_4	J point depression secondary to catecholamines II
When $K^+ \leq 2.8$, 80% have ECG changes			PR interval and ST segment occupy the same curve

TABLE 7–8. VARIOUS CLASSES AND MORPHOLOGIES OF ST-T WAVES AS SEEN IN LEAD V$_2$.[1]

	Normal ST segment (asymmetric upsloping ST segment with concavity, slight ST segment elevation)
	Abnormal ST segment elevation or lack of normal upward concavity in the first part of the ST-T segment (as seen in LVH or acute ischemia or injury)
	ST-T segment typical of acute or recent myocardial infarction, ie, the ST-T segment appears as though a thumb were pushed up into it
	Negative amplitudes in the latter part of the ST-T segment (may be seen in ischemia or old infarction)
	Negative T wave (may be a nonspecific sign, but may be seen in ischemia or old MI)
	Downward sloping in the first part of the ST-T segment (consider ischemia, digitalis, or hypokalemia)
	Flat ST-T segment (a nonspecific sign)

Nonspecific ST segment or T wave abnormalities
By definition, nonspecific abnormalities of either the ST segment (ones that are only slightly depressed or abnormal in contour) or T wave (ones that are either 10% the height of the R wave that produced it, or are either flat or slightly inverted) do not conform to the characteristic waveforms found above or elsewhere.

[1] *Adapted from Edenbrandt L, Devine B, Macfarlane PW: Classification of electrocardiographic ST-T segments—human expert vs. artificial neural network. J Electrocardiol 1992;25:167.*

Abnormal U Waves

Abnormal U waves have increased amplitude or merge with abnormal T waves and produce T–U fusion. Criteria include an amplitude ≥1.5 mm or a U wave that is as tall as the T wave that immediately precedes it.

Causes: Hypokalemia, digitalis, antiarrhythmic drugs.

Inverted U Waves

These are best seen in leads V_{4-6}.

Causes: LVH, acute ischemia.

Table 7–9 summarizes various classes and morphologies of ST–T–U abnormalities as seen in lead V_4.

N. QT INTERVAL

A prolonged QT interval conveys adverse outcomes. The QT interval is inversely related to the heart rate. QT interval corrections for heart rate often use Bazett's formula, defined as the observed QT interval divided by the square root of the R–R interval in seconds. A corrected QT interval of ≥440 ms is abnormal.

Use of the QT Nomogram (Hodges Correction)

Measure the QT interval in either lead V_2 or V_3, where the end of the T wave can usually be clearly distinguished from the beginning of the U wave. If the rate is regular, use the mean rate of the QRS complexes. If the rate is irregular, calculate the rate from the immediately prior R-R cycle, because this cycle determines the subsequent QT interval. Use the numbers you have obtained to classify the QT interval using the nomogram on p 331. Or remember that at heart rates of ≥40 bpm, an observed QT interval ≥480 ms is abnormal.

Prolonged QT Interval

The four major causes of a prolonged QT interval are as follows:

A. **Electrolyte Abnormalities:** Hypokalemia, hypocalcemia
B. **Drugs:** Also associated with torsade de pointes.
   Class Ia antiarrhythmic agents: Quinidine, procainamide, disopyramide
   Class Ic agents: Propafenone
   Class III agents: Amiodarone, bretylium, N-acetylprocainamide, sotalol

**TABLE 7–9. VARIOUS CLASSES AND MORPHOLOGIES OF ST-T-U ABNORMALITIES
AS SEEN IN LEAD V₄.**

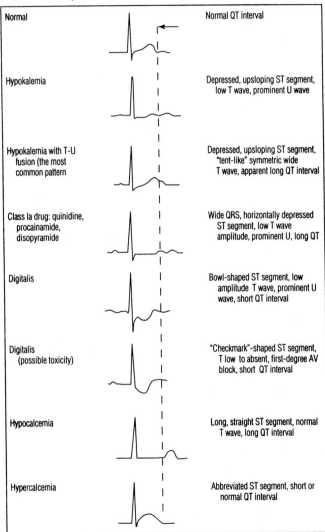

Normal	Normal QT interval
Hypokalemia	Depressed, upsloping ST segment, low T wave, prominent U wave
Hypokalemia with T-U fusion (the most common pattern)	Depressed, upsloping ST segment, "tent-like" symmetric wide T wave, apparent long QT interval
Class Ia drug: quinidine, procainamide, disopyramide	Wide QRS, horizontally depressed ST segment, low T wave amplitude, prominent U, long QT
Digitalis	Bowl-shaped ST segment, low amplitude T wave, prominent U wave, short QT interval
Digitalis (possible toxicity)	"Checkmark"-shaped ST segment, T low to absent, first-degree AV block, short QT interval
Hypocalcemia	Long, straight ST segment, normal T wave, long QT interval
Hypercalcemia	Abbreviated ST segment, short or normal QT interval

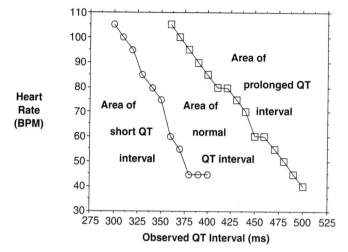

Antibiotics: Erythromycin, trimethoprim-sulfamethoxazole

Antifungals: Ketoconazole, itraconazole

Chemotherapeutics: Pentamidine, perhaps anthracyclines

Psychotropic agents: Tricyclic and heterocyclic antidepressants, phenothiazines, haloperidol

Toxins and poisons: Organophosphate insecticides

Miscellaneous: Cisapride, prednisone, probucol, chloral hydrate

C. Congenital Long QT Syndromes: Though rare, a congenital long QT syndrome should be considered in any young patient who presents with syncope or presyncope.

D. Miscellaneous Causes:

Third-degree and sometimes second-degree AV block

At the cessation of ventricular pacing

LVH (usually minor degrees of lengthening)

Myocardial infarction (in the evolutionary stages where there are marked repolarization abnormalities)

Significant active myocardial ischemia

Cerebrovascular accident (subarachnoid hemorrhage)

Hypothermia

Short QT Interval

The four causes of a short QT interval are hypercalcemia, digitalis, thyrotoxicosis, and increased sympathetic tone.

O. MISCELLANEOUS ABNORMALITIES

Right-Left Arm Cable Reversal Versus Mirror Image Dextrocardia

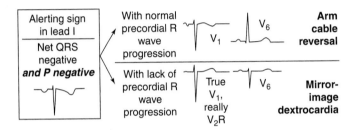

Misplacement of the Right Leg Cable

This error should not occur but it does occur nevertheless. It produces a "far field" signal when one of the bipolar leads (I, II, or III) records the signal between the left and right legs. The lead appears to have no signal except for a tiny deflection representing the QRS complex. There are usually no discernible P waves or T waves. RL–RA cable reversal is shown here.

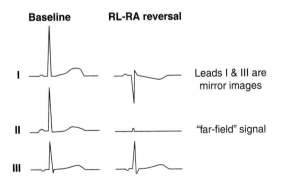

Early Repolarization Normal Variant ST–T Abnormality

Early repolarization normal variant ST-T abnormality

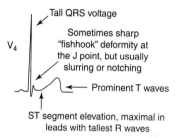

V₄

Tall QRS voltage

Sometimes sharp "fishhook" deformity at the J point, but usually slurring or notching

Prominent T waves

ST segment elevation, maximal in leads with tallest R waves

Hypothermia

Hypothermia is usually characterized on the ECG by a slow rate, a long QT, and muscle tremor artifact. An Osborn wave is typically present.

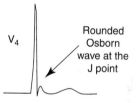

V₄

Rounded Osborn wave at the J point

Acute Pericarditis: Stage I
(With PR Segment Abnormalities)

There is usually widespread ST segment elevation with concomitant PR segment depression in the same leads. The PR segment in aVR protrudes above the baseline like a knuckle, reflecting atrial injury.

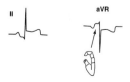

II   aVR

Differentiating Pericarditis From Early Repolarization

Only lead V_6 is used. If the indicated amplitude ratio A/B is $\geq 25\%$, suspect pericarditis. If A/B $< 25\%$, suspect early repolarization.

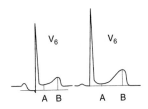

Wolff-Parkinson-White Pattern

The WPW pattern is most commonly manifest as an absent PR segment and initial slurring of the QRS complex in any lead. The lead with the best sensitivity is V_4.

V_4

commonly
tall R waves

A. **Left Lateral Accessory Pathway:** This typical WPW pattern mimics lateral or posterior myocardial infarction.

I, aVL

V_1

B. **Posteroseptal Accessory Pathway:** This typical WPW pattern mimics inferoposterior myocardial infarction.

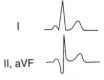

COPD Pattern, Lead II

The P wave amplitude in the inferior leads is equal to that of the QRS complexes.

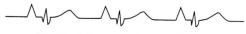

Prominent P waves with low QRS voltage

REFERENCES

Brady WJ et al: Electrocardiographic diagnosis of acute myocardial infarction. Emerg Med Clin North Am 2001; 19:295.

Brugada P et al: A new approach to the differential diagnosis of a regular tachycardia with a wide QRS complex. Circulation 1991; 83:1649.

Channer K et al: ABS of clinical electrocardiography. Myocardial ischemia. BMJ 2002; 324:1023.

Chauhan VS et al: Supraventricular tachycardia. Med Clin North Am 2001; 85:193.

Edhouse J, Morris F: Broad complex tachycardia. Part 1. BMJ 2002; 324:719.

Evans GT Jr: ECG Interpretation Cribsheets, 4th ed. Ring Mountain Press, 1999.

Haisty WK Jr et al: Performance of the automated complete Selvester QRS scoring system in normal subjects and patients with single and multiple myocardial infarctions. J Am Coll Cardiol 1992; 19:341.

Kusumoto FM: Arrhythmias. In *Cardiovascular Pathophysiology*, FM Kusumoto (editor). Fence Creek Publishing, 1999.

8

Diagnostic Algorithms

Stephen J. McPhee, MD, Diana Nicoll, MD, PhD, MPA, and Michael Pignone, MD, MPH

HOW TO USE THIS SECTION

This section contains useful algorithms, arranged alphabetically by subject, for difficult diagnostic challenges. A conventional algorithm layout is displayed below. Diagnostic tests are enclosed in ovals; diagnoses are in bold italics; and treatment recommendations in rectangles.

Abbreviations used throughout this section include the following:

$$
\begin{aligned}
\text{N} &= \text{Normal} \\
\text{Abn} &= \text{Abnormal} \\
\text{Pos} &= \text{Positive} \\
\text{Neg} &= \text{Negative} \\
\text{Occ} &= \text{Occasional} \\
\uparrow &= \text{Increased or high} \\
\downarrow &= \text{Decreased or low}
\end{aligned}
$$

SUSPECTED DIAGNOSIS/CLINICAL SITUATION

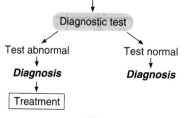

n

Contents

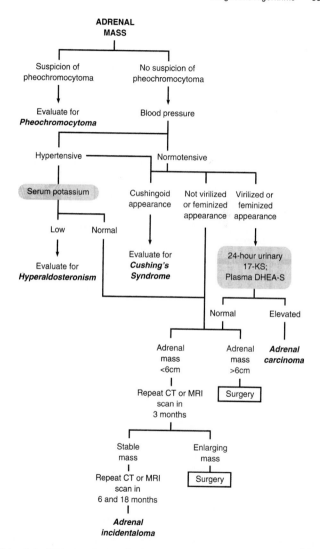

Figure 8–1. ADRENAL MASS: Diagnostic evaluation. **CT** = computed tomography; **DHEA-S** = dehydroepiandrosterone sulfate; **17-KS** = 17-ketosteroids; **MRI** = magnetic resonance imaging. *Modified, with permission, from Greene HL, Johnson WP, Lemcke GE [editors]. Decision-making in Medicine, 2nd ed. Mosby, 1998.)*

ADRENOCORTICAL INSUFFICIENCY SUSPECTED

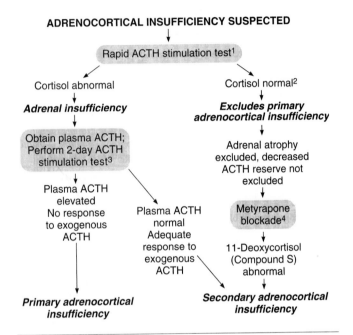

[1] In the rapid ACTH stimulation test, a baseline cortisol sample is obtained; cosyntropin, 10–25 μg, is given IM or IV; and plasma cortisol samples are obtained 30 or 60 minutes later.
[2] The normal response is a cortisol increment >7 μg/dL. If a cortisol level of >18 μg/dL is obtained, the response is normal regardless of the increment.
[3] Administer ACTH, 250 μg IV every 8 hours, as a continuous infusion for 48 hours, and measure daily urinary 17-hydroxycorticosteroids (17-OHCS) or free cortisol excretion and plasma cortisol. Urinary 17-OHCS excretion of >27 mg during the first 24 hours and >47 mg during the second 24 hours is normal. Plasma cortisol >20 μg/dL at 30 or 60 minutes after infusion is begun and >25 μg/dL 6–8 hours later is normal.
[4] Metyrapone blockade is performed by giving 2–2.5 g metyrapone orally at 12 midnight. Draw cortisol and 11-deoxycortisol levels at 8 AM. 11-Deoxycortisol level <7 μg/dL indicates secondary adrenal insufficiency (as long as there is adequate blockade of cortisol synthesis [cortisol level <10 μg/dL]).

Figure 8–2. ADRENOCORTICAL INSUFFICIENCY: Laboratory evaluation of suspected adrenocortical insufficiency. **ACTH** = adrenocorticotropic hormone. *(Modified, with permission, from Baxter JD, Tyrrell JB: The adrenal cortex. In: Endocrinology and Metabolism, 3rd ed. Felig P, Baxter JD, Frohman LA [editors]. McGraw-Hill, 1995; and from Harvey AM et al: The Principles and Practice of Medicine, 22nd ed. Originally published by Appleton & Lange. Copyright © 1988 by The McGraw-Hill Companies, Inc.)*

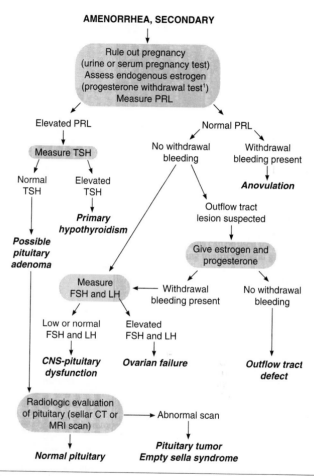

AMENORRHEA, SECONDARY

[1] Give medroxyprogesterone 5–10 mg orally once daily for 5 days. If withdrawal bleeding ensues thereafter, endogenous estrogen is adequate.

Figure 8–3. AMENORRHEA. Diagnostic evaluation of secondary amenorrhea. **PRL** = prolactin; **TSH** = thyroid-stimulating hormone; **FSH** = follicle-stimulating hormone; **LH** = luteinizing hormone; **CT** = computed tomography; **MRI** = magnetic resonance imaging. *(Modified, with permission, from Greenspan FS, Baxter JD [editors]: Basic & Clinical Endocrinology, 4th ed. Originally published by Appleton & Lange. Copyright © 1994 by The McGraw-Hill Companies, Inc.)*

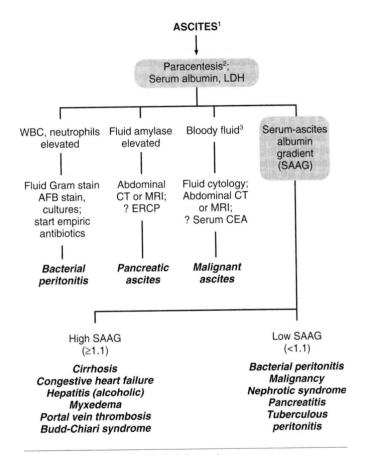

ASCITES[1]

Paracentesis[2];
Serum albumin, LDH

| WBC, neutrophils elevated | Fluid amylase elevated | Bloody fluid[3] | Serum-ascites albumin gradient (SAAG) |

Fluid Gram stain AFB stain, cultures; start empiric antibiotics

Bacterial peritonitis

Abdominal CT or MRI; ? ERCP

Pancreatic ascites

Fluid cytology; Abdominal CT or MRI; ? Serum CEA

Malignant ascites

High SAAG (≥1.1)

Cirrhosis
Congestive heart failure
Hepatitis (alcoholic)
Myxedema
Portal vein thrombosis
Budd-Chiari syndrome

Low SAAG (<1.1)

Bacterial peritonitis
Malignancy
Nephrotic syndrome
Pancreatitis
Tuberculous peritonitis

[1] On physical examination and/or abdominal ultrasound.
[2] Send ascitic fluid for albumin, amylase, glucose, cell count and differential, Gram stain, AFB stain, bacterial and other cultures, and cytology. See Table 9–4 p 364, for interpretation.
[3] On nontraumatic paracentesis.

Figure 8–4. ASCITES: Diagnostic evaluation. **CEA** = carcinoembryonic antigen, serum; **CT** = computed tomography; **ERCP** = endoscopic retrograde cholangiopancreatography; **LDH** = lactate dehydrogenase; **MRI** = magnetic resonance imaging; **SAAG** = serum-ascites albumin gradient;? = consider. *(Modified with permission, from Ferri FF: Clinical Advisor: Instant Diagnosis and Treatment, 4th ed. Mosby, 2002.)*

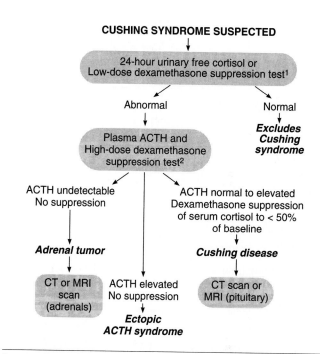

CUSHING SYNDROME SUSPECTED

24-hour urinary free cortisol or
Low-dose dexamethasone suppression test[1]

Abnormal → Plasma ACTH and High-dose dexamethasone suppression test[2]

Normal
Excludes Cushing syndrome

ACTH undetectable
No suppression

Adrenal tumor

CT or MRI scan (adrenals)

ACTH elevated
No suppression

Ectopic ACTH syndrome

ACTH normal to elevated
Dexamethasone suppression
of serum cortisol to < 50%
of baseline

Cushing disease

CT scan or MRI (pituitary)

---

[1] Low dose: Give 1 mg dexamethasone at 11 PM; draw serum cortisol at 8 AM. Normally, AM cortisol is <5 µg/dL.
[2] High dose: Give 8 mg dexamethasone at 11 PM; draw serum cortisol at 8 AM or collect 24-hour urinary free cortisol. Normally, AM cortisol is <5 µg/dL or 24-hour urinary free cortisol is <20 µg.

Figure 8–5. CUSHING SYNDROME: Diagnostic evaluation of Cushing syndrome. **ACTH** = adrenocorticotropic hormone; **CT** = computed tomography; **MRI** = magnetic resonance imaging. *(Modified, with permission, from Baxter JD, Tyrrell JB: The adrenal cortex. In: Endocrinology and Metabolism, 3rd ed. Felig P, Baxter JD, Frohman LA [editors]. McGraw-Hill, 1995; from Harvey AM et al [editors]: The Principles and Practice of Medicine, 22nd ed. Appleton & Lange, 1988; and from Greenspan FS, Baxter JD [editors]: Basic & Clinical Endocrinology, 4th ed. Originally published by Appleton & Lange. Copyright © 1994 by The McGraw-Hill Companies, Inc.)*

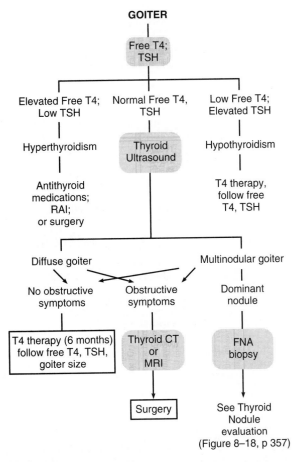

Figure 8–6. GOITER: Diagnostic evaluation and management strategy. **CT** = computed tomography; **FNA** = fine-needle aspiration; **MRI** = magnetic resonance imaging; **RAI** = radioactive iodine; **T4** = L-thyroxine; **TSH** = thyroid-stimulating hormone. *(Modified, with permission, from Goldman L, Bennett JC [editors]. Cecil Textbook of Medicine, 21st ed. Saunders, 2000.)*

HIRSUTISM

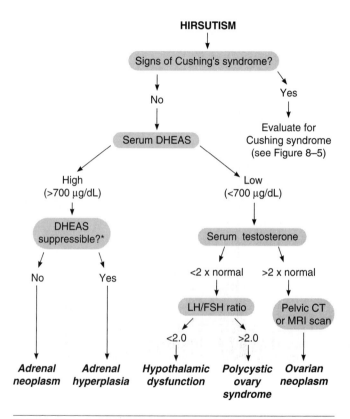

(*DHEAS <170 µg/dL after dexamethasone 0.5 mg orally every 6 hours for 5 days, with DHEAS repeated on the fifth day.)

Figure 8–7. HIRSUTISM: Evaluation of hirsutism in females. Exceptions occur that do not fit this algorithm. **CT** = computed tomography; **DHEAS** = dehydroepiandrosterone sulfate; **FSH** = follicle-stimulating hormone; **LH** = luteinizing hormone. (*Reproduced, with permission, from Fitzgerald PA [editor]:* Handbook of Clinical Endocrinology, *2nd ed. Originally published by Appleton & Lange. Copyright © 1992 by The McGraw-Hill Companies, Inc.*)

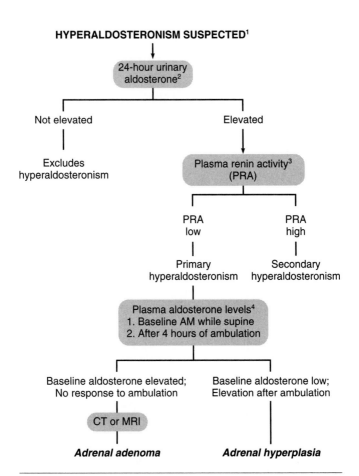

HYPERALDOSTERONISM SUSPECTED[1]

24-hour urinary aldosterone[2]

Not elevated → Excludes hyperaldosteronism

Elevated → Plasma renin activity[3] (PRA)

PRA low → Primary hyperaldosteronism

PRA high → Secondary hyperaldosteronism

Plasma aldosterone levels[4]
1. Baseline AM while supine
2. After 4 hours of ambulation

Baseline aldosterone elevated; No response to ambulation → CT or MRI → **Adrenal adenoma**

Baseline aldosterone low; Elevation after ambulation → **Adrenal hyperplasia**

---

[1] Usually, hypertension plus spontaneous (non-diuretic-related) hypokalemia.
[2] On high-sodium diet (120 meq Na+/d for ≥ 3 days), see p 45.
[3] On low-sodium diet (30–75 meq Na+/d), standing after ambulation, see p 158.
[4] See p 44.

Figure 8–8. HYPERALDOSTERONISM: Laboratory evaluation of suspected hyperaldosteronism. **CT** = computed tomography; **MRI** = magnetic resonance imaging; **PRA** = plasma renin activity. *(Modified, with permission, from Ferri F: Practical Guide to the Care of the Medical Patient, 5th ed. Mosby, 2001.)*

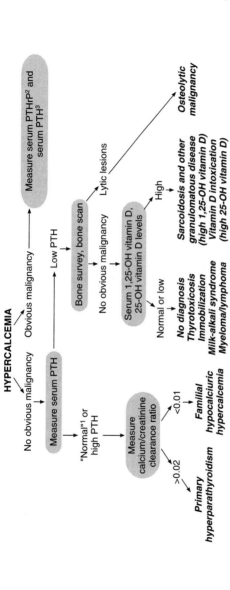

[1] "Normal" PTH in presence of hypercalcemia is inappropriate and indicative of primary hyperparathyroidism (see Parathyroid Hormone and Calcium Nomogram, Figure 10–8, p 416).

[2] PTH-related protein is high in solid tumors that cause hypercalcemia.

[3] To exclude coexistent primary hyperparathyroidism.

Figure 8–9. HYPERCALCEMIA: Diagnostic approach to hypercalcemia. **PTH** = parathyroid hormone. **PTHrP** = parathyroid hormone related protein. (*Modified, with permission, from Harvey AM et al [editors]: The Principles and Practice of Medicine, 22nd ed. Originally published by Appleton & Lange. Copyright © 1988 by The McGraw-Hill Companies, Inc.*)

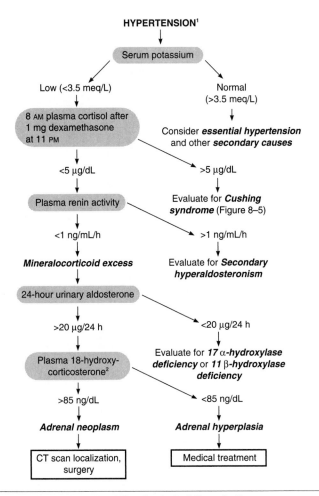

HYPERTENSION[1]

Serum potassium

Low (<3.5 meq/L) → 8 AM plasma cortisol after 1 mg dexamethasone at 11 PM

Normal (>3.5 meq/L) → Consider *essential hypertension* and other *secondary causes*

<5 µg/dL → Plasma renin activity

>5 µg/dL → Evaluate for *Cushing syndrome* (Figure 8–5)

<1 ng/mL/h → *Mineralocorticoid excess*

>1 ng/mL/h → Evaluate for *Secondary hyperaldosteronism*

Mineralocorticoid excess → 24-hour urinary aldosterone

>20 µg/24 h → Plasma 18-hydroxy-corticosterone[2]

<20 µg/24 h → Evaluate for *17 α-hydroxylase deficiency* or *11 β-hydroxylase deficiency*

>85 ng/dL → *Adrenal neoplasm*

<85 ng/dL → *Adrenal hyperplasia*

Adrenal neoplasm → CT scan localization, surgery

Adrenal hyperplasia → Medical treatment

---

[1] Studies are performed during a high-sodium intake (120 meq Na+/d).
[2] In addition, plasma aldosterone may be measured at 8 AM supine after overnight recumbency and after 4 hours of upright posture. See p 44.

Figure 8–10. HYPERTENSION WITH HYPOKALEMIA: Evaluation of secondary causes of hypertension associated with hypokalemia. *(Reproduced, with permission, from Fitzgerald PA [editor]: Handbook of Clinical Endocrinology, 2nd ed. Originally published by Appleton & Lange. Copyright © 1992 by The McGraw-Hill Companies, Inc.)*

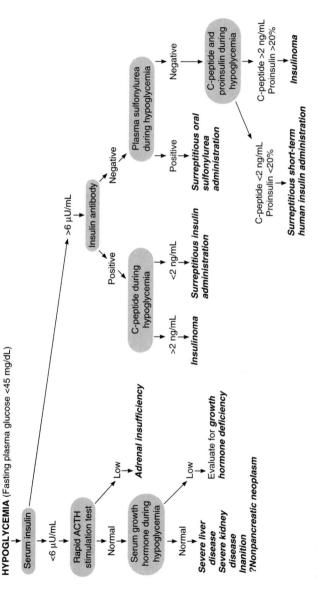

Figure 8–11. HYPOGLYCEMIA: Evaluation of fasting hypoglycemia in adults. *(Reproduced, with permission, from Fitzgerald PA [editor]: Handbook of Clinical Endocrinology, 2nd ed. Originally published by Appleton & Lange. Copyright © 1992 by The McGraw-Hill Companies, Inc.)*

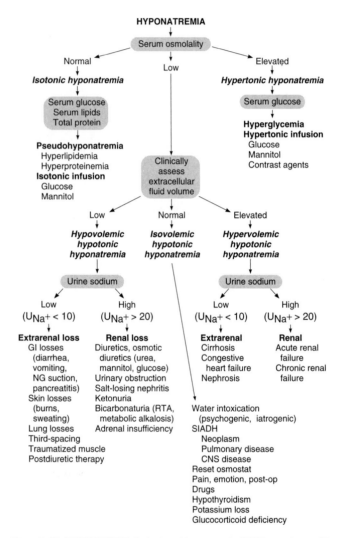

HYPONATREMIA

Serum osmolality

Normal → *Isotonic hyponatremia*

Serum glucose
Serum lipids
Total protein

Pseudohyponatremia
Hyperlipidemia
Hyperproteinemia
Isotonic infusion
Glucose
Mannitol

Low → Clinically assess extracellular fluid volume

Elevated → *Hypertonic hyponatremia*

Serum glucose

Hyperglycemia
Hypertonic infusion
Glucose
Mannitol
Contrast agents

Low → *Hypovolemic hypotonic hyponatremia*

Urine sodium

Low ($U_{Na^+} < 10$)
Extrarenal loss
GI losses (diarrhea, vomiting, NG suction, pancreatitis)
Skin losses (burns, sweating)
Lung losses
Third-spacing
Traumatized muscle
Postdiuretic therapy

High ($U_{Na^+} > 20$)
Renal loss
Diuretics, osmotic diuretics (urea, mannitol, glucose)
Urinary obstruction
Salt-losing nephritis
Ketonuria
Bicarbonaturia (RTA, metabolic alkalosis)
Adrenal insufficiency

Normal → *Isovolemic hypotonic hyponatremia*

Water intoxication (psychogenic, iatrogenic)
SIADH
    Neoplasm
    Pulmonary disease
    CNS disease
Reset osmostat
Pain, emotion, post-op
Drugs
Hypothyroidism
Potassium loss
Glucocorticoid deficiency

Elevated → *Hypervolemic hypotonic hyponatremia*

Urine sodium

Low ($U_{Na^+} < 10$)
Extrarenal
Cirrhosis
Congestive heart failure
Nephrosis

High ($U_{Na^+} > 20$)
Renal
Acute renal failure
Chronic renal failure

Figure 8–12. HYPONATREMIA: Evaluation of hyponatremia. **SIADH** = syndrome of inappropriate antidiuretic hormone; U_{Na^+} = urinary sodium (mg/dL). *(Adapted, with permission, from Narins RG et al: Diagnostic strategies in disorders of fluid, electrolyte and acid-base homeostasis. Am J Med 1982;72:496.)*

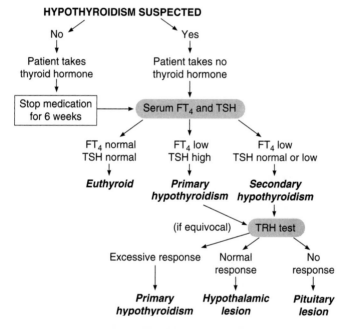

Figure 8–13. HYPOTHYROIDISM: Diagnostic approach to hypothyroidism. **FT$_4$** = free thyroxine; **TSH** = thyroid-stimulating hormone; **TRH** = thyroid-releasing hormone. *(Modified, with permission, from Greenspan FS, Gardner DG [editors]:* Basic & Clinical Endocrinology, *6th ed. Originally published by Appleton & Lange. Copyright © 2001 by The McGraw-Hill Companies, Inc.)*

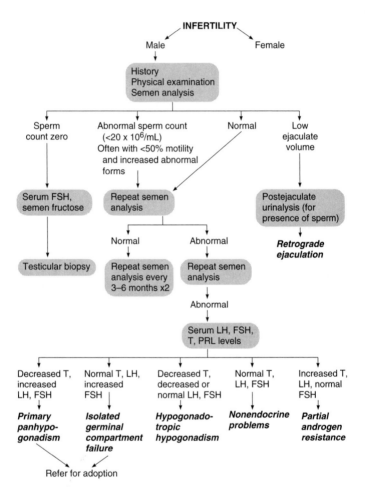

Figure 8–14. MALE INFERTILITY: Evaluation of male factor infertility. **FSH** = follicle-stimulating hormone; **LH** = luteinizing hormone; **PRL** = prolactin; **T** = testosterone. *(Adapted, with permission, from Swerdloff RS, Boyers SM: Evaluation of the male partner of an infertile couple: An algorithmic approach. JAMA 1982;247:2418. Copyright © 1982 by The American Medical Association.)*

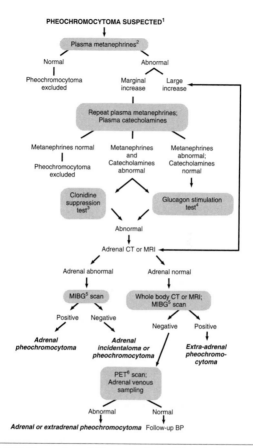

Plasma metanephrines[2]

Normal — Pheochromocytoma excluded

Abnormal

Marginal increase

Large increase

Repeat plasma metanephrines; Plasma catecholamines

Metanephrines normal — Pheochromocytoma excluded

Metanephrines and Catecholamines abnormal

Metanephrines abnormal; Catecholamines normal

Clonidine suppression test[3]

Glucagon stimulation test[4]

Abnormal

Adrenal CT or MRI

Adrenal abnormal

Adrenal normal

MIBG[5] scan

Whole body CT or MRI; MIBG[5] scan

Positive

Negative

Negative

Positive

Adrenal pheochromocytoma

Adrenal incidentaloma or pheochromocytoma

Extra-adrenal pheochromocytoma

PET[6] scan; Adrenal venous sampling

Abnormal

Normal

Adrenal or extradrenal pheochromocytoma

Follow-up BP

---

[1] Incidence of pheochromocytoma <0.1% among patients with hypertension.

[2] See p 126.

[3] Measure plasma norepinephrine after administering clonidine 0.15–0.3 mg orally. A >50% decrease in plasma norepinephrine to <2.96 nmol/L is a normal response; a lack of suppression indicates a pheochromocytoma. *Caution:* May precipitate severe hypotension. Perform with expert consultation only.

[4] Measure plasma norepinephrine after administering glucagon 1 mg intravenously. A >3-fold increase in plasma norepinephrine indicates a pheochromocytoma. *Caution:* May precipitate severe hypertension. Perform with expert consultation only.

[5] 131I- or 123I-labeled metaiodobenzylguanidine.

[6] 6-[18F]fluorodopamine positron emission tomography.

Figure 8–15. PHEOCHROMOCYTOMA: Diagnostic evaluation. **CT** = computed tomography; **MRI** = magnetic resonance imaging. *(Modified, with permission, from Pacak K et al: Recent advances in genetics, diagnosis, localization and treatment of pheochromocytoma. Ann Intern Med 2001;134;315.)*

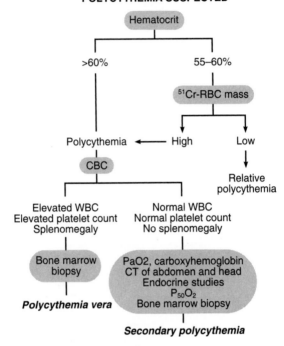

POLYCYTHEMIA SUSPECTED

Figure 8–16. POLYCYTHEMIA: Diagnostic evaluation. **CBC** = complete blood count; **CT** = computed tomography; **PaO₂** = partial pressure of oxygen in arterial blood; **P₅₀O₂** = partial pressure of oxygen at which hemoglobin is 50% saturated; **RBC** = red blood cell; **WBC** = white blood cell. *(Modified, with permission, from Stein JH [editor]. Internal Medicine, 5th ed. Mosby, 1998.)*

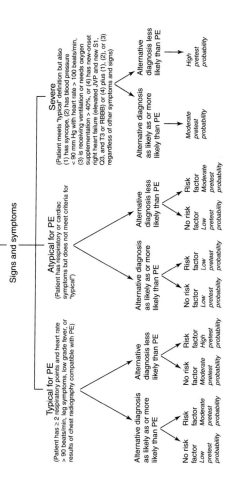

Figure 8–17A. ALGORITHM FOR THE CLINICAL MODEL TO DETERMINE THE PRETEST PROBABILITY OF PULMONARY EMBOLISM (PE): Respiratory points consist of dyspnea or worsening of chronic dyspnea, pleuritic chest pain, chest pain that is nonretrosternal and nonpleuritic, an arterial oxygen saturation <92% while breathing room air that corrects with oxygen supplementation <40%, hemoptysis, and pleural rub. Risk factors are surgery within 12 weeks, immobilization (complete bed rest) for 3 or more days in the 4 weeks before presentation, previous deep venous thrombosis or objectively diagnosed pulmonary embolism, fracture of a lower extremity and immobilization of the fracture within 12 weeks, strong family history of deep venous thrombosis or pulmonary embolism (two or more family members with objectively proved events or a first-degree relative with hereditary thrombophilia), cancer (treatment ongoing, within the past 6 months, or in the palliative stages), the postpartum period, and lower extremity paralysis. **JVP** = jugular venous pressure; **RBBB** = right bundle-branch block. See Figure 8–17B, p 356. *(Modified, with permission, from Wells PS et al: Use of a clinical model for safe management of patients with suspected pulmonary embolism. Ann Intern Med 1998;129:997.)*

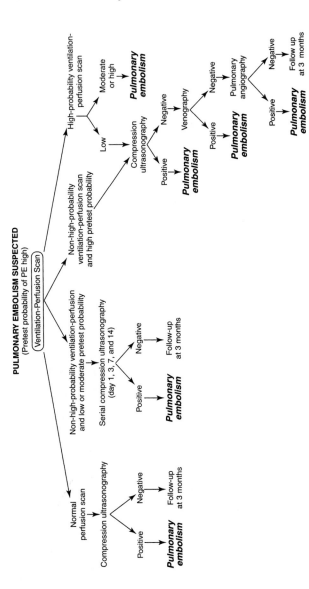

Figure 8–17B. DIAGNOSTIC STRATEGY USED IN PATIENTS WITH SUSPECTED PULMONARY EMBOLISM. See Figure 8–17A, p 355. *(Modified, with permission, from Wells PS et al: Use of a clinical model for safe management of patients with suspected pulmonary embolism. Ann Intern Med 1998;129:997.)*

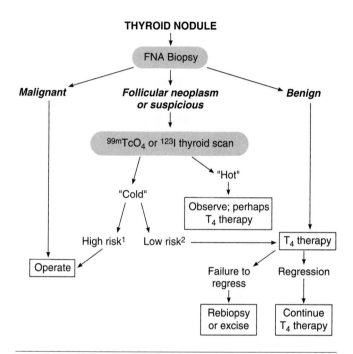

THYROID NODULE

FNA Biopsy

Malignant   *Follicular neoplasm or suspicious*   *Benign*

$^{99m}TcO_4$ or ^{123}I thyroid scan

"Cold"   "Hot"

Observe; perhaps T_4 therapy

High risk[1]   Low risk[2] T_4 therapy

Operate

Failure to regress   Regression

Rebiopsy or excise   Continue T_4 therapy

---

[1] High risk = child, young adult, male; solitary, firm nodule; family history of thyroid cancer; previous neck irradiation; recent growth of nodule; hoarseness, dysphagia, obstruction; vocal cord paralysis, lymphadenopathy.

[2] Low risk = older, female; soft nodule; multinodular goiter; family history of benign goiter; residence in endemic goiter area.

Figure 8–18. THYROID NODULE: Laboratory evaluation of a thyroid nodule. **FNA** = fine-needle aspiration; **T_4** = thyroxine. *(Modified, with permission, from Greenspan FS, Gardner DG [editors]: Basic & Clinical Endocrinology, 6th ed. Originally published by Appleton & Lange. Copyright © 2001 by The McGraw-Hill Companies, Inc.)*

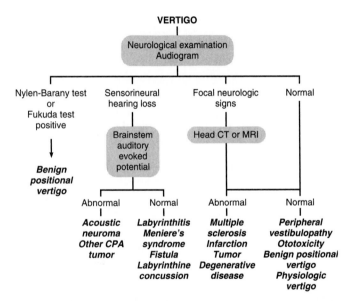

Figure 8–19. VERTIGO: Diagnostic evaluation. **CPA** = cerebellopontine angle; **CT** = computed tomography; **MRI** = magnetic resonance imaging. *(Modified, with permission, from Baloh RW: Hearing and equilibrium. (In Andreolli TE [editor]: Cecil Essentials of Medicine, 4th ed. Saunders, 1997.)*

9

Diagnostic Tests in Differential Diagnosis

Stephen J. McPhee, MD, Diana Nicoll, MD, PhD, MPA,
and Michael Pignone, MD, MPH

HOW TO USE THIS SECTION

This section shows how diagnostic tests can be helpful in differential diagnosis. Material is presented in tabular form, and tables are listed in alphabetical order by subject.

Abbreviations used throughout this section include the following:

$$
\begin{aligned}
\text{N} &= \text{Normal} \\
\text{Abn} &= \text{Abnormal} \\
\text{Pos} &= \text{Positive} \\
\text{Neg} &= \text{Negative} \\
\uparrow &= \text{Increased or high} \\
\downarrow &= \text{Decreased or low} \\
\text{Occ} &= \text{Occasional}
\end{aligned}
$$

Contents

TABLE 9-1. ACID–BASE DISTURBANCES: LABORATORY CHARACTERISTICS OF PRIMARY SINGLE DISTURBANCES OF ACID–BASE BALANCE.[1]

Disturbance	Acute Primary Change	Arterial pH	[K⁺] (meq/L)	Anion Gap[2] (meq)	Clinical Features
Normal	None	7.35–7.45	3.5–5.0	8–12	None.
Respiratory acidosis	PCO_2 retention	↓	↑	N	Dyspnea, polypnea, respiratory outflow obstruction, ↑ anterior-posterior chest diameter, musical rales, wheezes. In severe cases, stupor, disorientation, coma.
Respiratory alkalosis	PCO_2 depletion	↑	↓	N or ↓	Anxiety, breathlessness, frequent sighing, lungs usually clear to examination, positive Chvostek and Trousseau signs.
Metabolic acidosis	HCO_3^- depletion	↓	↑ or ↓	N or ↑	Weakness, air hunger, Kussmaul respiration, dry skin and mucous membranes. In severe cases, poor skin turgor, coma, hypotension, death.
Metabolic alkalosis	HCO_3^- retention	↑	↓	N	Weakness, positive Chvostek and Trousseau signs, hyporeflexia.

[1] Reproduced, with permission, from Harvey AM et al (editors): The Principles and Practice of Medicine, 22nd ed. Originally published by Appleton & Lange. Copyright © 1988 by The McGraw-Hill Companies, Inc.

[2] Anion gap = $[Na^+] - ([HCO_3^-] + [Cl^-]) = 8–12$ meq normally.

TABLE 9–2. ANEMIA: DIAGNOSIS OF COMMON ANEMIAS BASED ON RED BLOOD CELL (RBC) INDICES.[1]

Type of Anemia	MCV (fL)	MCHC (g/dL)	Common Causes	Common Laboratory Abnormalities	Other Clinical Findings
Microcytic, hypochromic	<80	<32	Iron deficiency	Low reticulocyte count, low serum and bone marrow iron, high TIBC.	Mucositis, blood loss.
			Thalassemias	Reticulocytosis, abnormal red cell morphology, normal serum iron levels.	Asian, African, or Mediterranean descent.
			Chronic lead poisoning	Basophilic stippling of RBCs, elevated lead and free erythrocyte protoporphyrin levels.	Peripheral neuropathy, history of exposure to lead.
			Sideroblastic anemia	High serum iron, ringed sideroblasts in bone marrow.	Population of hypochromic RBCs on smear.
Normocytic, normochromic	81–100	32–36	Acute blood loss	Fecal occult blood test positive.	Recent blood loss.
			Hemolysis	Haptoglobin low or absent, reticulocytosis, hyperbilirubinemia.	Hemoglobinuria, splenomegaly.
			Chronic disease[2]	Low serum iron, TIBC low or low normal.	Depends on cause.
Macrocytic, normochromic	>101[3]	>36	Vitamin B_{12} deficiency	Hypersegmented PMNs; low serum vitamin B_{12} levels; achlorhydria.	Peripheral neuropathy; glossitis.
			Folate deficiency	Hypersegmented PMNs; low folate levels.	Alcoholism; malnutrition.
			Liver disease	Mean corpuscular volume usually <120 fL; normal serum vitamin B_{12} and folate levels.	Signs of liver disease.
			Reticulocytosis	Marked (>15%) reticulocytosis.	Variable.

[1] Modified, with permission, from Saunders CE, Ho MT (editors): Current Emergency Diagnosis & Treatment, 4th ed. Originally published by Appleton & Lange. Copyright © 1992 by The McGraw-Hill Companies, Inc.

[2] May be microcytic, hypochromic.

[3] If MCV >120–130, vitamin B_{12} or folate deficiency is likely.

MCV = mean corpuscular volume; MCHC = mean corpuscular hemoglobin concentration; TIBC = total iron-binding capacity; serum; PMN = polymorphonuclear cell.

TABLE 9–3. ANEMIA, MICROCYTIC: LABORATORY EVALUATION OF MICROCYTIC, HYPOCHROMIC ANEMIAS.[1]

Diagnosis	MCV (fL)	Serum Iron (µg/dL)	Iron-Binding Capacity (µg/dL)	Transferrin Saturation (%)	Serum Ferritin (µg/L)	Free Erythrocyte Protoporphyrin (µg/dL)	Basophilic Stippling	Bone Marrow Iron Stores
Normal	80–100	50–175	250–460	16–60	16–300	<35	Absent	Present
Iron deficiency anemia	↓	<30	↑	<16	<12	↑	Absent	Absent
Anemia of chronic disease	N or ↓	<30	N or ↓	N or ↓	N or ↑	↑	Absent	Present
Thalassemia minor	↓	N	N	N	N	N	Usually present	Present

[1] Modified, with permission, from Harvey AM et al (editors): The Principles and Practice of Medicine, 22nd ed. Originally published by Appleton & Lange. Copyright © 1988 by The McGraw-Hill Companies, Inc.

TABLE 9–4. ASCITES: ASCITIC FLUID PROFILES IN VARIOUS DISEASE STATES.[1]

Diagnosis	Appearance	Fluid Protein (g/dL)	Serum-Ascites Albumin Gradient (SAAG)	Fluid Glucose (mg/dL)	WBC and Differential (per μL)	RBC (per μL)	Bacteriologic Gram Stain and Culture	Cytology	Comments
Normal	Clear	<3.0		Equal to plasma glucose	<250	Few or none	Neg	Neg	
TRANSUDATES[2]									
Cirrhosis	Clear	<3.0	High[3]	N	<250, MN	Few	Neg	Neg	Occasionally turbid, rarely bloody. Fluid LDH/serum LDH ratio <0.6
Congestive heart failure	Clear	<2.5	High[3]	N	<250, MN	Few	Neg	Neg	
Nephrotic syndrome	Clear	<2.5	Low[4]	N	<250, MN	Few	Neg	Neg	
Pseudomyxoma peritonei	Gelatinous	<2.5		N	<250	Few	Neg	Occ Pos	
EXUDATES[5]									
Bacterial peritonitis	Cloudy	>3.0	Low[4]	<50 with perforation	>500, PMN	Few	Pos	Neg	Blood cultures frequently positive.
Tuberculous peritonitis	Clear	>3.0	Low[4]	<60	>500, MN	Few, occasionally many	Stain Pos in 25%; culture Pos in 65%	Neg	Occasionally chylous. Peritoneal biopsy positive in 65%.

Malignancy	Clear or bloody	>3.0	Low⁴	<60	>500, MN, PMN	Many	Neg	Pos in 60–90%	Occasionally chylous. Fluid LDH/Serum LDH ratio >0.6. Peritoneal biopsy diagnostic.
Pancreatitis	Clear or bloody	>2.5	Low⁴	N	>500, MN, PMN	Many	Neg	Neg	Occasionally chylous Fluid amylase > 1000 IU/L, sometimes >10,000 IU/L Fluid amylase > serum amylase
Chylous ascites	Turbid	Varies, often >2.5		N	Few	Few	Neg	Neg	Fluid TG > 400 mg/dL (turbid) Fluid TG > serum TG

¹ Modified, with permission, from Harvey AM et al (editors): The Principles and Practice of Medicine, 22nd ed. Originally published by Appleton & Lange. Copyright © 1988 by The McGraw-Hill Companies, Inc.; and from Schiff L, Schiff ER (editors): Diseases of the Liver, 7th ed. Lippincott, 1993.

² Transudates have protein concentration <2.5–3.0 g/dL; fluid LDH/serum LDH ratio <0.6 (may be useful in difficult cases).

³ High = ≥1.1.

⁴ Low = <1.1.

⁵ Exudates have fluid protein concentration >2.5–3.0 g/dL; fluid LDH/serum LDH ratio >0.6 (may be useful in difficult cases).

MN = mononuclear cells; **PMN** = polymorphonuclear cells; **TG** = triglycerides.

TABLE 9–5. AUTOANTIBODIES: ASSOCIATIONS WITH CONNECTIVE TISSUE DISEASES.[1]

Suspected Disease State	Test	Primary Disease Association (Sensitivity, Specificity)	Other Disease Associations (Sensitivity)	Comments
CREST syndrome	Anti-centromere antibody	CREST (70–90%, high)	Scleroderma (10–15%), Raynaud disease (10–30%).	Predictive value of a positive test is >95% for scleroderma or related disease (CREST, Raynaud). Diagnosis of CREST is made clinically.
Systemic lupus erythematosus	Anti-nuclear antibody (ANA)	SLE (>95%, low)	RA (30–50%), discoid lupus, scleroderma (60%), drug-induced lupus (100%), Sjögren syndrome (80%), miscellaneous inflammatory disorders.	Often used as a screening test; a negative test virtually excludes SLE; a positive test, while nonspecific, increases posttest probability. Titer does not correlate with disease activity.
	Anti-double-stranded-DNA antibody (anti-ds-DNA)	SLE (60–70%, high)	Lupus nephritis, rarely RA, CTD, usually in low titer.	Predictive value of a positive test is >90% for SLE if present in high titer; a decreasing titer may correlate with worsening renal disease. Titer generally correlates with disease activity.
	Anti-Smith antibody (anti-Sm)	SLE (30–40%, high)		SLE specific. A positive test substantially increases posttest probability of SLE. Test rarely indicated.
Mixed connective tissue disease (MCTD)	Anti-ribonucleoprotein antibody (RNP)	MCTD (95–100%, low) Scleroderma (20–30%, low)	SLE (30%), Sjögren syndrome, RA (10%), discoid lupus (20–30%).	A negative test essentially excludes MCTD; a positive test in high titer, while nonspecific, increases posttest probability of MCTD.

Rheumatoid arthritis (RA)	Rheumatoid factor (RF)	Rheumatoid arthritis (50–90%)	Other rheumatic diseases, chronic infections, some malignancies, some healthy individuals, elderly patients.	Titer does not correlate with disease activity.
Scleroderma	Anti-Scl-70 antibody	Scleroderma (15–20%, high)		Predictive value of a positive test is >95% for scleroderma.
Sjögren syndrome	Anti-SS-A/Ro antibody	Sjögren syndrome (60–70%, low)	SLE (30–40%), RA (10%), subacute cutaneous lupus, vasculitis.	Useful in counseling women of childbearing age with known CTD, because a positive test is associated with a small but real risk of neonatal SLE and congenital heart block.
Wegener granulomatosis	Anti-neutrophil cyto-plasmic antibody (ANCA)	Wegener granulomatosis (systemic necrotizing vas-culitis) (56–96%, high)	Crescentic glomerulonephritis or other systemic vasculitis (eg, polyarteritis nodosa).	Ability of this assay to reflect disease activity remains unclear.

[1] Modified, with permission, from Harvey AM et al (editors): The Principles and Practice of Medicine, 22nd ed. Appleton & Lange, 1988; from White RH, Robbins DL: Clinical significance and interpretation of antinuclear antibodies. West J Med 1987;147:210; and from Tan EM: Autoantibodies to nuclear antigens (ANA): Their immunobiology and medicine. Adv Immunol 1982;33:173.

RA = rheumatoid arthritis; **SLE** = systemic lupus erythematosus; **CTD** = connective tissue disease; **MCTD** = mixed connective tissue disease; **SSA** = Sjögren syndrome A antibody; **CREST** = calcinosis, Raynaud phenomenon, esophageal dysmotility, sclerodactyly and telangiectasia.

TABLE 9-6. CEREBROSPINAL FLUID (CSF): CSF PROFILES IN CENTRAL NERVOUS SYSTEM DISEASE.

Diagnosis	Appearance	Opening Pressure (mm H_2O)	RBC (per µL)	WBC & Diff (per µL)	CSF Glucose (mg/dL)	CSF Protein (mg/dL)	Smears	Culture	Comments
Normal	Clear, colorless	70–200	0	≤5 MN, 0 PMN	45–85	15–45	Neg	Neg	
Bacterial meningitis	Cloudy	↑↑↑	0	200–20,000, mostly PMN	<45	>50	Gram stain Pos	Pos	PMN predominance may be seen early in course.
Tuberculous meningitis	N or cloudy	↑↑↑	0	100–1000, mostly MN	<45	>50	AFB stain Pos	±	Counterimmunoelectrophoresis or latex agglutination may be diagnostic. CSF and serum cryptococcal antigen positive in cryptococcal meningitis.
Fungal meningitis	N or cloudy	N or ↑	0	100–1000, mostly MN	<45	>50		±	
Viral (aseptic) meningitis	N	N or ↑	0	100–1000, mostly MN	45–85	N or ↑	Neg	Neg	RBC count may be elevated in herpes simplex encephalitis. Glucose may be decreased in herpes simplex or mumps infections. Viral cultures may be helpful.

Parasitic meningitis	N or cloudy	N or ↑	0	100–1000, mostly MN, E	<45	N or ↑	Amebae may be seen on wet smear	±	
Carcinomatous meningitis	N or cloudy	N or ↑	0	N or 100–1000, mostly MN	<45	N or ↑	Cytology Pos	Neg	
Cerebral lupus erythematosus	N	N or ↑	0	N or ↑, mostly MN	N	N or ↑	Neg	Neg	
Subarachnoid hemorrhage	Pink-red, supernatant yellow	↑	↑ crenated or fresh	N or 100–1000, mostly PMN	N or ↓	N or ↑	Neg	Neg	Blood in all tubes equally. Pleocytosis and low glucose sometimes seen several days after subarachnoid hemorrhage, reflecting chemical meningitis caused by subarachnoid blood.
"Traumatic" tap	Bloody, supernatant clear	N	↑↑↑ fresh	↑	N	↑	Neg	Neg	Most blood in tube #1, least blood in tube #4.

(continued)

TABLE 9–6 (CONTINUED).

Diagnosis	Appearance	Opening Pressure (mm H$_2$O)	RBC (per µL)	WBC & Diff (per µL)	CSF Glucose (mg/dL)	CSF Protein (mg/dL)	Smears	Culture	Comments
Spirochetal, early, acute syphilitic meningitis	Clear to turbid	↑	0	25–2000, mostly MN	15–75	>50	Neg	Neg	PMN may predominate early. Positive serum RPR or VDRL. CSF VDRL insensitive. If clinical suspicion is high, institute treatment despite negative CSF VDRL.
Late CNS syphilis	Clear	Usually N	0	N or ↑	N	N or ↑	Neg	Neg	CSF VDRL insensitive.
"Neighborhood" meningeal reaction	Clear or turbid, often xanthochromic	Variable, usually N	Variable	↑	N	N or ↑	Neg	Usually Neg	May occur in mastoiditis, brain abscess, sinusitis, septic thrombophlebitis, brain tumor, intrathecal drug therapy.
Hepatic encephalopathy	N	N	0	≤5	N	N	Neg	Neg	CSF glutamine >15 mg/dL.
Uremia	N	Usually ↑	0	N or ↑	N or ↑	N or ↑	Neg	Neg	
Diabetic coma	N	Low	0	N or ↑	↑	N	Neg	Neg	

MN = mononuclear cells (lymphocytes or monocytes); ***PMN*** = polymorphonuclear cells; ***E*** = eosinophils; ***CNS*** = central nervous system; ***WBC*** = white blood cells.

TABLE 9–7. CLOTTING DISORDERS: LABORATORY EVALUATION. [1]

Suspected Diagnosis	Platelet Count	PT	PTT	TT	Further Diagnostic Tests
Idiopathic thrombocytopenic purpura, drug sensitivity, bone marrow depression	↓	N	N	N	Platelet antibody, marrow aspirate.
Disseminated intravascular coagulation	↓	↑	↑	↑	Fibrinogen assays, fibrin D-dimers.
Platelet function defect, salicylates, or uremia	N	N	N	N	Bleeding time, platelet aggregation, blood urea nitrogen, creatinine.
von Willebrand disease	N	N	↑ or N	N	Bleeding time, factor VIII assay, factor VIII antigen.
Factor VII deficiency or inhibitor	N	↑	N	N	Factor VII assay (normal plasma should correct PT if no inhibitor is present).
Factor V, X, II, I deficiencies as in liver disease or with anticoagulants	N	↑	↑	N or ↑	Liver function tests.
Factor VIII (hemophilia), IX, XI, or XII deficiencies or inhibitor	N	N	↑	N	Inhibitor screen, individual factor assays.
Factor XIII deficiency	N	N	N	N	Urea stabilizing test, factor XIII assay.

[1] Modified, with permission, from Tierney LM Jr, McPhee SJ, Papadakis MA (editors): Current Medical Diagnosis & Treatment 1996. *Originally published by Appleton & Lange. Copyright © 1996 by the McGraw-Hill Companies, Inc.;* and from Harvey AM et al. (editors): The Principles and Practice of Medicine, 22nd ed. *Originally published by Appleton & Lange. Copyright © 1988 by The McGraw-Hill Companies, Inc.*

Note: In approaching patients with bleeding disorders, try to distinguish clinically between platelet disorders (eg, patient has petechiae, mucosal bleeding) and factor deficiency states (eg, patient has hemarthrosis).

PT = prothrombin time; **PTT** = activated partial thromboplastin time; **TT** = thrombin time.

TABLE 9–8. GENETIC DISEASES DIAGNOSED BY MOLECULAR DIAGNOSTIC TECHNIQUES.

Test/Range/Collection	Physiologic Basis	Interpretation	Comments
Breast cancer *BRCA1* and *BRCA2* **mutations** Blood Lavender $$$$	Mutations in two genes, *BRCA1* and *BRCA2*, are the major cause of familial early-onset breast cancer. A mutation in either gene confers an 80–90% lifetime risk of breast cancer. Although many mutations have been reported in *BRCA1* and *BRCA2*, three mutations found in Ashkenazi Jews have carrier frequencies high enough to warrant a preliminary screen prior to comprehensive and expensive testing such as DNA sequencing.	This assay will detect the 185 del AG and 5382 ins C mutations in *BRCA1* and the 6174 del T mutation in *BRCA2*. These three mutations have a combined carrier frequency of approximately 1.7% in the Ashkenazi Jewish population.	Oncogene 2000;19:6159. Semin Cancer Biol 2001;11:375.
Cystic fibrosis mutation PCR + reverse dot blot Blood Lavender $$$$	Cystic fibrosis is caused by a mutation in the cystic fibrosis transmembrane regulator gene (CFTR). Over 800 mutations have been found, with the most common being ΔF508, present in 68% of cases.	Test specificity approaches 100%, so a positive result should be considered diagnostic of a cystic fibrosis mutation. Because of the wide range of mutations, an assay for the ΔF508 mutation alone is 68% sensitive. Screening for 64 mutations provides a sensitivity of 70–95% in all U.S. ethnic groups except Asians, and >81% when the U.S. population is considered as a whole. The test can distinguish between heterozygous carriers and homozygous patients.	Cystic fibrosis is the most common inherited disease in North American Caucasians, affecting one in 2500 births. Caucasians have a carrier frequency of one in 25. The disease is autosomal recessive. Carrier screening might be offered to individuals and couples in high-risk groups (eg, Ashkenazi Jews, central or northern Europeans, one partner with cystic fibrosis, and individuals with a family history of cystic fibrosis) who seek preconception counseling, infertility care, or prenatal care. Clin Perinatol 2001;28:383. Genet Med 2001;3:168. Pediatrics 2001;107:280. Clin Chem 2002;48:1121.

Deafness nonsyndromic recessive *Connexin 26* mutations Blood Lavender or blue $$$$	The connexins are a family of proteins present in gap junctions of adherent cells. A common frameshift-mutation (35 del G) in *connexin 26*, found to occur at a carrier frequency of 1 in 35 to 1 in 79 in Europe, segregates world-wide in families with nonsyndromic recessive deafness. Another frameshift mutation (167 delT) is present at a carrier frequency of 1 in 25 among Ashkenazi-Jewish individuals.	This test detects both mutations. Both are deleterious when they occur either in homozygous or compound hetero-zygous forms.	Brain Res Rev 2000;32:181. J R Soc Med 2002;95:171.
Dementia, frontotemporal (FTD) *tau* gene mutations Blood Lavender $$$$	The microtubule-associated protein, tau, located on chromosome 17q21, coassembles with tubulin to form microtubules. Tau is mostly found in axons and when hyperphosphorylated appears to form tangles of paired heli-cal filaments, which can damage the neuronal cytoskeleton and lead to neurodegeneration. Mutations in the gene encoding tau are found in individ-uals with frontotemporal dementia and pallidopontonigral degeneration.	This test detects three mutations, two mis-sense mutations commonly found in the *tau* gene (P301L, A279L), and a splice isoform mutant (IVS 10, 14C to T).	Annu Rev Neurosci 2001;24:1121. Clin Neurol Neurosci Rep 2001;1:413. Med Clin North Am 2002;86:501.

(continued)

TABLE 9–8 (CONTINUED).

Test/Range/Collection	Physiologic Basis	Interpretation	Comments
Factor V (Leiden) mutation (activated protein C resistance) Blood Lavender or blue $$$$	The Leiden mutation is a single nucleotide base substitution leading to an amino acid substitution (glutamine replaces arginine) at one of the sites where coagulation factor V is cleaved by activated protein C. The mutation causes factor V to be partially resistant to protein C, which is involved in inhibiting coagulation. Factor V mutations may be present in up to half of the cases of unexplained venous thrombosis and are seen in 96% of patients with activated protein C resistance.	**Positive in:** Hypercoagulability secondary to factor V mutation (specificity approaches 100%).	The presence of mutation is only a risk factor for thrombosis, not an absolute marker for disease. Homozygotes have a 50- to 100-fold increase in risk of thrombosis (relative to the general population), and heterozygotes have a 7-fold increase in risk. The current PCR and reverse dot blot assay only detects the Leiden mutation of factor V; other mutations may yet be discovered. There is also increased risk of thrombosis in carriers of the prothrombin G → A[20210] variant and in methylenetetrahydrofolate reductase deficiency. Chest 2000;118:1405. Arch Intern Med 2001;161:1051. Arch Pathol Lab Med 2002;126;577.
Fragile X syndrome PCR, Southern blot Blood, cultured amniocytes Lavender $$$$	Fragile X syndrome results from a mutation in the familial mental retardation-1 gene *(FMRI)*, located at Xq27.3. Fully symptomatic patients have abnormal methylation of the gene (which blocks transcription) during oogenesis. The gene contains a variable number of repeating CGG sequences and, as the number of sequences increases, the probability of abnormal methylation increases. The number of copies increases with subsequent generations so that women who are unaffected carriers may have offspring who are affected.	Normal patients have 6–52 CGG repeat sequences. Patients with 52–230 repeat sequences are asymptomatic carriers. Patients with more than 230 repeat sequences are very likely to have abnormal methylation and to be symptomatic.	Fragile X syndrome is the most common cause of inherited mental retardation, occurring in one in 1000–1500 men and one in 2000–2500 women. Full mutations can show variable penetration in females, but most such women will be at least mildly retarded. Genet Test 2000;4:289. Diagn Mol Pathol 2001;10:34. Expert Rev Mol Diagn 2001;1:226. Health Technol Assess 2001;5:1.

Hemochromatosis, hereditary Blood Lavender $$$$	83% of hereditary hemochromatosis is caused by a G to A substitution at nucleotide 845 of the HLA-H gene. The carrier frequency among Europeans is 10%. Thus, 1 in 400 individuals will be homozygous for this mutation and may be affected with hemochromatosis.	Clin Chem 2001;47:1147. Curr Opin Hematol 2001;8:98. Annu Rev Public Health 2000;21:65.
Hemophilia A Southern blot Blood, cultured amniocytes Lavender $$$$	Approximately half of severe hemophilia A cases are caused by an inversion mutation within the factor VIII gene. The resulting rearrangement of *BCL1* sites can be detected by Southern blot hybridization assays.	Test specificity approaches 100%, so a positive result should be considered diagnostic of a hemophilia A inversion mutation. Because of a variety of mutations, however, test sensitivity is only about 50%.	Hemophilia A is one of the most common X-linked diseases in humans, affecting one in 5000 men. Haemophilia 2001;7:20. J Biochem Biophys Meth 2001;47:39. J Postgrad Med 2001;47:274. Thromb Haemost 2001;85:560.
Huntington disease PCR + Southern blot Blood, cultured amniocytes, or buccal cells Lavender $$$$	Huntington disease is an inherited neurodegenerative disorder associated with an autosomal dominant mutation on chromosome 4. The disease is highly penetrant, but symptoms (disordered movements, cognitive decline, and emotional disturbance) are often expressed until middle age. The mutation results in the expansion of a CAG trinucleotide repeat sequence within the gene.	Normal patients will have fewer than 34 CAG repeats, while patients with disease usually have more than 37 repeats and may have 80 or more. Occasional affected patients can be seen with "high normal" (32–34) numbers of repeats. Tests showing 34–37 repeats are indeterminate.	Huntington disease testing involves ethical dilemmas. Counseling is recommended prior to testing. Hum Mutat 1999;13:232. Clin Genet 2001;60:442.

(continued)

TABLE 9–8 (CONTINUED).

Test/Range/Collection	Physiologic Basis	Interpretation	Comments
Prader-Willi syndrome Angelman syndrome Blood Lavender $$$$	Prader-Willi syndrome (PWS) and Angelman (AS) syndrome are clinically different diseases related at the molecular level. They are caused by loss of function mutations in two chromosomal regions located close to each other on chromosome 15. An interstitial deletion of 15q11–13 is found in about 70% of patients with PWS or AS. PWS results when the deletion affects the paternal chromosome and AS, when it affects the maternal chromosome. A DNA probe from the affected region is used to determine the origin of the deletion by Southern blot analysis. In about 33% of patients with PWS and 20–30% with AS, no deletion can be found. Instead, uniparental disomy (UPD) may be found resulting in either two maternal or two paternal copies of chromosome 15. In 1–2% of patients with PWS and 20% of patients with AS, neither a deletion nor UPD can be found.	This test detects both the deletion and UPD defects in PWS and AS.	Annu Rev Genomics Hum Genet 2001;2:153. Brain Res Bull 2002;57:109.

| **α-Thalassemia**

PCR + Southern blot

Blood, cultured amniocytes, chorionic villi

Lavender
$$$$ | A deletion mutation in the α-globin gene region of chromosome 16 due to unequal crossing-over events can lead to defective synthesis of the α-globin chain of hemoglobin. Normally, there are two copies of the α-globin gene on each chromosome 16, and the severity of disease increases with the number of defective genes. | This assay is highly specific (approaches 100%). Sensitivity, however, can vary because detection of different mutations may require the use of different probes. α-Thalassemia due to point mutations may not be detected. | Patients with one deleted gene are usually normal or very slightly anemic; patients with two deletions usually have a hypochromic microcytic anemia; patients with three deletions have elevated hemoglobin H and a moderately severe hemolytic anemia; patients with four deletions generally die in utero with hydrops fetalis (see Table 9–21).
The most clinically significant situations arise when each parent is a carrier for a deletion that encompasses both α-globin genes, as seen mostly in South East Asian and Filipino populations. Each offspring of such carriers has a 25% risk of hydrops fetalis.
Less deleterious effects arise from chromosomes of Mediterranean and black ancestries. These chromosomes usually carry one α-globin gene deletion per chromosome. Offspring of carriers of a two α-globin gene deletion and single α-gene deletion are at risk for HbH disease.

Am J Hematol 1998;58:306.
Baillieres Clin Haematol 1998;11:215.
Br J Haematol 2000;108:295. |

(continued)

TABLE 9–8 (CONTINUED).

Test/Range/Collection	Physiologic Basis	Interpretation	Comments
β-Thalassemia PCR + reverse dot blot Blood, chorionic villi, cultured amniocytes Lavender $$$$	β-Thalassemia results from a mutation in the gene encoding the β-globin subunit of hemoglobin A (which is composed of a pair of α-chains and a pair of β-chains). A relative excess of α-globin chains precipitates within red blood cells, causing hemolysis and anemia. Over 300 different mutations have been described; testing usually covers a panel of the more common mutations. The test can distinguish between heterozygous and homozygous individuals.	Test specificity approaches 100%, so a positive result should be considered diagnostic of a thalassemia mutation. Because of the large number of mutations, sensitivity can be poor. A panel with the 43 most common mutations has a sensitivity that approaches 95%.	β-Thalassemia is very common; about 3% of the world's population are carriers. The incidence is increased in persons of Mediterranean, African, and Asian descent. The mutations may vary from population to population, and different testing panels may be needed for patients of different ethnicities (see Table 9–22). Baillieres Clin Haematol 1998;11:215. Prenat Diagn 1999;19:428. Hum Mutat 2002;19:287.

¹ Adapted, with permission, from Wall J, Chehab F, Kan YW: Clinical Laboratory Manual. UCSF, 1996, and updated with permission, 2002.
PCR (polymerase chain reaction) is a method for amplifying the amount of a particular DNA sequence in a specimen, facilitating detection by hybridization-based assay (ie, Southern blot, reverse dot blot).
Southern blot is a molecular hybridization technique whereby DNA is extracted from the sample and digested by different restriction enzymes. The resulting fragments are separated by electrophoresis and identified by labeled probes. **Reverse dot blot** is a molecular hybridization technique in which a specific oligonucleotide probe is bound to a solid membrane prior to reaction with PCR-amplified DNA.
$$$$ = >$100.00.

TABLE 9–9. HEPATIC FUNCTION TESTS.[1]

Clinical Condition	Direct Bilirubin (mg/dL)	Indirect Bilirubin (mg/dL)	Urine Bilirubin	Serum Albumin & Total Protein (g/dL)	Alkaline Phosphatase (IU/L)	Prothrombin time (seconds)	ALT (SGPT); AST (SGOT) (IU/L)
Normal	0.1–0.3	0.2–0.7	None	Albumin, 3.4–4.7 Total protein, 6.0–8.0	30–115 (lab specific)	11–15 seconds. After vitamin K, 15% increase within 24 hours.	ALT, 5–35; AST, 5–40 (lab specific)
Hepatocellular jaundice (eg, viral, alcoholic hepatitis)	↑↑	↑	↑	↓ Albumin	N to ↑	Prolonged if damage is severe. Does not respond to parenteral vitamin K.	Increased in hepatocellular damage, viral hepatitises; AST/ALT ratio often >2:1 in alcoholic hepatitis
Uncomplicated obstructive jaundice (eg, common bile duct obstruction)	↑↑	↑	↑	N	↑	Prolonged if obstruction marked but responds to parenteral vitamin K.	N to minimally ↑
Hemolysis	N	↑	None	N	N	N	N
Gilbert syndrome	↑↑	↑	None	N	N	N	N
Intrahepatic cholestasis (drug induced)	↑↑	↑	↑	N	↑↑	N	AST N or ↑; ALT N or ↑
Primary biliary cirrhosis	↑↑	↑	↑	N ↑ globulin	↑↑	N or ↑	↑

[1] Modified, with permission, from Tierney LM Jr, McPhee SJ, Papadakis MA (editors): Current Medical Diagnosis & Treatment 1996. *Originally published by Appleton & Lange. Copyright © 1996 by The McGraw-Hill Companies, Inc.; and from Harvey AM et al (editors): The Principles and Practice of Medicine, 22nd ed. Originally published by Appleton & Lange. Copyright © 1988 by The McGraw-Hill Companies, Inc.*
AST = aspartate aminotransferase; **ALT** = alanine aminotransferase.

TABLE 9–10. HEPATIC FUNCTION AND NUTRITION OR PROTHROMBIN TIME: RELATIONSHIP TO OPERATIVE DEATH RATE AFTER PORTACAVAL SHUNT.

	Group		
	A	B	C
Child's criteria			
Operative death rate	2%	10%	50%
Serum bilirubin (mg/dL)	<2	2–3	>3
Serum albumin (g/dL)	>3.5	3.0–3.5	<3
Ascites	None	Easily controlled	Poorly controlled
Encephalopathy	None	Minimal	Advanced
Nutrition[1]	Excellent	Good	Poor

Pugh modification[1]
    Prothrombin time
        (seconds prolonged)
	1–4	4–6	>6

[1] In the Pugh modification of Child's criteria, prothrombin time is substituted for nutrition.

TABLE 9–11. HYPERLIPIDEMIA: CHARACTERISTICS AND LABORATORY FINDINGS IN PRIMARY HYPERLIPIDEMIA.[1]

Lipoprotein Disorder	Lipoprotein Abnormalities or Defect	Appearance of Serum[2]	Cholesterol (mg/dL)	Triglyceride (mg/dL)	Clinical Presentation	Comments	Risk of Athero- sclerosis
None	None	Clear	<200	<165			Nil
Familial hyper- cholesterolemia	LDL elevated; decreased or lack of LDL receptors in liver	Clear	Usually 300– 600 but may be higher; LDL choles- terol high	Normal	Xanthelasma, tendon and skin xantho- mas, accelerated atherosclerosis. Detectable in childhood.	Onset at all ages. Consider hypo- thyroidism, nephrotic syn- drome, hepatic obstruction.	↑↑
Familial combined hyperlipidemia	LDL or VLDL elevated	Turbid or clear	Usually 250– 600; LDL cholesterol high	Usually 200–600	Accelerated athero- sclerosis. Associ- ated with obesity or diabetes.	Cholesterol or triglyc- eride or both may be elevated—at different times and in different mem- bers of the family.	↑↑
Familial hyper- triglyceridemia	VLDL elevated	Turbid	Typically normal	200–5000	Eruptive xanthomas. Triglycerides, if high enough, may cause pancreatitis.	Consider nephrotic syndrome, hypo- thyroidism, alco- holism, glycogen storage disease, oral contra- ceptives.	Nil

(continued)

TABLE 9-11 (CONTINUED).

Lipoprotein Disorder	Lipoprotein Abnormalities or Defect	Appearance of Serum[2]	Cholesterol (mg/dL)	Triglyceride (mg/dL)	Clinical Presentation	Comments	Risk of Atherosclerosis
Hyper-chylomicronemia	Chylomicrons elevated; deficiency of lipoprotein lipase or, less commonly, of C-II apolipoprotein	Creamy, separates into creamy supernate and clear infranate	Increased	Often 1000-10,000; chylomicrons	Eruptive xanthomas, lipemia retinalis, recurrent abdominal pain, hepatosplenomegaly, pancreatitis.	Onset in infancy or childhood. Aggravated by high fat intake, diabetes, alcohol.	Nil
Mixed hyper-triglyceridemia	VLDL and chylomicrons elevated	Creamy, separates into creamy supernate and turbid infranate	300-1000	Usually 500->10,000; chylomicrons high	Recurrent abdominal pain, hepatosplenomegaly, eruptive xanthomas; glucose intolerance	Symptoms begin in adult life. Sensitive to dietary fat. Alcohol and diabetes aggravate.	Nil to ↑
Dysbetalipoproteinemia (type III)	VLDL, IDL elevated; apolipoprotein E dysfunction	Turbid	200-500	200-500	Palmar xanthoma typical; other xanthomas common.	Aggravated by alcohol, estrogen.	↑↑

[1] Modified, with permission, from Schroeder SA et al (editors): Current Medical Diagnosis & Treatment 1991. *Originally published by Appleton & Lange. Copyright © 1991 by The McGraw-Hill Companies, Inc.; from Harvey AM et al (editors): The Principles and Practice of Medicine, 22nd ed. Originally published by Appleton & Lange. Copyright © 1988 by The McGraw-Hill Companies; and from Siperstein M, 1996. The collaboration of Dr. Marvin D. Siperstein is gratefully acknowledged.*

[2] Refrigerated serum overnight at 4°C.

Key: LDL = low-density lipoprotein, calculated as: Total cholesterol—HDL cholesterol—[Triglycerides/5]; **VLDL** = very low density lipoprotein; **IDL** = intermediate density lipoprotein.

TABLE 9–12. THE OSMOLAL GAP IN TOXICOLOGY.[1]

The osmolal gap (Δ osm) is determined by subtracting the calculated serum osmolality from the measured serum osmolality.

$$\begin{array}{l}\text{Calculated} \\ \text{osmolality (osm)} \\ \text{(mosm/kg } H_2O)\end{array} = 2\left(Na^+[meq/L]\right) + \frac{\text{Glucose (mg/dL)}}{18} + \frac{\text{BUN (mg/dL)}}{2.8}$$

$$\text{Osmolal gap } (\Delta \text{ osm}) = \text{Measured osmolality} - \text{Calculated osmolality}$$

Serum osmolality may be increased by contributions of circulating alcohols and other low-molecular-weight substances. Since these substances are not included in the calculated osmolality, there will be an osmolal gap directly proportional to their serum concentration and inversely proportional to their molecular weight:

$$\text{Serum concentration (mg/dL)} \approx \Delta \text{ osm} \times \frac{\text{Molecular weight of toxin}}{10}$$

For ethanol (the most common cause of Δ osm), a gap of 30 mosm/kg H_2O indicates an ethanol level of:

$$30 \times \frac{46}{10} = 138 \text{ mg/dL}$$

See the following for lethal concentrations of alcohols and their corresponding osmolal gaps.

LETHAL CONCENTRATIONS OF ALCOHOLS AND THEIR CORRESPONDING OSMOLAL GAPS

	Molecular Weight	Lethal Concentration (mg/dL)	Corresponding Osmolal Gap (mosm/kg H_2O)
Ethanol	46	350	75
Methanol	32	80	25
Ethylene glycol	62	200	35
Isopropanol	60	350	60

Note: *Most laboratories use the freezing-point method for calculating osmolality. If the vaporization point method is used, alcohols are driven off and their contribution to osmolality is lost.*
[1] *Modified, with permission, from:* Tierney LM Jr, McPhee SJ, Papadakis MA (editors): Current Medical Diagnosis & Treatment 2003. *McGraw-Hill, 2003.*
Na$^+$ = *sodium;* ***BUN*** = *blood urea nitrogen.*

TABLE 9–13. PLEURAL FLUID: PLEURAL FLUID PROFILES IN VARIOUS DISEASE STATES.[1]

Diagnosis	Gross Appearance	Protein (g/dL)	Glucose[2] (mg/dL)	WBC and Differential (per μL)	RBC (per μL)	Microscopic Exam	Culture	Comments
Normal	Clear	1.0–1.5	Equal to serum	≤1000, mostly MN	0 or Few	Neg	Neg	
TRANSUDATES[3]								
Congestive heart failure	Serous	<3; sometimes ≥3	Equal to serum	<1000	<10,000	Neg	Neg	Most common cause of pleural effusion. Effusion right-sided in 55–70% of patients.
Nephrotic syndrome	Serous	<3	Equal to serum	<1000	<1000	Neg	Neg	Occurs in 20% of patients. Cause is low protein osmotic pressure.
Hepatic cirrhosis	Serous	<3	Equal to serum	<1000	<1000	Neg	Neg	From movement of ascites across diaphragm. Treatment of underlying ascites usually sufficient.
EXUDATES[3]								
Tuberculosis	Usually serous; can be bloody	90% ≥3; may exceed 5 g/dL	Equal to serum; Occ <60	500–10,000, mostly MN	<10,000	Concentrate Pos for AFB in <50%	May yield MTb	PPD usually positive; pleural biopsy positive; eosinophils (>10%) or mesothelial cells (>5%) make diagnosis unlikely.
Malignancy	Usually turbid, bloody; Occ serous	90% ≥3	Equal to serum; <60 in 15% of cases	1000–10,000 mostly MN	>100,000	Pos cytology in 50%	Neg	Eosinophils uncommon; fluid tends to reaccumulate after removal.

			Glucose[2]					
Empyema	Turbid to purulent	≥3	Less than serum, often <20	25,000–100,000, mostly PMN	<5000	Pos	Pos	Drainage necessary; putrid odor suggests anaerobic infection.
Parapneumonic effusion, uncomplicated	Clear to turbid	≥3	Equal to serum	5000–25,000, mostly PMN	<5000	Neg	Neg	Tube thoracostomy unnecessary; associated infiltrate on chest x-ray; fluid pH ≥7.2.
Pulmonary embolism, infarction	Serous to grossly bloody	≥3	Equal to serum	1000–50,000, MN or PMN	100–>100,000	Neg	Neg	Variable findings; 25% are transudates.
Rheumatoid arthritis or other collagen-vascular disease	Turbid or yellow-green	≥3	Very low (<40 in most); in RA, 5–20 mg/dL	1000–20,000, mostly MN	<1000	Neg	Neg	Rapid clotting time; secondary empyema common.
Pancreatitis	Turbid to sero-sanguineous	≥3	Equal to serum	1000–50,000, mostly PMN	1000–10,000	Neg	Neg	Effusion usually left-sided; high amylase level.
Esophageal rupture	Turbid to purulent; red-brown	≥3	Usually low	<5000–over 50,000, mostly PMN	<5000	Pos	Pos	Effusion usually left-sided; high fluid amylase level (salivary); pneumothorax in 25% of cases; pH <6.0 strongly suggests diagnosis.

1 Modified, with permission, from Therapy of pleural effusion. A statement by the Committee on Therapy. Am Rev Respir Dis 1968;97:479; Tierney LM Jr., McPhee SJ, Papadakis MA (editors): Current Medical Diagnosis & Treatment 2003. McGraw Hill, 2003, and Way LW (editor): Current Surgical Diagnosis & Treatment. 10th ed. Originally published by Appleton & Lange. Copyright © 1974 by The McGraw-Hill Companies, Inc.

2 Glucose of pleural fluid in comparison to serum glucose.

3 Exudative pleural effusions meet at least one of the following criteria: (1) pleural fluid protein/serum protein ratio >0.5; (2) pleural fluid LDH/serum LDH ratio >0.6; and (3) pleural fluid LDH >$\frac{2}{3}$ upper normal limit for serum LDH. Transudative pleural effusions meet none of these criteria. Transudative effusions also occur in myxedema and sarcoidosis.

MN = mononuclear cells (lymphocytes or monocytes); PMN = polymorphonuclear cells; AFB = acid-fast bacilli; MTb = Mycobacterium tuberculosis.

TABLE 9–14. PRENATAL DIAGNOSTIC METHODS: AMNIOCENTESIS AND CHORIONIC VILLUS SAMPLING.[1]

Method	Procedure	Laboratory Analysis	Waiting Time for Results	Advantages	Disadvantages
Amniocentesis	Between the 12th and 16th weeks, and by the transabdominal approach, 10–30 mL of amniotic fluid is removed for cytologic and biochemical analysis. Preceding ultrasound locates the placenta and identifies twinning and missed abortion.	**1. Amniotic fluid** • Alpha-fetoprotein • Limited biochemical analysis • Virus isolation studies **2. Amniotic cell culture** • Chromosomal analysis	3–4 weeks	Over 40 years of experience.	Therapeutic abortion, if indicated, must be done in the second trimester. (RhoGam should be given to Rh-negative mothers to prevent sensitization.) Risks (approximately 1%): • Fetal: puncture or abortion. • Maternal: infection or bleeding.
Chorionic villus sampling	Between the 8th and 12th week, and with constant ultrasound guidance, the trophoblastic cells of the chorionic villi are obtained by transcervical or transabdominal endoscopic needle biopsy or aspiration.	**1. Direct cell analysis** • Chromosomal studies **2. Cell culture** • Limited biochemical analysis	1–10 days	Over 20 years of experience. Therapeutic abortion, if indicated, can be done in the first trimester.	Risks (approximately 3%) • Fetal: abortion. • Maternal: bleeding and infection (uncommon).

[1] Modified, with permission, from Schroeder SA et al (editors): Current Medical Diagnosis & Treatment 1990. Originally published by Appleton & Lange. Copyright © 1990 by The McGraw-Hill Companies, Inc.

TABLE 9–15. PULMONARY FUNCTION TESTS: INTERPRETATION IN OBSTRUCTIVE AND RESTRICTIVE PULMONARY DISEASE. [1]

Tests	Units	Definition	Obstructive Disease	Restrictive Disease
SPIROMETRY				
Forced vital capacity (FVC)	L	The volume that can be forcefully expelled from the lungs after maximal inspiration.	N or ↓	↓
Forced expiratory volume in 1 second (FEV_1)	L	The volume expelled in the first second of the FVC maneuver.	↓	N or ↓
FEV_1/FVC	%		↓	N or ↑
Forced expiratory flow from 25%–75% of the forced vital capacity (FEF 25%–75%)	L/sec	The maximal midexpiratory airflow rate.	↓	N or ↓
Peak expiratory flow rate (PEFR)	L/sec	The maximal airflow rate achieved in the FVC maneuver.	↓	N or ↑
Maximum voluntary ventilation (MVV)	L/min	The maximum volume that can be breathed in 1 minute (usually measured for 15 seconds and multiplied by 4).	↓	N or ↓
LUNG VOLUMES				
Slow vital capacity (SVC)	L	The volume that can be slowly exhaled after maximal inspiration.	N or ↓	↓
Total lung capacity (TLC)	L	The volume in the lungs after a maximal inspiration.	N or ↑	↓
Functional residual capacity (FRC)	L	The volume in the lungs at the end of a normal tidal expiration.	↑	N or ↓
Expiratory reserve volume (ERV)	L	The volume representing the difference between FRC and RV.	N or ↓	N or ↓
Residual volume (RV)	L	The volume remaining in the lungs after maximal expiration.	↑	N or ↑
RV/TLC ratio	...		↑	N or ↑

[1] Modified, with permission, from Tierney LM Jr, McPhee SJ, Papadakis MA (editors): Current Medical Diagnosis & Treatment 2003. McGraw-Hill, 2003.
N = normal; ↓ = less than predicted; ↑ = greater than predicted. Normal values vary according to subject sex, age, body size, and ethnicity.

TABLE 9–16. RANSON'S CRITERIA FOR SEVERITY OF ACUTE PANCREATITIS.[1]

Criteria present at diagnosis or admission
  Age over 55 years
  White blood cell count >16,000/μL
  Blood glucose >200 mg/dL
  Serum LDH >350 IU/L (laboratory specific)
  AST (SGOT) >250 IU/L (laboratory specific)

Criteria developing during first 48 hours
  Hematocrit fall >10%
  BUN rise >5 mg/dL
  Serum calcium <8 mg/dL
  Arterial PO_2 <60 mm Hg
  Base deficit >4 meq/L
  Estimated fluid sequestration >6 L

**MORTALITY RATES CORRELATE WITH THE NUMBER
OF CRITERIA PRESENT**

Number of Criteria	Mortality
0–2	1%
3–4	16%
5–6	40%
7–8	100%

[1] *Modified from Way LW (editor):* Current Surgical Diagnosis & Treatment, *10th ed. Originally published by Appleton & Lange. Copyright © 1994 by the McGraw-Hill Companies, Inc. 1994.* **LDH** = *lactic dehydrogenase;* **AST** = *aspartate dehydrogenase;* **BUN** = *blood urea nitrogen.*

TABLE 9-17. CLASSIFICATION AND DIFFERENTIAL DIAGNOSIS OF RENAL FAILURE. [1]

Classification	Prerenal Azotemia	Postrenal Azotemia	Acute Tubular Necrosis (Oliguric or Polyuric)	Intrinsic Renal Disease	
				Acute Glomerulonephritis	Acute Interstitial Nephritis
Etiology	Poor renal perfusion	Obstruction of the urinary tract	Ischemia, nephrotoxins	Poststreptococcal; collagen-vascular disease	Allergic reaction; drug reaction
Urinary indices					
Serum BUN: Cr ratio	>20:1	>20:1	<20:1	>20:1	<20:1
U_{Na^+} (meq/L)	<20	Variable	>20	<20	Variable
FE_{Na^+} (%)	<1	Variable	>1	<1	<1; >1
Urine osmolality (mosm/kg)	>500	<400	250–300	Variable	Variable
Urinary sediment	Benign, or hyaline casts	Normal or red cells, white cells, or crystals	Granular casts, renal tubular cells	Dysmorphic red cells and red cell casts	White cells, white cell casts, with or without eosinophils

[1] Reproduced, with permission, from Tierney LM Jr., McPhee SJ, Papadakis MA (editors): Current Medical Diagnosis & Treatment 2003. McGraw-Hill, 2003.

$$FE_{Na^+} = \left(\cfrac{\cfrac{Urine\ Na^+}{Plasma\ Na^+}}{\cfrac{Urine\ Creatinine}{Plasma\ Creatinine}} \right) \times 100$$

U_{Na^+} = urine sodium.

TABLE 9–18. RENAL TUBULAR ACIDOSIS (RTA): LABORATORY DIAGNOSIS OF RENAL TUBULAR ACIDOSIS.[1]

Clinical Condition	Renal Defect	GFR	Serum [HCO_3] (meq/L)	Serum [K^+] (meq/L)	Minimal Urine pH	Associated Disease States	Treatment
Normal	None	N	24–28	3.5–5	4.8–5.2	None	None
Proximal RTA (type II)	Proximal H^+ secretion	N	15–18	→	<5.5	Drugs, Fanconi syndrome, various genetic disorders, dysproteinemic states, secondary hyperparathyroidism, toxins (heavy metals), tubulointerstitial diseases, nephrotic syndrome, paroxysmal nocturnal hemoglobinuria.	$NaHCO_3$ or $KHCO_3$ (10–15 meq/kg/d), thiazides.
Classic distal RTA (type I)	Distal H^+ secretion	N	20–23	→	>5.5	Various genetic disorders, autoimmune diseases, nephrocalcinosis, drugs, toxins, tubulointerstitial diseases, hepatic cirrhosis, empty sella syndrome.	$NaHCO_3$ (1–3 meq/kg/d).
Buffer deficiency distal RTA (type III)	Distal NH_3 delivery	→	15–18	N	<5.5	Chronic renal insufficiency, renal osteodystrophy, severe hypophosphatemia.	$NaHCO_3$ (1–3 meq/kg/d).
Generalized distal RTA (type IV)	Distal Na^+ reabsorption, K^+ secretion, and H^+ secretion	→	24–28	←	<5.5	Primary mineralocorticoid deficiency (eg, Addison disease), hyporeninemic hypoaldosteronism (diabetes mellitus, tubulointerstitial diseases, nephrosclerosis, drugs), salt-wasting mineralocorticoid-resistant hyperkalemia.	Fludrocortisone (0.1–0.5 mg/d), dietary K^+ restriction, furosemide (40–160 mg/d), $NaHCO_3$ (1–3 meq/kg/d).

[1] Modified, with permission, from Cogan MG: Fluid & Electrolytes: Physiology & Pathophysiology. Originally published by Appleton & Lange. Copyright © 1991 by the McGraw-Hill Companies, Inc.

GFR = glomerular filtration rate.

TABLE 9–19. SYNOVIAL FLUID: CLASSIFICATION OF SYNOVIAL (JOINT) FLUID.[1]

Type of Joint Fluid	Volume (mL)	Viscosity	Appearance	WBC (per µL)	PMNs	Gram Stain & Culture	Glucose	Comments
Normal	<3.5	High	Clear, light yellow	<200	<25%	Neg	Equal to serum	Protein 2.0–3.5 g/dL.
Non-inflammatory (Class I)	Often >3.5	High	Clear, light yellow	200–2000	<25%	Neg	Equal to serum	Degenerative joint disease, trauma, avascular necrosis, osteochondritis dissecans; osteochondromatosis, neuropathic arthropathy, subsiding or early inflammation, hypertrophic osteoarthropathy, pigmented villonodular synovitis.
Inflammatory (Class II)	Often >3.5	Low	Cloudy to opaque, dark yellow	3000–100,000	≥50%	Neg	>25, but lower than serum	Protein >3 g/dL. Rheumatoid arthritis, acute crystal-induced synovitis (gout, pseudogout), Reiter syndrome, ankylosing spondylitis, psoriatic arthritis, sarcoidosis, arthritis accompanying ulcerative colitis and Crohn disease, rheumatic fever, SLE, scleroderma; tuberculous, viral, or mycotic infections. Crystals diagnostic of gout or pseudogout: gout (urate) crystals show negative birefringence; pseudogout (calcium pyrophosphate) show positive birefringence when red compensator filter is used with polarized light microscopy.

(continued)

TABLE 9–19 (CONTINUED).

Type of Joint Fluid	Volume (mL)	Viscosity	Appearance	WBC (per μL)	PMNs	Gram Stain & Culture	Glucose	Comments
Inflammatory (Class II) (Continued)								Phagocytic inclusions in PMNs suggest rheumatoid arthritis (RA cells). Phagocytosis of leukocytes by macrophages seen in Reiter syndrome.
Purulent (Class III)	Often >3.5	Low	Cloudy to opaque, dark yellow to green	Usually >40,000, often >100,000	≥75%	Usually positive	<25, much lower than serum	Pyogenic bacterial infection (eg, *N gonorrhoeae, S aureus*). Bacteria on culture or Gram-stained smear. Commonest exception: gonococci seen in only about 25% of cases. WBC count and % PMN lower with infections caused by organisms of low virulence or if antibiotic therapy already started.
Hemorrhagic (Class IV)	Often >3.5	Variable	Cloudy, pink to red	Usually >2000	30%	Neg	Equal to serum	Trauma with or without fracture, hemophilia or other hemorrhagic diathesis, neuropathic arthropathy, pigmented villonodular synovitis, synovioma, hemangioma and other benign neoplasms. Many RBCs found also. Fat globules strongly suggest intra-articular fracture.

[1] Modified, with permission, from Rodnan GP: *Primer on the rheumatic diseases: Appendix III.* JAMA 1973;224(5):802–803. Copyright © 1973 by American Medical Association.

TABLE 9-20. SYPHILIS: LABORATORY DIAGNOSIS IN UNTREATED PATIENTS.[1]

Stage	Onset After Exposure	Persistence	Clinical Findings	Sensitivity of VDRL or RPR[2] (%)	Sensitivity of FTA-ABS[3] (%)	Sensitivity of MHA-TP[4] (%)
Primary	21 days (range 10–90)	2–12 wk	Chancre	72	91	50–60
Secondary	6 wk–6 mo	1–3 mo	Rash, condylomata lata, mucous patches, fever, lymphadenopathy, patchy alopecia	100	100	100
Early latent	<1 yr	Up to 1 yr	Relapses of secondary syphilis	73	97	98
Late latent	>1 yr	Lifelong unless tertiary syphilis appears	Clinically silent	73	97	98
Tertiary	1 yr until death	Until death	Dementia, tabes dorsalis, aortitis, aortic aneurysm, gummas	77	99	98

[1] Modified, with permission, from Harvey AM et al (editors): The Principles and Practice of Medicine, 22nd ed. Originally published by Appleton & Lange. Copyright © 1988 by The McGraw-Hill Companies, Inc.

[2] VDRL is a slide flocculation test for nonspecific (anticardiolipin) antibodies, used for screening, quantitation of titer, and monitoring response to treatment; RPR is an agglutination test for nonspecific antibodies, used primarily for screening.

[3] FTA-ABS is an immunofluorescence test for treponemal antibodies utilizing serum absorbed for nonpathogenic treponemes, used for confirmation of infection, not routine screening.

[4] MHA-TP is a microhemagglutination test similar to the FTA-ABS, but one which can be quantitated and automated.

VDRL = Venereal Disease Research Laboratories test; **RPR** = rapid plasma reagin test; **FTA-ABS** = fluorescent treponemal antibody absorption test; **MHA-TP** = microhemagglutination assay for T pallidum.

TABLE 9–21. ALPHA-THALASSEMIA SYNDROMES.[1,2]

Syndrome	Alpha Globin Genes	Hematocrit	MCV (fL)
Normal	4	N	N
Silent carrier	3	N	N
Thalassemia minor	2	32–40%	60–75
Hemoglobin H disease	1	22–32%	60–75
Hydrops fetalis	0	Fetal death occurs in utero	

[1] *Modified, with permission, from Tiemey LM Jr, McPhee SJ, Papadakis MA (editors):* Current Medical Diagnosis & Treatment 2003. *McGraw-Hill, 2003.*
[2] *Alpha thalassemias are due primarily to deletion in the alpha globin gene on chromosome 16.*

TABLE 9–22. BETA-THALASSEMIA SYNDROMES: FINDINGS ON HEMOGLOBIN ELECTROPHORESIS.[1,2]

Syndrome	Beta Globin Genes	Hb A[3]	Hb A$_2$[4]	Hb F[5]
Normal	Homozygous beta	97–99%	1–3%	<1%
Thalassemia minor	Heterozygous beta[0][6]	80–95%	4–8%	1–5%
	Heterozygous beta[+][7]	80–95%	4–8%	1–5%
Thalassemia intermedia	Homozygous beta[+] (mild)	0–30%	0–10%	6–100%
Thalassemia major	Homozygous beta[0]	0%	4–10%	90–96%
	Homozygous beta[+]	0–10%	4–10%	90–96%

[1] *Modified, with permission, from Tierney LM Jr. McPhee SJ, Papadakis MA (editors):* Current Medical Diagnosis & Treatment 2003. *McGraw-Hill, 2003.*
[2] *Beta thalassemias are usually caused by point mutations in the beta globin gene on chromosome 11 that result in premature chain terminations or defective RNA transcription, leading to reduced or absent beta globin chain synthesis.*
[3] *Hb A is composed of two alpha chains and two beta chains:* $\alpha_2\beta_2$
[4] *Hb A$_2$ is composed of two alpha chains and two delta chains:* $\alpha_2\delta_2$.
[5] *Hb F is composed of two alpha chains and two gamma chains:* $\alpha_2\gamma_2$.
[6] *Beta[0] refers to defects that result in absent globin chain synthesis.*
[7] *Beta[+] refers to defects that cause reduced globin chain synthesis.*

TABLE 9–23. THYROID FUNCTION TESTS.[1]

Condition	Total T_4 (μg/dL)	Free T_4 (ng/dL)	Total T_3 (ng/dL)	Sensitive Serum TSH (RIA) (μU/mL)	RAI (^{131}I) Uptake (at 24 hours)	Comments and Treatment
Normal[2]	5–12	Varies with method	95–190	0.3–5	10–30%	
Hyperthyroidism	↑	↑	↑	↓	↑	In TRH stimulation test, TSH shows no response. Thyroid scan shows increased diffuse activity (Grave disease) versus "hot" areas (hyperfunctioning nodules). Thyroperoxidase (TPO) and thyroid-stimulating hormone receptor antibodies (TSH-R Ab [stim]) elevated in Graves disease.
Hypothyroidism	↓	↓		Usually ↑ (primary[3] hypothyroidism, rarely ↓ (secondary[4] hypothyroidism)	N or ↓	TRH stimulation test shows exaggerated response in primary hypothyroidism. In secondary hypothyroidism, TRH test helps to differentiate pituitary from hypothalamic disorders. In pituitary lesions, TSH fails to rise after TRH; in hypothalamic lesion, TSH rises but response is delayed. Antithyroglobulin and thyroperoxidase (TPO) antibodies elevated in Hashimoto's thyroiditis.
HYPOTHYROIDISM ON REPLACEMENT						
T_4 replacement	N	N	V	N or ↓	↓	TSH ↓ with 0.1–0.2 mg T_4 daily.
T_3 replacement	↓	↓	V	N or ↓	↓	TSH ↓ with 50 μg T_3 daily.
Euthyroid following injection of radiocontrast dye	N	N or ↑	N	N	↓	Effects may persist for 2 weeks or longer.

(continued)

TABLE 9–23 (CONTINUED).

Condition	Total T$_4$ (µg/dL)	Free T$_4$ (ng/dL)	Total T$_3$ (ng/dL)	Sensitive Serum TSH (RIA) (µU/mL)	RAI (^{123}I) Uptake (at 24 hours)	Comments and Treatment
PREGNANCY						
Hyperthyroid	↑	↑	↑	↓		Effects may persist for 6–10 weeks post-partum. RAI uptake contraindicated in pregnancy.
Euthyroid	↑	N	↑	N		
Hypothyroid	N or ↓	↓		↑		
Oral contraceptives, estrogens, methadone, heroin	↑	N	↑	N	N	Increased serum thyroid-binding globulin.
Glucocorticoids, androgens, phenytoin, asparaginase, salicylates (high dose)	↓	N	N or ↓	N	N	Decreased serum thyroid-binding globulin.
Nephrotic syndrome	↓	N	N or ↓	N	N	Loss of thyroid-binding globulin accounts for serum T$_4$ decrease.
Iodine deficiency	N	N	N	N	↑	Extremely rare in USA.
Iodine ingestion	N	N	N	N	↓	Excess iodine may cause hypothyroidism or hyperthyroidism in susceptible individuals.

Laboratory Test Results	Most Common Diagnosis	Other Common Diagnoses	Comment
Low TSH Elevated free T_3 or T_4	Graves disease	Multinodular goiter Toxic nodule Transient thyroiditis	
Low TSH Normal free T_3 or T_4	Subclinical hyperthyroidism	Thyroxine ingestion	
Low or normal TSH Low free T_3 or T_4	Nonthyroidal illness[5]	Recent treatment for hyperthyroidism Secondary (pituitary) hypothyroidism	
Elevated TSH Low free T_4 or T_3	Chronic autoimmune thyroiditis (Hashimoto disease)	Hypothyroid phase of transient thyroiditis Previous neck irradiation or thyroid surgery Iodine deficiency Drugs (amiodarone)	
Elevated TSH Normal free T_4 and T_3	Subclinical autoimmune thyroiditis	Heterophile antibody Incomplete treatment for hypothyroidism	
Normal or elevated TSH Elevated free T_4 or T_3	None	Interfering antibodies Intermittent T_4 therapy TSH-secreting pituitary tumor	

Adapted, with permission, from Dayan, Lancet 2001;357:619.

[1] *Normal values vary with laboratory.*
[2] *Thyroid (end-organ) failure.*
[3] *Pituitary or hypothalamic lesions.*
[5] *Commonly referred to as "euthyroid sick."*

N = *normal;* **V** = *variable.*

TABLE 9-24. TRANSFUSION: SUMMARY CHART OF BLOOD COMPONENTS.[1]

Component	Major Indications	Action	Not Indicated For	Special Precautions	Hazards[2]	Rate of Infusion
Whole blood	Symptomatic anemia with large volume deficit	Restoration of oxygen-carrying capacity, restoration of blood volume	Condition responsive to specific component	Must be ABO identical Labile coagulation factors deteriorate within 24 hours after collection	Infectious diseases; septic/toxic, allergic, febrile reactions; circulatory overload; GVHD	For massive loss, as fast as patient can tolerate
Red blood cells; red blood cells with adenine-saline added[3]	Symptomatic anemia	Restoration of oxygen-carrying capacity	Pharmacologically treatable anemia Coagulation deficiency	Must be ABO compatible	Infectious diseases; septic/toxic, allergic, febrile reactions; GVHD	As patient can tolerate, but less than 4 hours
Red blood cells, leukocyte-reduced	Symptomatic anemia, febrile reactions from leukocyte antibodies or cytokines, prevention of platelet refractoriness due to alloimmunization	Restoration of oxygen-carrying capacity	Pharmacologically treatable anemia Coagulation deficiency	Must be ABO compatible	Infectious diseases; septic/toxic, allergic reactions (unless plasma also removed, eg, by washing); GVHD	As patient can tolerate, but less than 4 hours
Fresh-frozen plasma[3]	Deficit of labile and stable plasma coagulation factors and TTP	Source of labile and nonlabile plasma factors	Condition responsive to volume replacement	Must be ABO compatible	Infectious diseases, allergic reactions, circulatory overload	Less than 4 hours
Liquid plasma; plasma; and thawed plasma	Deficit of stable coagulation factors	Source of nonlabile plasma factors	Deficit of labile coagulation factors or volume replacement	Must be ABO compatible	Infectious diseases, allergic reactions	Less than 4 hours

Cryoprecipitate AHF	Hemophilia A,[4] von Willebrand's disease,[4] hypo-fibrinogenemia, factor XIII deficiency	Provides factor VIII, fibrinogen, von Willebrand factor, factor XIII	Deficit of any plasma protein other than those enriched in cryoprecipitated AHF	Frequent repeat doses may be necessary for factor VIII	Infectious diseases; allergic reactions	Less than 4 hours
Platelets; platelets from pheresis[5]	Bleeding from thrombocytopenia or platelet function abnormality	Improves hemostasis	Plasma coagulation deficits and some conditions with rapid platelet destruction (eg, ITP)	Should not use some microaggregate filters (check manufacturer's instructions)	Infectious diseases; septic/toxic, allergic, febrile reactions; GVHD	Less than 4 hours
Granulocytes from pheresis	Neutropenia with infection	Provides granulocytes	Infection responsive to antibiotics	Must be ABO compatible; do not use depth-type microaggregate filters or leuko-depletion filters	Infectious diseases; allergic, febrile reactions; GVHD	One unit over 2–4 hours. Observe closely for reactions.

[1] From American Association of Blood Banks, American Red Cross, American Blood Centers. Circular of information for the use of human blood and blood components. Bethesda: American Association of Blood Banks 1999, 13th ed.

[2] For all cellular components, there is a risk the recipient may become alloimmunized.

[3] Solvent detergent pooled plasma is an alternative in which some viruses are inactivated, but clotting factor composition is changed.

[4] When virus-inactivated concentrates are not available.

[5] Red blood cells and platelets may be processed in a manner that yields leukocyte-reduced components. The main indications for leukocyte-reduced components are prevention of febrile, nonhemolytic transfusion reactions and prevention of leukocyte alloimmunization. Risks are the same as for standard components except for reduced risk of febrile reactions.

AHF = antihemophilic factor; **GVHD** = graft-versus-host disease; **ITP** = idiopathic thrombocytopenic purpura; **TTP** = thrombotic thrombocytopenic purpura.

TABLE 9–25. URINE COMPOSITION URINALYSIS: FINDINGS IN COMMON DISEASE STATES.[1]

Disease	Daily Volume	Specific Gravity	Protein[2] (mg/dL)	Esterase	Nitrite	RBC	WBC	Casts	Other Microscopic Findings
Normal	600–2500 mL	1.003–1.030	0–trace (0–30)	Neg	Neg	0 or Occ	0 or Occ	0 or Occ	Hyaline casts
Fever	→	←	Trace or 1+ (<30)	Neg	Neg	0	Occ	0 or Occ	Hyaline casts, tubular cells
Congestive heart failure	→	← (varies)	1–2+ (30–100)	Neg	Neg	None or 1+	0	1+	Hyaline and granular casts
Eclampsia	→	←	3–4+ (30–2000)	Neg	Neg	None or 1+	0	3–4+	Hyaline casts
Diabetic coma	← or →	←	1+ (30)	Neg	Neg	0	0	0 or 1+	Hyaline casts
Acute glomerulonephritis	→	←	2–4+ (100–2000)	Pos	Neg	1–4+	1–4+	2–4+	Blood; RBC, cellular, granular, and hyaline casts; renal tubular epithelium

Nephrotic syndrome	N or ↓	N or ↑	4+ (>2000)	Neg	Neg	1–2+	0	4+	Granular, waxy, hyaline, and fatty casts; fatty tubular cells
Chronic renal failure	↑ or ↓	Low; invariable	1–2+ (30–100)	Neg	Neg	Occ or 1+	0	1–3+	Granular, hyaline, fatty, and broad casts
Connective tissue disorders	N, ↑ or ↓	N or ↓	1–4+ (30–2000)	Neg	Neg	1–4+	0 or Occ	1–4+	Blood, cellular, granular, hyaline, waxy, fatty, and broad casts; fatty tubular cells; telescoped sediment
Pyelonephritis	N or ↓	N or ↓	1–2+ (30–100)	Pos	Pos	0 or 1+	4+	0 or 1+	WBC casts and hyaline casts; many pus cells; bacteria
Hypertension	N or ↑	N or ↓	None or 1+ (<30)	Neg	Neg	0 or Occ	0 or Occ	0 or 1+	Hyaline and granular casts

[1] Modified, with permission, from Krupp MA et al (editors): Physician's Handbook, 21st ed. Originally published by Appleton & Lange. Copyright © 1985 by The McGraw-Hill Companies, Inc.
[2] Protein concentration in mg/dL is listed in parentheses.

TABLE 9-26. VAGINAL DISCHARGE: LABORATORY EVALUATION.[1]

Diagnosis	pH	Odor With KOH (Positive "Whiff" Test)	Epithelial Cells	WBCs	Organisms	KOH Prep	Gram Stain	Comments
Normal	<4.5	No	N	Occ	Variable, large rods not adherent to epithelial cells	Neg	Gram-positive rods	
Trichomonas vaginalis vaginitis	>4.5	Yes	N	↑	Motile, flagellated organisms	Neg	Flagellated organisms	
Bacterial vaginosis (*Gardnerella vaginalis*)	>4.5	Yes	Clue cells[2]	Occ	Coccobacilli adherent to epithelial cells	Neg	Gram-negative coccobacilli	
Candida albicans vaginitis	<4.5	No	N	Occ slightly increased	Budding yeast or hyphae	Budding yeast or hyphae	Budding yeast or hyphae	Usually white "cottage cheese" curd
Mucopurulent cervicitis (*N gonorrhoeae*)	Variable, usually >4.5	No	N	↑	Variable	Neg	Intracellular gram-negative diplococci	

[1] Modified, with permission, from Kelly KG: Tests on vaginal discharge. In: Walker HK et al (editors): Clinical Methods: The History, Physical and Laboratory Examinations, 3rd ed. Butterworths, 1990.

[2] Epithelial cells covered with bacteria to the extent that cell nuclear borders are obscured.

TABLE 9-27. VALVULAR HEART DISEASE: DIAGNOSTIC EVALUATION OF CARDIAC VALVULAR DISEASE.[1]

Diagnosis	Chest X-Ray	ECG	Echocardiography	Comments
MITRAL STENOSIS (MS) Rheumatic disease	Straight left heart border. Large LA sharply indenting esophagus. Elevation of left main bronchus. Calcification occ seen in MV.	Broad negative phase of biphasic P in V_1. Tall peaked P waves, right axis deviation, or RVH appear if pulmonary hypertension is present.	**M-Mode:** Thickened, immobile MV with anterior and posterior leaflets moving together. Slow early diastolic filling slope. LA enlargement. Normal to small LV. **2D:** Maximum diastolic orifice size reduced. Reduced subvalvular apparatus. Foreshortened, variable thickening of other valves. **Doppler:** Prolonged pressure half-time across MV. Indirect evidence of pulmonary hypertension.	"Critical" MS is usually defined as a valve area <1.0 cm². Balloon valvuloplasty has high initial success rates and higher patency rates than for AS. Open commissurotomy can be effective. Valve replacement is indicated when severe regurgitation is present. Catheterization can confirm echo results.
MITRAL REGURGITATION (MR) Myxomatous degeneration (MV prolapse) Infective endocarditis Subvalvular dysfunction Rheumatic disease	Enlarged LV and LA.	Left axis deviation or frank LVH. P waves broad, tall, or notched, with broad negative phase in V_1.	**M-Mode and 2D:** Thickened MV in rheumatic disease. MV prolapse; flail leaflet or vegetations may be seen. Enlarged LV. **Doppler:** Regurgitant flow mapped into LA. Indirect evidence of pulmonary hypertension.	In nonrheumatic MR, valvuloplasty without valve replacement is increasingly successful. Acute MR (endocarditis, ruptured chordae) requires emergent valve replacement. Catheterization is the best assessment of regurgitation.
AORTIC STENOSIS (AS) Calcific (especially in congenitally bicuspid valve) Rheumatic disease	Concentric LVH. Prominent ascending aorta, small knob. Calcified valve common.	LVH.	**M-Mode:** Dense persistent echoes of the AoV with poor leaflet excursion. LVH with preserved contractile function. **2D:** Poststenotic dilatation of the aorta with restricted opening of the leaflets. Bicuspid AoV in about 30%.	"Critical" AS is usually defined as a valve area <0.7 cm² or a peak systolic gradient of >50 mm Hg. Catheterization is definitive diagnostic test.

(continued)

TABLE 9–27 (CONTINUED).

Diagnosis	Chest X-Ray	ECG	Echocardiography	Comments
AORTIC STENOSIS (AS), continued			**Doppler:** Increased transvalvular flow velocity, yielding calculated gradient.	Prognosis without surgery is less than 50% survival at 3 yr when CHF, syncope, or angina occur. Balloon valvuloplasty has a high restenosis rate.
AORTIC REGURGITATION (AR) Bicuspid valves Infective endocarditis Hypertension Rheumatic disease Aorta/aortic root disease	Moderate to severe LV enlargement. Prominent aortic knob.	LVH.	**M-Mode:** Diastolic vibrations of the anterior leaflet of the MV and septum. Early closure of the valve when severe. Dilated LV with normal or decreased contractility. **2D:** May show vegetations in endocarditis, bicuspid valve, or root dilatation. **Doppler:** Demonstrates regurgitation. Estimates severity.	Aortography at catheterization can demonstrate AR. Acute incompetence leads to LV failure and requires AoV replacement.
TRICUSPID STENOSIS (TS) Rheumatic disease	Enlarged RA only.	Tall, peaked P waves. Normal axis.	**M-Mode and 2D:** TV thickening. Decreased early diastolic filling slope of the TV. MV also usually abnormal. **Doppler:** Prolonged pressure half-time across TV.	Right heart catheterization is diagnostic. Valvulotomy may lead to success, but TV replacement is usually needed.
TRICUSPID REGURGITATION (TR) RV overload (pulmonary hypertension) Inferior infarction Infective endocarditis	Enlarged RA and RV.	Right axis deviation usual.	**M-Mode and 2D:** Enlarged RV. MV often abnormal and may prolapse. **Doppler:** Regurgitant flow mapped into RA and venae cavae. RV systolic pressure estimated.	RA and jugular pressure tracings show a prominent V wave and rapid Y descent. Replacement of TV is rarely done. Valvuloplasty is often preferred.

[1] Modified, with permission, from Tierney LM Jr, McPhee SJ, Papadakis MA (editors): Current Medical Diagnosis & Treatment 2003. McGraw Hill, 2003.
RA = right atrium; **RV** = right ventricle; **LA** = left atrium; **LV** = left ventricle; **AoV** = aortic valve; **MV** = mitral valve; **TV** = tricuspid valve; **LVH** = left ventricular hypertrophy; **RVH** = right ventricular hypertrophy; **CHF** = congestive heart failure.

TABLE 9–28. WHITE BLOOD CELLS: WHITE BLOOD CELL COUNT AND DIFFERENTIAL.[1]

Cells	Range ($10^3/\mu L$)	Increased in	Decreased in
WBC count (total)	3.4–10.0	Infection, hematologic malignancy.	Decreased production (aplastic anemia, folate or B_{12} deficiency, drugs [eg, ethanol, chloramphenicol]); decreased survival (sepsis, hypersplenism, drugs).
Neutrophils	1.8–6.8	Infection (bacterial or early viral), acute stress, acute and chronic inflammation, tumors, drugs, diabetic ketoacidosis, leukemia (rare).	Aplastic anemia, drug-induced neutropenia (eg, chloramphenicol, phenothiazines, antithyroid drugs, sulfonamide), folate or B_{12} deficiency, Chédiak-Higashi syndrome, malignant lymphoproliferative disease, physiologic (in children up to age 4 years).
Lymphocytes	0.9–2.9	Viral infection (especially infectious mononucleosis, pertussis), thyrotoxicosis, adrenal insufficiency, ALL and CLL, chronic infection, drug and allergic reactions, autoimmune diseases.	Immune deficiency syndromes (HIV).
Monocytes	0.1–0.6	Inflammation, infection, malignancy, tuberculosis, myeloproliferative disorders.	Depleted in overwhelming bacterial infection.
Eosinophils	0.0–0.4	Allergic states, drug sensitivity reactions, skin disorders, tissue invasion by parasites, polyarteritis nodosa, hypersensitivity response to malignancy (eg, Hodgkin disease), pulmonary infiltrative disease, disseminated eosinophilic hypersensitivity disease.	Acute and chronic inflammation, stress, drugs (corticosteroids).
Basophils	0.0–0.1	Hypersensitivity reactions, drugs, myeloproliferative disorders (eg, CML), myelofibrosis.	

[1] In the automated differential, 10,000 WBCs are classified on the basis of size and peroxidase staining as neutrophils, monocytes, or eosinophils (peroxidase-positive) and as lymphocytes or large unstained cells (LUC), which are peroxidase-negative. LUCs, larger than normal lymphocytes, may be atypical lymphocytes or peroxidase-negative blasts. Basophils are identified using two-angle light scattering, based on their singular resistance to lysis.

The reproducibility of 100-cell manual differentials is notoriously poor. Review of blood smears is useful to visually identify rare abnormal cells, blasts, nucleated RBCs, morphologic abnormalities (eg, hypersegmentation, toxic granulation, sickle cells, target cells, spherocytes, basophilic stippling) and to look for rouleaux (stacking of red cells due to increased globulins) and clumped platelets).

WBC differential is unlikely to be abnormal with a normal WBC count or to be changed if the total WBC count is unchanged.

ALL = Acute lymphocytic leukemia; **CLL** = Chronic lymphocytic leukemia; **CML** = Chronic myelocytic leukemia.

10

Nomograms & Reference Material

Stephen J. McPhee, MD, Diana Nicoll, MD, PhD, MPA,
and Michael Pignone, MD, MPH

HOW TO USE THIS SECTION

This section contains useful nomograms and reference material. Material is presented in alphabetical order by subject.

Contents

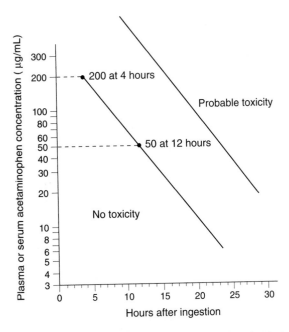

Figure 10–1. ACETAMINOPHEN TOXICITY: Nomogram for prediction of acetaminophen hepatotoxicity following acute overdosage. The upper line defines serum acetaminophen concentrations known to be associated with hepatotoxicity; the lower line defines serum levels 25% below those expected to cause hepatotoxicity. To give a margin for error, the lower line should be used as a guide to treatment. *(Modified and reproduced, with permission, from Rumack BH, Matthew H: Acetaminophen poisoning and toxicity. Pediatrics 1975;55:871. Reproduced by permission of Pediatrics. Copyright © 1975. Permission obtained also from Saunders CE, Ho MT [editors]:* Current Emergency Diagnosis & Treatment, *4th ed. Originally published by Appleton & Lange. Copyright © 1992 by The McGraw-Hill Companies, Inc.)*

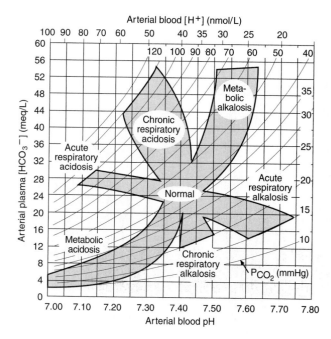

Figure 10–2. ACID–BASE NOMOGRAM: Shown are the 95% confidence limits of the normal respiratory and metabolic compensations for primary acid–base disturbances. *(Reproduced, with permission, from Cogan MG [editor]: Fluid and Electrolytes: Physiology & Pathophysiology. Originally published by Appleton & Lange. Copyright © 1991 by The McGraw-Hill Companies, Inc.)*

Peripheral nerve   **Nerve root**

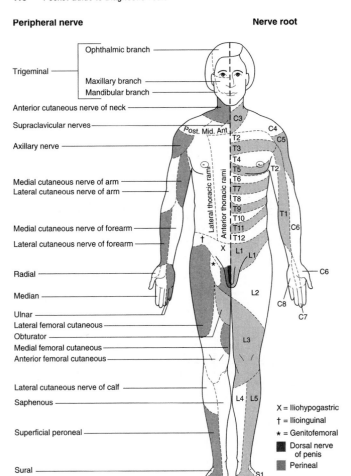

Trigeminal
- Ophthalmic branch
- Maxillary branch
- Mandibular branch

Anterior cutaneous nerve of neck

Supraclavicular nerves

Axillary nerve

Medial cutaneous nerve of arm
Lateral cutaneous nerve of arm

Medial cutaneous nerve of forearm
Lateral cutaneous nerve of forearm

Radial

Median

Ulnar
Lateral femoral cutaneous
Obturator
Medial femoral cutaneous
Anterior femoral cutaneous

Lateral cutaneous nerve of calf
Saphenous

Superficial peroneal

Sural
Lateral and medial plantar
Deep peroneal

Post. Mid. Ant.
Lateral thoracic rami
Anterior thoracic rami

C3
C4
C5
T2
T3
T4
T5
T6
T7
T8
T9
T10
T11
T12
T2
T1
C6
L1
L1
C6
L2
C8
C7
L3
L4 L5
S1

X = Iliohypogastric
† = Ilioinguinal
★ = Genitofemoral

■ Dorsal nerve of penis
▨ Perineal

Figure 10–3. DERMATOME CHART: Cutaneous innervation. The segmental or radicular (root) distribution is shown on the right side of the body, and the peripheral nerve distribution on the left side. **Above:** anterior view; **next page:** posterior view. *(Reproduced, with permission, from Aminoff MJ, Greenberg DA, Simon RP: Clinical Neurology, 3rd ed. Originally published by Appleton & Lange. Copyright © 1996 by The McGraw-Hill Companies, Inc.)*

Nerve root

Peripheral nerve

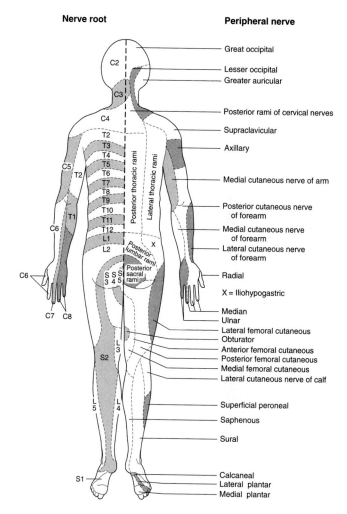

Figure 10–3. (*Continued*)

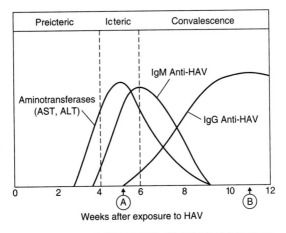

Figure 10–4. HEPATITIS A: Usual pattern of serologic changes in hepatitis A. **HA** = hepatitis A; **AST** = aspartate aminotransferase; **ALT** = alanine aminotransferase; **Anti-HAV** = hepatitis A virus antibody; **IgM** = immunoglobulin M; **IgG** = immunoglobulin G. *(Reproduced, with permission, from Harvey AM et al [editors]: The Principles and Practice of Medicine, 22nd ed. Originally published by Appleton & Lange. Copyright © 1988 by The McGraw-Hill Companies, Inc.)*

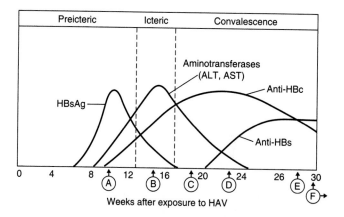

Weeks after exposure to HAV

Usual Patterns of Hepatitis B Antigens and Antibodies			
	HBsAg	Anti-HBc	Anti-HBs
A Very early	+	+ or −	−
B Acute	+	+	−
C Active HB with high titer Anti-HBc ("window")	−	+	−
D Convalescence	−	+	+
E Recovery	−	+ or −	+
F Chronic carrier	+	+	−

Figure 10–5. HEPATITIS B: Usual pattern of serologic changes in hepatitis B (HB). **HBV** = hepatitis B virus; **HBsAg** = hepatitis B surface antigen; **Anti-HBc** = hepatitis B core antibody; **Anti-HBs** = hepatitis B surface antibody; **AST** = aspartate aminotransferase; **ALT** = alanine aminotransferase. *(Modified and reproduced, with permission, from Harvey AM et al [editors]: The Principles and Practice of Medicine, 22nd ed. Originally published by Appleton & Lange. Copyright © 1988 by The McGraw-Hill Companies, Inc.)*

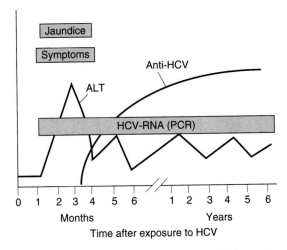

Figure 10–6. HEPATITIS C: The typical course of chronic hepatitis C. **ALT** = alanine aminotransferase; **Anti-HCV** = antibody to hepatitis C virus by enzyme immunoassay; **HCV RNA [PCR]** = hepatitis C viral RNA by polymerase chain reaction. *(Reproduced, with permission, from Tierney LM Jr, McPhee SJ, Papadakis MA [editors]:* Current Medical Diagnosis & Treatment 2003. *McGraw-Hill, 2003.)*

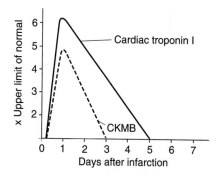

Figure 10–7. MYOCARDIAL ENZYMES: Time course of serum enzyme concentrations after a typical myocardial infarction. **CKMB** = isoenzyme of creatine kinase.

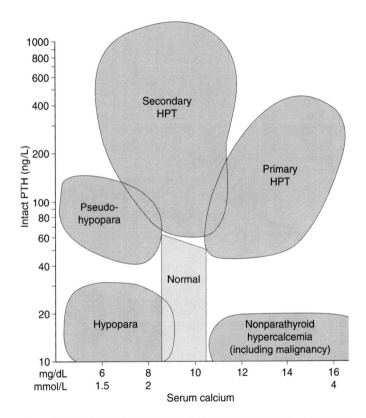

Figure 10–8. PARATHYROID HORMONE AND CALCIUM NOMOGRAM. Relationship between serum intact parathyroid hormone (PTH) and serum calcium levels in patients with hypoparathyroidism, pseudohypoparathyroidism, nonparathyroid hypercalcemia, primary hyperparathyroidism, and secondary hyperparathyroidism. **HPT** = hyperparathyroidism. *(Courtesy of GJ Strewler.)*

SPIROGRAM

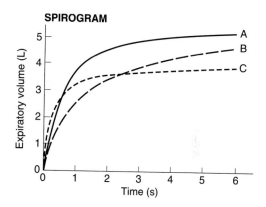

EXPIRATORY FLOW-VOLUME CURVE

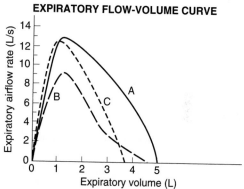

Figure 10–9. PULMONARY FUNCTION TESTS: SPIROMETRY. Representative spirograms (upper panel) and expiratory flow-volume curves (lower panel) for normal **(A),** obstructive **(B),** and restrictive **(C)** patterns. *(Reproduced, with permission, from Tierney LM Jr, McPhee SJ, Papadakis MA [editors]:* Current Medical Diagnosis & Treatment 2003. *McGraw-Hill, 2003.)*

Nomogram and Procedure for Rapid Evaluation of Endogenous Creatinine Clearance

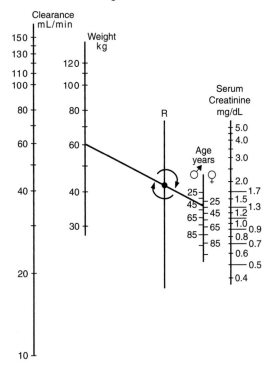

Figure 10–10. RENAL FAILURE: ESTIMATED CREATININE CLEARANCE. Siersback-Nielsen nomogram for estimation of creatinine clearance from serum creatinine.

  (1) Identify the axis point along the reference line (R) around which the relation between the patient's serum creatinine and creatinine clearance rotates. To do so, place a straightedge so as to connect the patient's age (in years, for male or female) with the patient's weight (in kilograms).
  (2) Put a dot along the reference line where the rule and line intersect.
  (3) Rotate the ruler to connect the patient's serum creatinine and this dot, and determine where the ruler falls along the line, estimating the patient's creatinine clearance.

Note: This nomogram is based on the assumption that an increase in weight represents an increase in lean body mass. Substantial error in the estimate occurs when a weight increase reflects obesity rather than increased lean body mass. In addition, the nomogram yields a much more accurate estimate in the presence of moderate to moderately severe renal impairment than in the presence of normal renal function. It should also not be relied upon in severe renal insufficiency (eg, serum creatinine >5 mg/dL or creatinine clearance <15 mL/min). *(Modified, with permission, from Harvey AM et al [editors):* The Principles and Practice of Medicine, *22nd ed. Originally published by Appleton & Lange. Copyright © 1988 by The McGraw-Hill Companies, Inc.)*

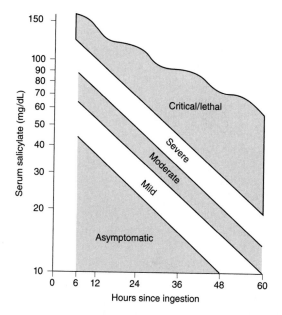

Figure 10–11. SALICYLATE TOXICITY: Nomogram for determining severity of salicylate intoxication. Absorption kinetics assume acute ingestion of non–enteric-coated aspirin preparation. *(Modified and reproduced, with permission, from Done AK: Significance of measurements of salicylate in blood in cases of acute ingestion. Pediatrics 1960;26:800. Permission obtained also from Saunders CE, Ho MT [editors]: Current Emergency Diagnosis & Treatment, 4th ed. Originally published by Appleton & Lange. Copyright © 1992 by The McGraw-Hill Companies, Inc.)*

Index

NOTE: A *t* following a page number indicates tabular material, and an *f* following a page number indicates a figure.